DRY AREA AGRICULTURE, FOOD SCIENCE AND HUMAN NUTRITION

Pergamon Titles of Related Interest

ASAP ANIMAL PRODUCTION IN AUSTRALIA
Carter FAMINE IN AFRICA
Gordon CONTROLLED BREEDING IN FARM ANIMALS
Lockhart INTRODUCTION TO CROP HUSBANDRY
Nash CROP CONSERVATION & STORAGE
Perpich BIOTECHNOLOGY IN SOCIETY
Vose CROP BREEDING: A CONTEMPORARY BASIS

Journals of Related Interest*

BIOTECHNOLOGY ADVANCES
CURRENT ADVANCES IN PLANT SCIENCE
ENVIRONMENTAL & EXPERIMENTAL BOTANY
JOURNAL OF RURAL STUDIES
NUTRITION RESEARCH
OUTLOOK ON AGRICULTURE
PROGRESS IN FOOD & NUTRITION SCIENCE

***Sample copies available on request**

DRY AREA AGRICULTURE, FOOD SCIENCE AND HUMAN NUTRITION

Edited by

David F. Nygaard
Farming Systems Program, ICARDA, Aleppo, Syria and Agricultural Development Council, 725 Park Avenue, New York

Peter L. Pellett
Professor of Human Nutrition, University of Massachusetts, Amherst, MA

Proceedings of a Workshop held at the University of Aleppo, Aleppo, Syria
February 21-25, 1982

Sponsored by

The International Center for Agricultural Research in the Dry Areas (ICARDA)
and
The United Nations University (UNU)

PERGAMON PRESS
New York Oxford Toronto Sydney Frankfurt

Pergamon Press Offices:

U.S.A.	Pergamon Press Inc., Maxwell House, Fairview Park, Elmsford, New York 10523, U.S.A.
U.K.	Pergamon Press Ltd., Headington Hill Hall, Oxford OX3 0BW, England
CANADA	Pergamon Press Canada Ltd., Suite 104, 150 Consumers Road, Willowdale, Ontario M2J 1P9, Canada
AUSTRALIA	Pergamon Press (Aust.) Pty. Ltd., P.O. Box 544, Potts Point, NSW 2011, Australia
FEDERAL REPUBLIC OF GERMANY	Pergamon Press GmbH, Hammerweg 6, D-6242 Kronberg-Taunus, Federal Republic of Germany
BRAZIL	Pergamon Editora Ltda., Rua Eça de Queiros, 346, CEP 04011, São Paulo, Brazil
JAPAN	Pergamon Press Ltd., 8th Floor, Matsuoka Central Building, 1-7-1 Nishishinjuku, Shinjuku, Tokyo 160, Japan
PEOPLE'S REPUBLIC OF CHINA	Pergamon Press, Qianmen Hotel, Beijing, People's Republic of China

---

First printing 1986

Library of Congress Cataloging in Publication Data
Main entry under title:

Dry area agriculture, food science, and human nutrition.

Bibliography: p.
Includes index.
1. Arid regions agriculture--Congresses. 2. Food supply--Congresses. 3. Nutrition--Congresses.
I. Nygaard, David F. II. Pellett, Peter L.
III. International Center for Agricultural Research in the Dry Areas. IV. United Nations University.
S612.2.D79 1986 363.8 86-707
ISBN 0-08-033996-4

In order to make this volume available as economically and as rapidly as possible, the authors' typescripts have been reproduced in their original forms. This method unfortunately has its typographical limitations but it is hoped that they in no way distract the reader.

Printed in Great Britain by A. Wheaton & Co. Ltd., Exeter

TABLE OF CONTENTS

FOREWORD

In 1975, the first Advisory Group of the World Hunger Programme of the United Nations University noted that there was a neglect of food and nutrition considerations in agricultural planning and research. They also discussed the general failure of nutritionists to adapt their dietary recommendations to the practices, customs, and potential of local agriculture. Therefore, this group proposed a series of workshops to encourage dialogue and collaboration of agriculturalists, food scientists, and nutritionists to focus on the major agricultural regions of the world. As a result, such meetings have been held at six locations: International Institute of Tropical Agriculture (IITA), Ibadan, Nigeria (1977); International Rice Research Institute (IRRI), Los Banos, Philippines (1978); Institute of Nutrition of Central America and Panama (INCAP), Guatemala City; International Center for Tropical Agriculture (CIAT), Palmira, Colombia; and International Maize and Wheat Improvement Center (CIMMYT), Londres, Mexico (1979); and International Crops Research Institute for the Semi-Arid Tropics (ICRISAT), Hyderabad, India (1981).

In each case, agricultural scientists, including agronomists, plant breeders, and economists met with leaders in the areas of nutrition and food science to discuss common interests and arrive at specific recommendations for improving communication and cooperation among these scientists. While each of the workshops has had a particular character and focus, all have been effective in highlighting neglected issues, clarifying misunderstandings among the disciplines involved, and promoting better allocation of research expenditures. The records and recommendations of these workshops reveal a growing sophistication in interdisciplinary dialogue and a broadening of the viewpoints represented.

The United Nations University was particularly pleased to be a part of this seventh workshop, the first in the Middle East, and co-sponsor it with ICARDA. The interactions of agriculture, food and nutrition in a region in which farmers face low and variable rainfall are complex and unique. Because of the interdisciplinary nature of ICARDA's research programme, it was a most appropriate environment to begin this dialogue.

ICARDA has four research programmes: The Farming Systems Programme, the Cereal Improvement Programme, the Food Legume Improvement Programme, and the Pasture and Forage Improvement Programme. The formulation and development of each of these programmes have given careful attention to existing agricultural practices, to the impact of changing these practices on farming families and agricultural areas, and to the interactions of the many components that are being studied. In doing so, ICARDA hopes to be able to avoid many of the problems associated with previous agricultural development projects, for example projects that increase production but lower the nutritional quality of the diet, reduce employment opportunities, or increase prices of basic foodstuffs.

Scientists from countries in the ICARDA region are also aware of these issues. It was a pleasure for ICARDA to join hands with the United Nations University and enable scientists from the region to come together in an environment conducive to promoting discussion, action, and progress in the field of development.

The value of this undertaking can be seen in these proceedings. We believe that it was successful in that an unusual workshop format was tried and produced a spirit of good will and cooperation that, in turn, led us in new directions for research and programme activities. These are captured in this document. It therefore has relevance for not only the Middle East but for other regions trying to cope with problems of achieving balanced economic and agricultural development that contributes to improved nutrition and health for their populations.

Mohamed A. Nour
Director General
ICARDA

Nevin S. Scrimshaw
Director
Food, Nutrition and Poverty Programme
The United Nations University

PREFACE

This publication is an attempt to capture two rather independent themes. The first is a presentation of the proceedings of a workshop where discussions, aimed to identify economic development problems, particularly in rural areas, and to survey the status and effectiveness of efforts of researchers and development agencies to find solutions to these problems.

The second is a recording of the results of a conscientious effort to foster a dialogue among a multidisciplinary group of people. It is increasingly recognized by researchers involved in economic development that development problems are complex. The solutions are also complex and efforts to find them require the efforts of multidisciplinary teams. However, it is not easy to get such teams together and operating effectively. We believe that the first step in organizing multidisciplinary research is to create an effective means to communicate. We feel that this was achieved in that a surprisingly good environment existed in which ideas from scientists of different specializations were expressed and discussed.

The meeting originated from a visit by Dr. Samir Miladi and Dr. Peter L. Pellett to ICARDA in December, 1980 on behalf of the World Hunger Programme (now the Subprogramme on Food, Nutrition and Poverty) of the United Nations University. They held discussions with the Directorate and Programme Leaders at ICARDA and plans were laid to hold a workshop. The workshop was financed by ICARDA and the United Nations University and was held in cooperation with the University of Aleppo.

The organizing committee was chaired by Dr. David Nygaard, head of the Farming Systems Program at ICARDA. Members of the committee included Dr. Samir Miladi, Dr. Ibrahim Nahal (University of Aleppo) and Drs. Habib Ibrahim, K.B. Singh, Mohamed Salah Mekni and Bhal Somaroo of ICARDA. The workshop was held from 21 to 25 February, 1982.

It was comprised of six half-day sessions and a seventh session to formulate recommendations. Each session consisted of the presentation of two (and in one session, three) prepared papers followed by an open discussion. To encourage interdisciplinary communication, the time allotted to discussion was equal to the time given to the speakers.

There was a general consensus among the workshop participants that, because of the high quality of both the papers and the discussions, the workshop proceedings should be published in order to share the deliberations with others. There was also a feeling that the spirit as well as the letter of the discussion sessions should be captured in the publication, since the workshop was very successful and, therefore, rather unusual in achieving truly interdisciplinary communication.

Our task as editors was to attempt to meet both of these criteria -- to produce a useful document on the subject area while capturing the essence and ambiance of the discussions. Thus, these proceedings follow the same order as the workshop. Each set of papers is presented followed by the opening comments of the discussion leader and then a transcript of the discussion.

The papers were revised during the editing process, but in no case were substantial changes made. The comments of the discussion leaders were transcribed and edited, but again there was no change in substance. The editing of discussions themselves was much more difficult and as some changes were made, the procedure followed deserves to be clarified. The discussions were transcribed from tapes of the sessions and edited initially for grammatical and other errors in language use. In the majority of instances, the order of intervention was not altered, although sometimes comments may have been moved forward to fit with other comments on the same subject.

It should be noted that, throughout the discussion, rapporteurs kept written records of all interventions and speakers were encouraged to provide brief written versions of their questions or answers. A few interventions or parts of them that were not pertinent to the subject being discussed, or were not clear, were dropped.

On occasion, the editors contacted the speaker to clarify a point, but since this was not feasible for all of the dialogue, some editorial changes have been made. Extreme care was taken in comparing summaries with transcripts and in listening to the original tapes of the discussions, and we believe that we have produced as true a record of the discussion as was possible. If errors have been made in attribution we must take full responsibility.

Throughout the discussions, first names were frequently used in referring to other speakers, together with the use of titles, courtesy and otherwise, such as Doctor or Professor. In our summaries, in order to make it easier for the reader, first names and titles have been dropped and speakers are merely referred to by their family names. No discourtesy is intended and we can assure readers that all actual discussions were friendly.

Grateful thanks are due to all speakers, participants and members of the organizing committee, especially to Samir Miladi for his enthusiastic organizational activities and for his personal contacts in facilitating the bringing together of outstanding scientists both from the region and from international organizations.

Mesdames Rosie Keatinge, Mary Nygaard and Margaret Allan were responsible for transcribing the tapes. Ms. Marcia Boyagi not only typed and retyped these, she was responsible for most of the communications related to the workshop and to this publication. Thanks also to Jane Dittrich and M.I.T. We hope the quality of this publication represents the excellent contributions of all these people who made it possible.

David Nygaard and Peter L. Pellett
Aleppo, Syria and
Amherst, Massachusetts,

PARTICIPANTS

AHMED EL ACHKAR	Faculty of Economics and Commerce, Aleppo University, Aleppo, SYRIA
HAROLD ALDERMAN	International Food Policy Research Institute (IFPRI), c/o Ford Foundation, P.O. Box 2344, Cairo, EGYPT
ABDALLA EL MUBARAK ALI	Food Science and Technology, Food Research Center, P.O. Box 213, Khartoum, SUDAN
ALISTER ALLAN	Farming Systems Program, The International Center for Agricultural Research in the Dry Areas (ICARDA), Aleppo, SYRIA
MOHAMED AMIR-HUSSIEN	Nutrition Requirement and Growth Department, Nutrition Institute, 16, Kasr El-Aini Street, Cairo, EGYPT
RICARDO BRESSANI	Division of Food and Agricultural Sciences, Institute of Nutrition of Central America and Panama (INCAP), Apartado Postal 1188, Guateala City, Guatemala, Central America
PETER COOPER	Farming Systems Program, ICARDA
WILLIAM ERSKINE	Food Legumes Improvement Program, ICARDA
JOHN D. GERHART	Representative for North Africa and the Middle East, c/o Ford Foundation, P.O. Box 2344, Cairo EGYPT
HASSAN M. GHAZAL	Faculty of Agriculture, University of Aleppo, Aleppo, SYRIA
PETER GOLDSWORTHY	Deputy Director General, Research, ICARDA
HABIB M. HALILA	Field Crops, Institut National Recherche Agronomique d'Tunisie, (INRAT), 2080 Ariana, Tunis, TUNISIA
GEOFFRY HAWTIN	Deputy Director General, International Cooperation, ICARDA
IBRAHIM HAYANI	Farming Systems Program, ICARDA
LEILA HUSSEIN	Human Nutrition and Food Technology, National Research Center, Giza,
PAUL LUNVEN*	Food Policy and Nutrition Division, Food and Agriculture Organization of the United Nations, Via delle Terme di caracalla, 00100 Rome, ITALY
S.K. MAJUMDER*	Central Food Technological Research Institute (CFTRI), Mysore, INDIA

MOHAMED MANSOUR	Department of Applied Nutrition, National Nutrition Institute, 11 Rue Aristude Briand, Bab Saadoun, Tunis, TUNISIA
AHMED MAZID	Research, Farming Systems Program, ICARDA
MOHAMED SALAH MEKNI	Cereal Improvement Program, ICARDA
SAMIR MILADI	UNU Regional Coordinator, P.O. Box 863, Tunis, TUNISIA
CYHTHIA MYNTTI	Anthropology Program Office, Ford Foundation, P.O. Box 2344, Cairo, EGYPT
MOHAMED MILOUDI NACHIT	Cereal Improvement Program, ICARDA
IBRAHIM NAHAL	Vice Rector for Academic Affairs, University of Aleppo, Aleppo, SYRIA
THOMAS NORDBLOM	Agricultural Economics, Farming Systems Program, ICARDA
MOHAMED ABDULLA NOUR	Director General, ICARDA
DAVID F. NYGAARD	Farming Systems Program, ICARDA
STELIOS PAPACHRISTODOULOU	Agricultural Economics Section, Agricultural Research Institue, Nicosia, CYPRUS
HUSAIN A.B. PARPIA	Development Studies Division, The United Nations University, Toho Seimei Building, 15-1 Shibuya 2-chome, Shibuya-ku, Tokyo 150, JAPAN
PETER L. PELLETT	Department of Food Science and Nutrition, University of Massachusetts, Amherst, Massachusetts 01003, USA
PER PINSTRUP ANDERSEN	International Food Policy Research Institute (IFPRI), 1776 Massachusetts Avenue N.W., Washington, D.C. 20036, USA
YOUSEF SABET	Farming Systems Program, ICARDA
MAHMUD SALAMEH	Food and Nutrition, Department of Agricultural Affairs, Damascus, SYRIA
ABDUL BARI SALKINI	Farming Systems Program, ICARDA
CHAFIK SALLAH	Assistant Program Officer, Economist, UNICEF, c/o UNDP, Damascus, SYRIA
MOHAN SAXENA	Food Legumes Improvement Program, ICARDA
FAROUK EL SAYED	Food Legumes Improvement, ICARDA
NEVIN S. SCRIMSHAW	Programme Director, Food, Nutrition and Poverty Programme, The United Nations University, Cambridge

	Programme Office, Massachusetts Institute of Technology, 20A-201, Cambridge, Massachusetts 02139, USA
K.B. SINGH	Food Legumes Improvement Program, ICARDA
KUTLU SOMEL	Farming Systems Program, ICARDA
JIT SRIVASTAVA	Cereal Improvement Program, ICARDA
RICHARD STEWART	Training and Communication Program, ICARDA
RAJA I. TANNOUS*	Faculty of Agriculture and Food Science, American University of Beirut, Beirut, LEBANON
EUAN F. THOMSON	Livestock Division, Farming Systems Program, ICARDA
PHILIP C. WILLIAMS	Grain Technology, Canadian Grain Commission/ICARDA, Grain Research Laboratory, 1404-303 Main Street, Winnipeg, Manitoba R3c 3G8, CANADA
FAYEZ EL YASSIN	Animal Nutrition, Dean, Faculty of Agriculture, University of Aleppo, Aleppo, SYRIA

*Not in attendance

SECTION I

MALNUTRITION AND HUNGER

GLOBAL PERSPECTIVES OF HUNGER AND MALNUTRITION

PETER L. PELLETT

INTRODUCTION

Hunger and malnutrition have been prevalent throughout human history. Famines, i.e., catastrophic mass undernutrition, occurred frequently in Europe until recently. These, however, appear to have been of relatively limited scale compared to those in Africa and Asia in which countless millions have perished.

Apart from the tragic emergencies of famine there has been much hunger and malnutrition throughout the world at the best of times and both are widespread still. Because of the enormous increase in world population, equally true statements are made that, in absolute numbers, more are well fed or more are starving than ever before. Similarly bald, unhelpful statements may be made that so many tens or hundreds of millions are currently suffering from hunger or malnutrition. Other than the shock value to the uninformed, such statements do little to help understand or alleviate the problem. Re-examination of the numbers suffering from malnutrition (1) indicate that fewer are at risk than previously thought.

Using various techniques and criteria for assessment of nutritional status, which will be discussed below, regional and country data of much more general usefulness can be constructed. However, before these are discussed it is of value to consider the multifactorial origins of hunger and malnutrition.

CAUSATION OF HUNGER AND MALNUTRITION

General views on the causation of malnutrition have undergone considerable change over the last two decades. It is now increasingly recognized that malnutrition may be caused less by nutrient deficiency as such and more by many interrelated social, political, and economic factors; the widespread prevalence of malnutrition is usually a symptom of a very sick society. Because of this multifactorial causation, solutions must also be multifaceted even if concepts such as the elimination of poverty and improvement of living standards are basic. Malnutrition affects the growth, development, and survival of children, and the health, activity, and well-being of adults. Conventional solutions in the form of specific programmes are usually inadequate to tackle problems, and their effects are transitory because they do not reach causes. Nutrition can be improved through upgrading the level of living -- particularly real income, food availability, environment, access to services -- of the malnourished; and in certain cases by preventing vulnerability to critical food shortage and famine. Solutions are therefore mostly outside the traditional field of nutrition but come through economic and social development.

While the term "malnutrition" strictly should include overnutrition and some of the diseases of affluence, it is often only used to mean the condition resulting from a deficient intake of energy or of a particular nutrient. Four especially important and broad causes of malnutrition are: i) a lack of knowledge about food, nutrition, and health, ii) an insufficient supply of the foods necessary for a balanced diet, often caused by production failure, iii) an uneven distribution of the available food (both among and within families), and iv) infectious diseases that are synergistic with malnutrition (2). These are tabulated in Table 1.

Hunger is often used synonymously with malnutrition. The terms are not identical but can overlap, and it would be unproductive to attempt exact delineation. Hunger has been defined (3) as the deterioration of health status and/or social and productive performance of individuals or populations subsisting on too low an intake of food. The major immediate cause of hunger is poverty. Other important causes, such as poor environmental sanitation, infections, and infestations are also related to poverty. The interplay of all these factors not only produces but perpetuates malnutrition and hunger. Poverty exists everywhere and is found even in countries of high apparent wealth as indicated by per capita Gross National Product. The problem of controlling hunger and malnutrition is difficult and complex, and success will depend on how effectively four major tasks are undertaken: increasing the supply of the right kind of food where it is needed, reducing poverty, improving the stability of food supplies, and decreasing the rate of population growth. These tasks, however, all lie more in the political sphere and less in the scientific.

Some of the varied causes of hunger are tabulated in Table 2, which originates from a recent UNU-WHP review on the causation of hunger (3). As indicated earlier, these causes range far more widely than the traditional concerns of nutrition, which, until relatively recently, were still centered on food and nutrients.

NUTRITIONAL STATUS EVALUATION

Evaluation of the nutritional status of populations can be derived from consideration of various levels of information, and these can be separated into two major categories, the first pertaining to agriculture and food availability, the second to the health of the population. Agriculture and food production data have limitations, but they can indicate approximate availability of food supplies to a population. Close examination of agricultural production data can also allow judgement on the success or failure of local agricultural techniques together with the role of food imports and exports in the society. The next level of information concerning food derives from dietary surveys and food consumption patterns within the society and provides data on socio-economic variables as well as on the marketing, distribution, and storage of foods. Dietary surveys are difficult to perform with accuracy, but give the most detailed information available on food consumption at the family level.

Health-related data are derived first at the regional or country level by using vital and health statistics. These identify the extent of risk to the community and identification of high-risk groups within the community. At a more individual level, nutritional assessment includes the measurement and description of the nutritional status of a population in relation to those socio-economic, demographic, and physiologic variables that can affect the nutrition of that population. These usually include anthropometric, biochemical, and clinical studies. Consideration of the results of such surveys can give information on the effects of nutrition on physical development, on the impairment of biochemical function, and of the deviation from health caused by malnutrition. Impairment of health can usually only be ascribed to malnutrition when corresponding food and nutrient intake information is available to correlate with the health data.

AGRICULTURAL AND FOOD DATA

At the world or regional level, analysis of food production and population growth trends provides an indication of the progress achieved by mankind in the struggle to feed itself. In general, the growth of world food production since the 1960s has been greater than that of the population, but the margin between the two has been shrinking. The state of food and agriculture has recently been reviewed (4). Trends are disquieting; while world food and agricultural production increased by an estimated 0.3 percent in 1979, this was the smallest annual rise since 1972, and in more than half of the developing countries production increase failed to match population growth. Although global aspects of food production are discussed in detail elsewhere (5), Tables 3 and 4 show food production and per capita food availability data for the world regions. The performance of Africa has been especially disappointing, with the rate of growth of food production in the 1970s being only three-fifths that in the previous decade. In the most seriously affected (MSA) countries, per capita food production actually fell by 0.3 percent a year after negligible increases in the 1960s.

The potential problems of some countries are shown more clearly in Table 5, which gives the annual rate of growth of food production in relation to population growth. For some countries, notably those towards the bottom right of the Table, food production is greater than population growth; others are in a much more serious situation where their population growth is exceeding, sometimes by a large degree, the increase in food production. For some of these, the causes are clearly the effects of war, liberation struggles, or internal conflicts and it could be reasonably hoped that when these crises are over, production will increase sharply. In others there are valid economic reasons on the grounds of comparative advantage to export agricultural or even food products and import the balance of food required. However, in certain countries, the high rates of populaton growth in the range of 3 to 4 percent per year far outweigh the growth of food production. As FAO remarked laconically, "There is no clear indication as to how and when the problem could be resolved" (4).

The FAO Food Balance Sheet and per capita Food Supply data now contain information from 164 countries and territories (6). A Food Balance Sheet presents a comprehensive picture of the pattern of a country's food supply during a specified reference period, but Food Balance Sheets, being derived statistics, are of course dependent upon the reliability of the underlying basic statistics of population, supply and utilization of foods, and of their nutritive value. Nevertheless, Food Balance Sheets tabulated regularly over a period of years will show the trends in overall national food supply; disclose changes that may have taken place in the types of foods consumed, i.e., the pattern of the diet; and reveal the extent to which the food supply of the country, as a whole, is adequate in relation to nutritional requirements.

Food Balance Sheets have been the main source of data used for the assessment and appraisal of the world food situation (1,7). In Table 6, estimates are shown for the number of persons on a world basis who can be considered as suffering from an inadequate food intake as defined by Basal Metabolic Rate (BMR). If an intake of food energy less than 1.2 x BMR is considered critical, some 455 million people subsisted below this critical minimum intake in 1972-74, an increase of some 10 percent since 1969-71. In this respect the Near East Region, which includes several countries in North Africa, is the only region that showed a decrease, albeit small, in the number of people estimated at risk during this period. Deductions of this type have limitations because of the physiological adaptation that can occur to low intakes.

DRA-B

While malnutrition is caused by the interplay of a large number of factors, the three main ones are food availability, socio-economic status, and total population, with all three being closely interrelated. In accordance with these factors, the incidence of malnutrition varies from one country to another, but world data can, nevertheless, be separated into three major groups. In the first lie the high-income countries with very low rates of population growth and high levels of food availability. The general pattern of malnutrition is one of overeating, resulting in obesity and possibly atherosclerosis. The second group comprises middle-income developing countries that have per capita incomes of about U.S. $1,000. These countries have high rates of population growth (about 2.8 percent annually), mainly because death rates have dropped more rapidly than birth rates. They generally have experienced rapid economic growth together with large increases in food availability. However, because of population growth and poor income and land distribution, food deprivation and widespread malnutrition continue in most. In addition, the richer parts of their populations may also suffer from the malnutrition of affluence. The third group includes the poorest countries with per capita GNPs in the order of U.S. $200. These are the countries in which hunger and malnutrition are most severe.

Population growth is a major determinant in per capita food availability, and the rate of growth varies greatly between regions. As is shown in Table 7, the population of the world increased in the 1970s at an annual rate of almost 2 percent and exceeded 4,000 million in 1977. Regional growth rates are 2.7 to 2.8 percent for Africa, Latin America, and the Near East in contrast to 0.6 to 1.0 percent for Western developed regions. Population growth puts tremendous pressures on many aspects of a nation's economy. A large number of infants and young children have to be fed and cared for. Later they will need to be educated and trained, and later still, jobs will be needed for them as they enter the labour force. Provision of health services is only one of many competing demands.

HEALTH AND MALNUTRITION

The last few years have not been favourable for the general world health situation (8); droughts and severe winters have reduced harvest yields; wars and civil unrest have destroyed crops, land, and housing; and rapid population growth has become a matter for serious concern. In addition to this, inflation has raised costs and inhibited the development of trade on a world basis. These circumstances have hindered health progress, but may perhaps have played an important part in shaping new thinking about development. No longer is it generally assumed that economic development and social development are distinct, and that economic progress should be the only goal.

Newer policies are emerging that are aimed more specifically at development to meet basic human social needs. Throughout the world, some 800 million people still live in conditions of abject deprivation with incomes too low to ensure basic nutrition and with little access to services essential to health and life. Less than one-third of all people in developing countries have safe water and adequate sewage disposal. Housing conditions and educational opportunities are still generally unsatisfactory and the number of illiterate adults is increasing. These data are mostly approximations because there is a lack of reliable information from many regions of the world. In general, however, there is a positive correlation between social and economic factors, well-being, and level of health. When a country is desperately poor and the people are individually poor, undernourished, and uneducated, and there are few public services, the health of the people is likewise poor (8). In the middle range, where there is enough money for countries to make decisions as to how it is spent, there will often be enormous variations in the proportions of people who are underfed, the proportions of children enrolled in school, the availability of public services, and the health of the people.

A major change in the world social situation that has come into sharper focus in the last decade has been the role of women in society. The increasing involvement of women in economic life in much of the world has influenced family lifestyles. The demand for day-care services for children has increased, and although these services still play a very minor role in developing societies, demand will probably increase in the decades ahead, and development of preschool care and education facilities will be required.

Leading directly from considerations of the role of women in society and the mother-child dyad (9) are general considerations of infant and early childhood mortality on a world and regional basis. Such data are shown in Table 8, where it can be seen that the differences between the developed and the less developed regions remain enormous. Not only is infant mortality higher, but also early childhood mortality (1-4 years) is considerably greater. The ratio between these two indices may be indicative of the general health status of the population, and ranges from above 20 for the more developed regions to less than 10 in certain less developed regions.

Some 120 million infants are born each year, and of these roughly 10 percent will die before reaching their first birthday and another 4 percent before their fifth birthday. Chances of survivial are extremely unevenly distributed through the world, with vast differences between regions. As indicated in Table 9, the ratios between the highest levels and the lowest levels reported on a world basis are enormous, ranging from 10 times as large for perinatal mortality to up to 200 times as large for maternal mortality. These differences are highly associated with socio-economic development, and it can be seen from Table 10 that both infant mortality and food energy availability are closely related to wealth, as measured by GNP. The underlying causes of perinatal deaths are linked to those of maternal deaths, i.e., poor health and nutritional status of the mother and complications of pregnancy and childbirth. Perinatal mortality is also closely associated with low birth weight defined as below 2500 g: this affects mortality in the whole first year of life and probably also for a few years afterwards (10,11) and will be discussed again later as a major world problem. Diarrhoeal diseases, closely followed by respiratory infections, are the leading cause of mortality and morbidity in infancy. Malnutrition as an underlying cause is responsible for almost 60 percent of infant deaths in some countries (12).

The single most effective measure for the prevention of malnutrition and protection against infection in infancy is breast-feeding (13,14). Data suggest that infant mortality rates in developing countries are five to ten times higher among infants who have not been breast-fed or who have been breast-fed for less than six months (8). Despite the marked advantages of breast-feeding, its popularity, as shown by the number of women who practice it and how long they do so, has declined significantly in many parts of the world. Historically this decline has been particularly marked in the developed countries, but there is now evidence suggesting that the prevalence and duration of breast-feeding may be increasing in these countries. In developing countries, where the value of breast-feeding is greatest and where larger proportions of infants are at risk of malnutrition and infections, large numbers of mothers do not breast-feed. Of those who do, many wean their infants before the age of six months. The prevalence and duration of breast-feeding among rural populations in developing countries, however, continue to be high, although in some cases nutritional and other health problems appear to be associated with the late introduction of appropriate and regular supplemental feeding.

Mortality at ages 1-4 years is much lower in all populations than infant mortality, but the infectious diseases of childhood such as measles and pertussis, as well as pneumonia, begin to appear in the second half of the first year or in the second year. When combined with malnutrition, these diseases can have high case fatality rates (12,15). An overall, general health indicator, which includes both consideration of infant mortality and childhood mortality, is life expectancy at birth. The values for this index differ considerably between the developed countries and the less developed countries. A life expectancy in excess of 70 years is common in most developed regions, whereas it may be below 50 in the poorer regions of the world, as illustrated in Table 11.

The major causes of mortality in children under five years in the less developed regions are primarily associated with excessive incidence of infectious, parasitic, and respiratory diseases. In recent years there has not been much progress in reducing either the incidence or prevalence of many diseases that plague developing countries. The threat posed by such diseases as malaria, schistosomiasis, cholera, and leishmanaisis has either not lessened or has actually increased (8). The incidence of food-borne diseases and certain zoonoses similarly seems to be increasing. To the ravages of these diseases must be added the debilitating and often fatal consequence of widespread nutritional deficiencies. Taken together, malnutrition and the infectious, parasitic, and respiratory diseases, that have been largely eliminated in the more developed countries, are still the principal sources of the suffering, disability, and death in the less developed regions. Inasmuch as the incidence of most of these conditions can be dramatically reduced at relatively modest cost, the suffering and death they cause must be counted as unnecessary and preventable.

MAJOR GLOBAL PROBLEMS OF MALNUTRITION

In Table 12, the characteristics of hunger and some of the more major world nutritional problems are shown. Problems other than these, such as scurvy, rickets, beri-beri, and pellagra still exist, but are generally less widespread than those conditions tabulated.

Hunger

The wide range of factors that can cause hunger has already been discussed. There is no doubt that the problem is widespread, but exact numbers are impossible to obtain because conditions that could be described as hunger vary from the gross manifestation of prolonged starvation to mild and apparently reversible growth failure. An important consideration, which is not discussed elsewhere, is the adverse effect of hunger on work capacity that has been observed both in field and laboratory experimentation.

The effect of hunger on individuals is variable and depends not only on the duration and severity of the deprivation, but also on the adaptive capacity of the individual. Among the major problems of malnutrition, the conditions of protein-energy malnutrition and the factors causing low birth-weight infants overlap to a considerable degree with hunger, so much so that they may become indistinguishable. Solutions to world problems of hunger are, even more obviously than for malnutrition, in the realms of politics and economics.

Protein-Energy Malnutrition

Estimates of the world prevalence of protein-energy malnutrition (PEM) have been made in recent years using large-scale survey data (12, 16-18) collected in Latin America, Africa, and Asia. It was concluded that there were some 9 million children with severe PEM and almost 90 million suffering from moderate PEM, giving a grand total of almost 100 million cases. Using the proportions estimated by Bengoa and Donoso (17), but using 1977 population estimates (Table 13), would indicate some 104 million cases in the total developing regions with almost 11 million in the Near East region. These numbers probably represent a minimum, since many children are reported to have died from or contracted an infectious disease when indeed malnutrition was the underlying or associated cause. In the second place, malnutrition is subject to seasonal variation, making timing and duration of the study important.

Conclusions on the prevalence of severe PEM are generally drawn from two types of data, the first being anthropometric where a criterion of less than 60 percent of a given reference weight for age was used; the second group of studies were based on clinical criteria to determine the degree of prevalence. In both sets of studies the prevalence of PEM ranged from about 4 percent of children examined in community surveys to about 30 percent in severely poverty-stricken areas. For infants and young children, the risk of dying is very closely related to the conditions of the environment in which they live. As discussed earlier, infants in low-income groups experience higher infant mortality rates than those in other income groups. Other factors of importance in the pathogenesis of PEM are family socio-economic status and place of residence, methods of infant feeding, environmental sanitation, housing conditions, and cultural beliefs and customs (19,20). Harfouche (19) estimates that 60 to 80 percent of all infant deaths occur in the post-neonatal period, the time when deaths are caused mainly by an interaction between infections and malnutrition (15).

PEM has been defined by WHO (21,22) as a range of pathological conditions arising from coincidental lack, in varying proportions, of protein and calories, occurring most frequently in infants and young children and commonly associated with infections. The conditions concerned can be said to range in severity from mild through moderate to severe. Certainly the mild, and probably also the moderate, degrees are subclinical and can only be detected by anthropometric and biochemical tests. The early stages are characterized by growth failure and possibly some retardation of mental development. Severe PEM may have several clinical forms that range in a graded fashion (22).

Two distinct syndromes occur at either end of the spectrum, marasmus and kwashiorkor; in between varying degrees of each are found in what is termed marasmic-kwashiorkor. A variety of biochemical tests have shown (23) that severe PEM in these various clinical forms constitutes a spectrum of both clinical signs and biochemical change, both being most marked in frank kwashiorkor and least evident in marasmus. Until relatively recently, kwashiorkor received the most attention, partly because of the large variety of biochemical abnormalities associated with it. More emphasis is now being placed on the socio-economic and political aspects of malnutrition, and research is increasingly being devoted to the clarification of energy and protein relationships in health and disease (24,25,26).

Severe protein-energy malnutrition can be diagnosed using both anthropometric and clinical criteria, but the mild and moderate forms are subclinical and can only be classified by anthropometric standards. These have frequently been based on a deficit in weight-for-age (27). While this has been of immense value, it is limited in that it is unable to distinguish between acute and chronic or present and past malnutrition. Recent expert committees on nutritional surveillance have recommended the use of weight-for-age and weight-for-height as primary indicators of nutritional status in children (28, 29).

Xerophthalmia and Vitamin A Deficiency

Hypovitaminosis A is considered to be the most common cause of blindness in the developing countries (30, 31). With the data available, however, it is not possible to estimate the prevalence of keratomalacia directly attributable to vitamin A deficiency. Subclinical hypovitaminosis A is not measurable at present in human subjects, but animal studies indicate that possible subclinical effects should not be ignored. The recommended procedure for identifying the "at risk" population involves a three-part survey to evaluate dietary intake, biochemical indices, and clinical signs. In the present state of knowledge, it is probable that none of these three procedures gives a truly satisfactory estimate of vitamin A status. Vitamin A activity in the human diet is obtained from preformed vitamin A (retinol) and from provitamin A (carotenoids). Of the latter, B-carotene has the highest vitamin A activity and is the most plentiful in human foods (32). Carotenes are active only after being converted into retinol during, or subsequent to, absorption through the intestinal wall. In the blood, retinol is transported in association with a specific protein, retinol-binding protein, whereas the carotenoids are associated with the lipid-bearing proteins.

One of the biochemical functions of retinol is maintenance of normal conditions in the mucous membranes; in the eye it functions in the visual process. One of the early symptons of vitamin A deficiency is impaired dark adaption (night blindness). Continued deficiency leads to damage of ocular tissues and eventually to blindness, particularly in young children. In addition to the preschool child, pregnant and lactating women also require higher intakes of vitamin A. In developing countries these groups are likely to eat diets that are limited in vitamin A-containing foods. Preformed vitamin A is found only in animal food products, which, in the poorest sections of the poor countries, are only consumed in small quantities by the vulnerable population groups. The food sources with vitamin A activity that are most likely to be available to such groups are the green and yellow vegetables, fruits and leaves that provide carotenes.

Even if vitamin A intake could be assessed with accuracy from dietary intakes in communities, this would be of little value without more precise knowledge of requirements for the vitamin. Adequate intakes are now being defined as "...a level sufficient to provide tissue needs while allowing a safe quantity to be stored in tissue reserves." Because the precise biochemical roles of vitamin A have yet to be characterized other than in the formation of visual pigment, and because this concept of a safe level of storage is relatively new, the vitamin A requirements of different age and sex groups are not firmly established. Information on the requirements of children is especially scarce.

The basic problems pertaining to vitamin A requirement are that: i) the established methodology is only useful in detecting frank deficiency states; ii) different amounts of vitamin A are required to support each of its various functions, and iii) vitamin A is metabolized at rates proportional to total body stores and not solely in response to tissue needs. A newer steady-state approach to the determination of vitamin A requirements was proposed in 1974 (33). The approach was first to define a minimally adequate total body reserve of vitamin A and then to determine the amounts of dietary vitamin A or carotene necessary to maintain it.

Biochemical assessment of vitamin A status is also necessary. The level of vitamin A stored in the liver is the best indicator of relative vitamin A status, but cannot be assayed directly in living human populations because biopsy procedures are far from risk-free and cannot be ethically justified for survey purposes. Blood levels of the vitamin are easily assayed, but provide little direct information about relative vitamin A status because they are homeostatically controlled at a relatively constant value beween the extremes of liver depletion or saturation. Even the more complex determination of plasma retinol-binding protein (RBP) gives little additional information, and its usefulness as an indicator for assessment purposes has not yet been sufficiently tested in human populations. Specific co-enzyme roles, like those of several of the water-soluble vitamins, have not as yet been fully identified for vitamin A, nor have any urinary metabolites that quantitatively relate to vitamin A status.

Even clinical assessment of vitamin A status is far from clear-cut. While there is general agreement that deficiency progressses from night blindness through xerophthalmia to irreversible keratomalacia, there is little detailed information on the progression of histological changes that accompany vitamin A deficiency. The problem is that in human populations these changes are influenced by additional dietary, physiological, and environmental factors. Criteria have been proposed for determining whether or not hypovitaminosis A is a significant public health problem and these are shown in Table 14. Such criteria are logical but difficult to apply in practice. The prevalence of clinical signs of xerophthalmia fluctuates seasonally, so a single survey may miss the peak occurrence and underestimate the magnitude of the problem. This means that surveys must be conducted repeatedly over an extended period, adding considerably to their cost.

There is a close link between vitamin A metabolism and protein metabolism. For normal synthesis and functioning of retinol transport proteins, namely RBP and PA (prealbumin), an adequate intake of good-quality protein is necessary (31). In severe protein deficiency, synthesis of carrier protein may be a limiting factor in the utilization of vitamin A. An inadequate intake of good-quality protein will impair vitamin A absorption from the alimentary tract, yet in spite of altered vitamin A absorption in severe protein deficiency, a substantial portion of a high-level oral dose of vitamin A seems to be absorbed in children; however, infections may impair absorption (34).

It seems likely that hypovitaminosis A as a public health problem will only be eliminated when all members of a society have access to a diet sufficient in vitamin A and also in other nutrients that interact in vitamin A metabolism. This goal will only be achieved following a general public upgrading of the level of development in these countries and a generally more equitable distribution of the benefits of development. Serious hypovitaminosis A rarely occurs in countries where protein-energy malnutrition of children is not also a problem. Underwood (31) emphasized that serious undernutrition as a public health problem does not exist where people have sufficient income to buy foods of their choice. However, money alone does not by itself eliminate malnutrition, as has also been observed for PEM (35).

Goitre and Iodine Deficiency

Endemic goitre is another disease entity that, in our present state of knowledge, could either be eliminated or reduced significantly. An example of what can be achieved comes from Paraguay. In the mid 1940s Paraguay had one of the highest rates of endemic goitre in the Americas, with an incidence ranging from 39 to 79 percent amongst school-aged children. Initially, iodine tablets were used, but in 1958 mandatory iodization of salt was decreed. Since that time various studies have been conducted, with the most recent showing national averages of 15.2 percent, 2.7 percent and 0.2 percent for grades 1, 2, and 3, respectively, as opposed to the 1956 levels of 42.5, 14.5, and 2.5 percent (36).

Kelly and Snedden, in their classic review of the prevalence and geographic distribution of endemic goitre in 1960 (37), wrote that, although the geographic distribution of goitre has not apparently altered in the past 100 years, the intensity of the disease has substantially declined in certain countries, particularly those that have enjoyed rising standards of living and an enlightened outlook on public health. In 1967, the joint FAO/WHO Expert Committee on Nutrition (38) declared that "...in spite of the fact that sufficient knowledge is now available to control goitre, the application of control measures has been very slow." Fifteen years later, one could write the same. The example of Paraguay, where goitre has almost been eliminated, could be followed by most other developing countries.

Iron Deficiency Anaemia

Iron deficiency is by far the commonest nutritional disorder and the most frequent cause of anaemia in both developing and affluent societies (39). It has been revealed from determination of serum ferritin levels that iron deficiency is not synonymous with anaemia. Anaemia is only a late and relatively uncommon manifestation of iron depletion. Before the appearance of pallor, easy fatigability and low haemoglobin, iron deficiency may cause other disordered functions. Iron deficiency is thus a major public health concern throughout the world, but more so in developing countries where detectable and significant effects on resistance to infections, morbidity and mortality, and physical work performance have been described.

Surveys have repeatedly affirmed the high world-wide prevalence of nutritional anaemias, especially in the less developed countries (40). One vulnerable population consists of women of reproductive age, particularly during pregnancy; another is infants and growing children. Prevalence studies in the Near East Region leave no doubt that nutritional anaemias are a most serious and widespread problem. Rao (41) has estimated that 20 to 25 percent of children, 20 to 40 percent of adult females, and up to 10 percent of adult males suffer from varying degrees of anaemia in the Near East Region. In vulnerable groups such as infants and pregnant and lactating women, the proportions with anaemia seem to reach 70 to 90 percent. These and other surveys have demonstrated that, while B_{12} and folate deficiency do have a role in the development of anaemias, this is relatively minor except possibly during pregnancy. Thus, for practical purposes, nutritional anaemia equates with iron deficiency anaemia.

Parasitic infestations relate closely to the problem of anaemia, because the blood loss they sometimes cause adds to potential existing food deficiencies. Problems exist in the diagnosis of mild iron deficiency because the normal distribution of the parameters overlaps the iron-deficient range. Further difficulties exist with the appropriate standard to use for the level of haemoglobin where anaemia should be diagnosed as present. Surveys in the United States have shown consistently lower values for haemoglobin in Blacks than in Whites (42). These differences appear to persist even when the populations are standardized for socio-economic and other differences.

Because of these and other problems, it is important that, when anaemia has been diagnosed solely from haemoglobin status, it should be confirmed as being truly iron deficiency anaemia by both FEP (43) determinations and also be determining the haemoglobin response to doses of oral ferrous salts. Theoretically, changing dietary patterns to increase the intake of iron or of foods that promote iron absorption, such as meat, fish, and those rich in ascorbic acid, will improve the iron balance. This, however, is difficult to perform in practice and is a long-term approach to the problem. An excellent recent review on nutritional anaemia, with the emphasis on its being a controllable public health problem (39), indicates that in regions where there is a high prevalence of anaemia there is unlikely to be any single public health solution to the problem, and it will be necessary to develop and combine a number of different approaches.

Low Birth-Weight Infants

The term "low birth weight" is ambiguous when used for developed countries, though it still has considerable relevance to developing countries. Low birth weight (LBW) includes all infants born with a weight of 2500 g or less. Within this classification, there are two main groups: i) Those whose low birth weight is due to short gestational age (prematurity), and ii) those whose gestational age is normal (foetal growth retardation). In developing countries as a whole, it is probable that the high prevalence of low birth weight is caused more by foetal growth retardation than by prematurity. Lechtig (44) estimated that about 22 million children throughout the world were born with low birth weight in 1975. WHO (Table 15) makes similar estimates (11). The incidence of low birth weight is closely correlated with socio-economic status; 90 percent of the countries that receive less than 2800 calories per capita/day showed a high incidence of low birth weight infants, and the underdeveloped countries as a whole contained 94 percent of all children with low birth weight.

Infants with low birth weight caused by retardation of foetal growth show a tendency toward hypoglycemia, hypothermia, frequent and severe infections, loss of subcutaneous fat and of skin turgescence, high mortality, and suboptimal postnatal development. A positive correlation between birth weight and physical postnatal growth has also been found (44). This is important because physical growth retardation is associated with psychomotor and mental development retardation and with reduced survival capacity. The low survival capacity associated with low birth weight appears primarily to be caused by lower resistance to infections and consequently a greater frequency and severity of infections. The problem, as yet, has not been widely studied in countries of the Near East Region but has been well studied in Latin America (44, 45). It was concluded from a longitudinal study that maternal nutrition both before and during pregnancy affects foetal development and survival (45). There appeared to be a minimum level of nutrients that had to be available in order to obtain adequate birth weight. There was an impact of a nutritional intervention for pregnant women with 25 to 84 g increments in birth weight per 10,000 additional calories ingested during pregnancy. The third meeting of the ACC/SCN Consultative Group on Maternal and Young Child Nutrition has recently reported on maternal nutrition in deprived populations and has made recommendations on possible remedial measures (46).

It would thus seem that, in common with other nutritional deficiency syndromes, while there are complex relationships, the basic solution is simple but takes on a politico-socio-economic dimension rather than a purely nutritional one. The prevalence and importance of low birth-weight infants throughout the whole Near East region needs much more intensive investigation and should be a priority activity for regional nutritional research.

Diseases of Affluence

Discussion of the diseases of affluence may at first sight seem out of place in a discussion of hunger and malnutrition. Heart diseases are the major causes of death in most industrialized countries, but the control of infectious diseases is now making them important sources of morbidity and mortality in many non-industrialized countries. Indeed, WHO tabulates heart disease as one of the three major causes of death for all age groups beyond adolescence in both developed and less developed countries. Recent data for Kuwait (47) show heart disease now to be the major cause of death. Much evidence, largely epidemiological, indicates that coronary heart disease (CHD) is preventable (48). There are also definite links between the several diseases of affluence, and prevalence of one can lead to prevalence of another. Causal relationships appear to exist in one direction or another between the diseases of diabetes and obesity, and the incidence of vascular disease.

The relationship between diet and heart disease has now been studied intensively for more than three decades. One provocative researcher/reviewer (49) concludes that we have come to the end of an era and rejects the diet-heart theory. In contrast, in the view of many, the evidence linking fatty diet to risk of CHD still appears sufficiently strong to recommend that steps should be taken to lower the fat content in the diet of many affluent countries. In the case of developing nations, this would imply attempting to prevent an unacceptable increase in fat intake.

The whole relationship is further complicated by the interrelationships between atherosclerosis, normal lipid metabolism, diabetes mellitus, and smoking. Nevertheless, epidemiological studies have laid the basis for a preventive approach to CHD.

On balance (48), evidence indicates that low-fat diets, cessation of smoking, and control of blood pressure should form the basis of a preventive programme. Other factors likely to produce a beneficial effect on CHD occurrence include reduction of obesity and increased physical activity. While nothing is absolutely certain within this complex field -- indeed in several surveys low serum cholesterol appears to correlate with increased incidence of certain cancers (50) -- the recent reductions in CHD rates in the United States probably follow from greater public awareness of the problem and increased physical activity, associated with recognition of the dangers of high fat diets and excessive smoking. Richer developing countries should recognize the potential problem and initiate preventive programmes that would be acceptable within the social norms of their societies.

POTENTIAL FOR ACTION

There are thus a number of major nutritional problems of which hunger, PEM, xerophthalmia, and LBW are the most serious and life-threatening, while goitre and iron deficiency anaemia are less serious but of generally wider prevalence. The measures for treatment and prevention of these nutritional diseases vary greatly; nutritional solutions (e.g., nutrient fortification) are possible for goitre and anaemia, but for PEM and LBW, the causes are primarily related to poverty and thus the solutions lie more in the social, economic, educational, and political spheres. Xerophthalmia is intermediate in this respect, with curative actions and medium-term prophylaxis needing direct use of vitamin A, while long-term prevention requires reduction of infectious diseases and poverty and wider consumption of a better diet.

It is thus easy to make general recommendations for nutritional measures such as iron or iodine fortification of food vehicles. In contrast, however, it is much more difficult, indeed impossible, for a nutrition scientist to make realistic recommendations to a country concerning better health for all or a balanced diet for all. These require the elimination or reduction of poverty and more equitable distribution of resources -- acts that are political and economic, not nutritional! Broad statements in this respect concerning social justice and dignity for all are often made and are usually acceptable but are almost meaningless. All that can be said by a nutritionist is that, while nutrition education can perhaps help people to be able to meet nutrient requirements at lower cost, rational solutions require simultaneous improvements in housing, distribution of money, education, and food availability.

We must assume that all governments desire progress for their people, but with political and social systems varying widely, the suggested means for achieving these aims differ from country to country and, of course, are also fully dependent on external economic, strategic, and political factors. Solutions to alleviate malnutrition require a balance between population growth and food production together with reduction of poverty. Governments must attempt to develop national plans concerning food (including food control), nutrition, and health. Such a plan could be termed National Nutrition Policy (51) and would require nutritional surveillance as a component (28, 52). The report of the United Nations Expert Committee on Methodology of Nutrition Surveillance (28) states that, "Surveillance should provide ongoing information about the nutritional conditions of the population and the factors that influence them." The new AID-funded project at Cornell University (53) is an attempt to improve and define procedures for nutritional surveillance or nutritional information systems in developing countries. Such surveillance can prevent major problems before they become serious.

"Health for all by the year 2000" was a goal proposed by the Director General of WHO in 1975. This was defined as an acceptable level of health evenly distributed throughout the world's population. The range of infant and maternal mortalities between the rich and poor parts of the world, and the differing life expectancies shown in Tables 9 to 11, indicate how far we are from that aim at present. Health must be considered in the light of its contribution to social development. For much of the world, the present situation means unemployment and underemployment, economic poverty, scarcity of worldly goods, a low level of education, poor housing, poor sanitation, malnutrition, ill health, social apathy, and a lack of will and initiative to make changes for the better. In this situation, conventional medical care benefits only a minority of individuals in the main cities, with the majority of the population, both urban and rural, receiving minimal or no benefits (8, 54).

There are several interrelated factors that can significantly affect the goal. These include demography, social and eocnomic trends, and the availability of health manpower. In general, prospects for the future are scarcely encouraging. In a discussion on the economic prospects for the developing world, Burki (55) pictures the advent of an age of global scarcity in a world of increasing population and reveals a remarkable and pessimistic consensus concerning future trends. The Independent Commission of International Development Issues (Brandt Commission) (56) was the synthesis of the results of various reports, but with emphasis on the policy initiatives that the world community could take to avert economic, political, and social disaster in the remaining decades of the century. One of the Commission conclusions was that the world economy is going through a significant and irreversible structural change, with the whole becoming increasingly interdependent. The developing countries as a whole were virtually self-sufficient in food in the 1950s; by 1970, 15 to 20 million tons of staple foods needed to be imported, but it is anticipated that by 1985, food will fall short of demand by about 45 million tons. The countries will then be importing approximately 11 percent of their food supply. Major changes leading to agrarian reform and rural development appear essential.

Life expectancy at birth, despite the well known limitations of this statistic, has proved to be possibly the most important single measure of the level of health of a population (8). WHO projections would place life expectancy at birth between 65 and 70 years for the developing countries by the year 2000 in contrast to the 55 years now. These projections used the rather more optimistic economic development indicators that were expected as recently as 1978. Circumstances have changed and they may no longer be acceptable (55). As indicated earlier, while the struggle against infectious and parasitic diseases must continue within the developing countries, health problems now typical of the developed countries such as cancer, cardiovascular diseases, mental illness, and accidents will become of major concern as countries move along the path of socio-economic development. Nonetheless, WHO (8) emphasizes that the dangers posed by infectious diseases should not be underestimated, and that unless the main causes of poverty and underdevelopment are removed, safe water and sanitation are made available for the whole population, and there is immunization of all children against the major infectious diseases, the situation will not improve.

Moral questions arise because of the increasing scarcity of food (57). Questions on whether there are universal rights such as the primary right of survival may receive less sympathy now than earlier, especially when such a right can be extended with logic to a basic right to access to resources, or even further to a moral right to do whatever is necessary to acquire and assure access to that most basic resource of all - food! The questions should be raised but the answers remain equivocal. Nevertheless, food, nutrition, and health are now part of the political spectrum and it is naive to assume otherwise: moral dimensions have a habit of becoming lost when political and national considerations arise. Even among those most committed to development, it is recognized that aid cannot be unlimited forever and self-help is, of course, essential. Nevertheless, much present political rhetoric concerning development is as unrealistic as was the advice given by the British government to the starving Irish in the 1840s (58) i.e., to become self-reliant and leave all provision of food to private enterprise and private traders.

While ongoing research is obviously essential, the fight against hunger and malnutrition is less limited by scientific criteria than by financial and political constraints. For the future, cooperation is essential between rich and poor, North and South and East and West, but real cooperation seems as far away as ever. It is difficult to be other than a pessimist when one sees the present state of the world and the resounding disinterest shown by many of the richer nations to the very reasonable and modest suggestions put forward by the Brandt Commission (56). Behind everything looms the traditional question of peace and war and the massive expenditures on armaments that take resources away from urgent needs. To quote from the Commission Report, "There is a real danger that in the year 2000 a large part of the world's population will still be living in poverty. The world may become over populated and will certainly be over urbanized. Mass starvation and the dangers of destruction may be growing steadily. The aims of the future must be to diminish the distance between the rich and poor nations, to do away with discrimination, to approach equality of opportunities step by step. This is not only a matter of striving for justice, which in itself would be important, but it is also sound self-interest not only for the poor and very poor nations, but for the better off as well."

REFERENCES

1. T.T. Poleman, "Quantifying the Nutrition Situation in Developing Countries," Food Res. Inst. Stud. XVIII(1):1 (1981).

2. M.C. Latham, "Human Nutrition in Tropical Africa," FAO Food and Nutrition Series No. 11, Rev. 1, FAO, Rome (1979).

3. U. Jonsson, "The Causes of Hunger," UNU Food and Nutrition Bulletin 3(2):1 (1981).

4. Food and Agriculture Organization, The State of Food and Agriculture, 1979, FAO Agricultural Series No. 10, FAO, Rome (1980).

5. M.A. Nour and D.F. Nygaard, "Perspectives for Food Production in the Middle East and North Africa," this volume.

6. Food and Agriculture Organization, "Food Balance Sheets, 1975-1977, Average and Per Caput Food Supplies," FAO, Rome (1980).

7. Food and Agriculture Organization, The Fourth World Food Survey, FAO Food and Nutrition Series No. 10, FAO, Rome (1977).

8. World Health Organization, Sixth Report on the World Health Situation, Part I. Global Analysis, WHO, Geneva, 1980.

9. L. Hambraeus and S. Sjolin (eds.) The Mother Child Dyad -Nutritional Aspects (Almquist and Wiksell International, Stockholm, Sweden, 1979).

10. World Health Organization, Division of Family Health. Low Birth Weight Infants, World Health Statistics Quarterly 31:74083 (1978).

11. World Health Organization, Division of Family Health, The Incidence of Low Birth Weight - A Critical Review of Available Information. World Health Statistics Quarterly 33(3):197-224 (1980).

12. J.M. Bengoa, "The State of World Nutrition," in M. Rechcigl, Jr., ed., Man, Food and Nutrition (CRC Press, Cleveland, Ohio, 1973).

13. D.B. Jelliffe and E.F.P. Jelliffe, "Cultural Traditions and Nutritional Practices Related to Pregnancy and Lactation," in L. Hambraeus and S. Sjolin, eds., The Mother Child Dyad - Nutritional Aspects (Almquist and Wiksell, Stockholm, Sweden, 1979).

14. S. Almoth and T. Greiner, "The Economic Value of Breast Feeding," FAO Food and Nutrition Paper No. 11, FAO, Rome (1979).

15. N.S. Scrimshaw, C.E. Taylor, and J.E. Gordon, Interactions of Nutrition and Infection, WHO Monograph Series No. 57 (WHO, Geneva, 1968).

16. J.M. Bengoa, "The Problem of Malnutrition," WHO Chronicle 28:3 (1974).

17. J.M. Bengoa and G. Donoso, "Prevalence of Protein-Calorie Malnutrition," PAG Bulletin 4(1):24 (1974).

18. R.R. Puffer and C.V. Serrano, Patterns of Mortality in Childhood: Report of the Inter-American Investigation of Mortality in ChildPAHO Scientific Publication No. 262 (Pan American Health Organization, Washington, D.C. 1973).

19. J.K. Harfouche, "Health Care Problems of the Young Child in a Developing Context," Bull. Wrld. Hlth. Org. 57(3):387 (1979).

20. D. Mamarbachi, P.L. Pellett, H.M. Basha, and F. Djani, "Observations on Nutritional Marasmus in a Newly Rich Nation," Ecol. Food Nutr. 9:43 (1980).

21. World Health Organization, Food and Nutrition Terminology, Terminology Circular No. 27 (WHO, Geneva, 1973).

22. D.S. McLaren, "Protein-Energy Malnutrition (P-#M): Classification, Pathogenesis, Prevalence and Prevention," in D.S. McLaren and D. Burman, eds., Textbook of Paediatric Nutrition (Churchill-Livingstone, Edinburgh and New York, 1976).

23. D.S. McLaren, P.L. Pellett, and W.W. Read, "A Simple Scoring System for Classifying the Severe Forms of Protein-Calorie Malnutrition in Early Childhood," Lancet i:533 (1967).

24. G.H. Beaton, D.H. Calloway, and J. Waterlow, "Protein-Energy Requirements: A Joint FAO/WHO Memorandum," Bull. Wrld. Hlth. Org. 57(1):65 (1979).

25. V. Viteri, R.G. Whitehead, and V.R. Young, eds., Protein-Energy Requirements Under Conditions Prevailing in Developing Countries: Current Knowledge and Research Needs (WHTR-1/UNUP-18) (The United Nations University Press, Tokyo, Japan, 1979).

26. B. Torun, V.R. Young, and W.M. Rand, eds., Protein-Energy Requirements of Developing Countries: Evaluation of New Data (WHTR/UNUP-295) (The United Nations University Press, Tokyo, Japan, 1981).

27. G. Gomez, R. Ramos-Galvan, S. Frenk, J.M. Cravioto, R. Chavez, and J. Vasquez, "Mortality in Third Degree Malnutrition," J. Trop. Pediat. 2:77 (1956).

28. World Health Organization, Methodology of Nutritional Surveillance, WHO Tech. Re. Ser. No. 593, WHO, Geneva (1976).

29. J.C. Waterlow, R. Buzina, W. Keller, J.M. Lane, M.Z. Nichaman, and J.M. Tanner, The Presentation and Use of Height and Weight Data for Comparing the Nutritional Status of Groups of Children under the Age of 10 Years," Bull. Wrld. Hlth. Org. 55(4) 489 (1977).

30. World Health Organization, Vitamin A Deficiency and Xerophthalmia, Report of a Joint WHO/USAID Meeting. WHO Tech. Rep. Ser. No. 590, WHO, Geneva (1976).

31. B.A. Underwood, "Hypovitaminosis-A and Its Control," Bull. Wrld. Hlth. Org. 56(4):525 (1978).

32. Food and Agriculture Organization and World Health Organization, Handbook on Human Nutritional Requirements, FAO Nutrition Studies No. 28 and WHO Monograph Ser. No. 61, (FAO Rome, and WHO Geneva, 1974).

33. S. Suthutvoravoot and J.A. Olson, "Plasma and Liver Concentrations of Vitamin A in a Normal Population of Urban Thai," Amer. J. Clin. Nutr. 27:883 (1974), and J.A. Olson, Wrld. Rev. Nutr. Dietet. 31:130 (1978).

34. M. Mansour, M.M. Mikhail, and Z. Farid, "Chronic Salmonella Septicemia and Malabsorption of Vitamin A," Amer. J. Clin. Nutr. 32:319 (1979).

35. P.L. Pellett, "Malnutrition, Wealth, and Development," UNU Food Nutr. Bull. 3(1):17 (1980).

36. F. Ojeda Villalba and H. Miranda, Prevention of endemic Goitre in Paraguay, Ministry of Public Health and Social Welfare, Paraguay (1978). Abstracted in Nutrition Planning 2(2):577 (1979).

37. F.C. Kelly and W.W. Snedden, Prevalence and Geographical Distribution of Endemic Goitre, Wrld. Hlth. Org. Monograph Ser. No. 44 (WHO, Geneva, 1960).

38. Joint FAO/WHO Expert Committee on Nutrition, Seventh Report, Wrld Hlth. Org. Tech. Rep. Ser. No. 377 (WHO, Geneva, 1967).

39. S.J. Baker, "Nutritional Anaemia - A Major Controllable Public Health Problem," Bull. Wrld. Hlth. Org. 56(5):659 (1978).

40. G.H. Beaton, "Epidemiology of Iron Deficiency Anaemia," in A. Jacobs and M. Worwood, eds., Iron in Biochemistry and Medicine (Academic Press, New York, 1974).

41. L.S. Rao, Panorama of Malnutrition in the Eastern Mediterranean Region. Report to Second Regional Seminar on Food and Nutrition, FAO, Cairo and WHO, Alexandria (1973).

42. P.R. Dallman, G.D. Barr, C.M. Allen, and R.H. Shinefield, "Hemoglobin Concentration in White, Black and Oriental Children: Is There a Need for Separate Criteria in Screening for Anemia?" Amer. J. Clin. Nutr. 31:377 (1978).

43. S. Piomelli, A. Brickman, and E. Carlos, "Rapid Diagnosis of Iron Deficiency by Measurement of Free Erythrocyte Porphyrins and Hemoglobin: The FEP/Hemoglobin Ratio," Pediatrics 57:136 (1976).

44. A. Lechtig, ed., "Prenatal and Perinatal Nutrition. Arch. Latinoámer. Nutric. XXVII, No. 2, Suppl. 1, Second Part (June, 1977; issued March, 1980).

45. A. Lechtig, H. Delgado, R. Martorell, and R.E. Klein, "Effects of Maternal Nutrition on the Mother Child Dyad," in L. Hambraeus and S. Sjoln, eds., The Mother Child Dyad - Nutritional Aspects (Almquist and Wiksell, Stockholm, Sweden, 1979).

46. Administrative Committee on Coordination - Subcommittee on Nutrition (ACC/SCN) Report of the Third Meeting of the ACC/SCN Consultative Group on Maternal and Young Child Nutrition, UNU Food Nutr. Bull. 3(1):20 (1981).

47. Department of Public Health and Planning, Ministry of Public Health, Kuwait. Vital and Health Statistics Division Annual Report (Kuwait, 1978).

48. M.G. Marmot, "Epidemiological Basis for Prevention of Coronary Heart Disease," Bull. Wrld. Hlth. Org. 57(3):331 (1979).

49. G.V. Mann, "Diet-heart: End of an Era," New Engl. J. Med. 297:644 (1977).

50. G.B. Kolata, "Data Sought on Low Cholesterol and Cancer," Science 211:1410 (1981).

51. J. Mayer and J. Dwyer, eds., Food and Nutrition Policy in a Changing World (Oxford University Press, New York, 1979).

52. J.P. Habicht, J.M. Lone, and A.J. McDowell, "National Nutrition Surveillance," Fed. Proc. 37:1181 (1978).

53. J. Mason and J.P. Habicht, "Nutritional Surveillance," in A.E. Harper and G.K. Davis, eds., Nutrition in Health and Disease and International Development. Symposia from the XIIth International Congress of Nutrition, San Diego, California, August 1981 (Alan R. Liss, New York, 1981).

54. H. Mahler, "Health for All by the Year 2000," WHO Chronicle 29:457 (1975).

55. S.J. Burki, "The Prospects for the Developing World: A Review of Recent Forecasts," Finance and Development 18(1):20 (1981).

56. W. Brandt, Chairman, North-South, A Programme for Survival. The Report of the Independent Commission on International Development Issues. (MIT Press, Cambridge, Massachusetts, 1980).

57. S.E. Stumpf, "The Moral Dimension of the World's Food Supply," Ann. Rev. Nutr. 1:1 (1981).

58. C. Woodham-Smith, The Great Hunger - Ireland 1845-1849 (Harper & Row, New York, 1962).

TABLE 1. Some Major Factors in the Causation of Malnutrition

1. Poor food production and supply, soil, climate, poor techniques, overpopulation.

2. Poor food distribution
   a. Within region: Poverty, transport
   b. Within family

3. Poor education
   Lack of knowledge on nutrition and health

4. Poor Health and Sanitation
   Infections and infestations, synergism

Source: Reference 2

TABLE 2. Some Symptoms and Causes of Hunger at Different Levels of Society

	Symptoms	Immediate Causes	Underlying Causes	Basic Causes
National	High infant mortality Malnutrition as the cause of deaths	Disease pattern Food intake pattern	Accessibility of health services Water and education services Production of fertilizers	Imperialism and Neocolonialism Power structure Political organization Soil and Climate Technology Historical Causes
Area Level	Low weight/age, etc. Low birth weights High infant mortality Malnutrition as the cause of deaths	Disease pattern Food intake pattern	Accessibility of health services Water and education services	Division of labour Exploitation Fiscal policy Political organization Soil and Climate Historical causes
Village level	Low weight/age, etc. Clinical signs of nutrient deficiency Low birth weights High infant mortality	Disease pattern Food intake pattern	Accessibility of health services Water and education services	Division of labour Exploitation Fiscal policy Political organization Knowledge and wisdom Historical causes
Household level	Clinical signs of nutrient deficiency Metabolic disorders Weight loss Apathy, etc.	Disease pattern Food intake pattern	Accessibility of health services Sanitary conditions Education Access to water	Division of labour Fiscal policy Power structure Religion Habits Traditional laws

Source: Reference 3

TABLE 3. Food Production and Food Energy Availability in World Regions.

	Africa	Far East	Latin America	Near East	Developing Nations	Developed Nations	World
Food Production Index 1979[1]	115	124	134	131	128	121	124
Annual Rate of % Increase 1970-79	1.6	2.9	3.5	3.5	3.0	2.2	2.5
Food Energy as % of Requirement							
1966	92	88	106	98	91	126	103
1977	95	94	108	109	100	133	110

1 1969-1971 Average = 100
Source: Reference 4

TABLE 4. FAO Index Number of Food (Crops and Livestock) Production Per Caput, Developing Regions and MSAs

	1975	1976	1977	1978	1979	Change 1978 to 1979	Annual rate of change 1961-70	1970-79
	.....1969-71 average = 100..					............%.............		
Developing market economies	101	101	102	103	100	-2.6	0.4	0.3
Africa	94	94	89	90	89	-0.9	-	-1.3
Far East	102	99	103	104	100	-4.3	0.2	0.4
Latin America	102	104	105	106	105	-0.3	0.7	0.8
Near East	106	109	104	106	103	-2.7	0.5	0.7
Asian centrally-planned economies	108	111	108	113	116	2.7	1.1	1.6
TOTAL DEVELOPING COUNTRIES	103	104	104	106	105	-0.9	0.6	0.7
MSA in Africa	94	93	91	91	90	-1.1	0.4	-1.2
MSA in Far East	100	96	101	101	95	-6.0	-0.1	-0.1
MSA in Latin America	95	98	98	101	103	2.0	1.0	
MSA in Near East	103	102	95	95	92	-3.0	0.2	-0.5
TOTAL MSA COUNTRIES	99	96	99	99	94	-4.8	0.1	-0.3

Source: Reference 4
MSA - Most Seriously Affected Countries.

TABLE 5. Annual Rate of Change of Food (Crops and Livestock) Production In Relation To Population Growth for Selected Developing Countries. 1970-79.

Population % / Food Production %	1.5 and below	1.6 to 2.0	2.1 to 2.5	2.6 to 3.0	3.1 to 3.5	3.6 & above
-3.0 and below			Kampuchea Dem.			
-2.9 to - 2.0	Barbados					
-1.9 to -0.1	Trinidad & Tobago		Mozambique, Congo	Morocco, Gambia, Namibia, Ghana, Mauritania	Algeria	
0.0 to 0.9	Uruguay, Gabon, Jamaica, Suriname, Cyprus	Samoa	Ethiopia, Lebanon, Angola, Guinea, Egypt	Togo, Peru, Somalia	Honduras, Iraq	Jordan
1.0 to 1.5		Chile, Yemen Ar. Rep.	Haiti, Nepal, Chad, Sierra Leone			
1.6 to 2.0		Cuba, Fiji, Mauritius	Lesotho, Madagascar, Bangladesh, Lao	Tanzania, Zaire, Uganda, Burma, Benin, Mongolia	Dominican Rep., Nigeria	Kenya
2.1 to 2.5		Guinea Bissau	Buthan, Guyana, Vietnam, Central Afr. Rep., India, Indonesia		Rhodesia, Malawi, Liberia	
2.6 to 3.0			Upper Volta, Burundi, Papua New Guinea	Afghanistan, Niger, Botswana, Mali		
3.1 to 3.5	China	Reunion	Cameroon, Yemen. Dem.	Swaziland, Rwanda, Paraguay	Mexico, Pakistan, Venezuela	
3.6 and above	Argentina	Sri Lanka, Korea Rep.	Tunisia, Costa Rica, Colombia	Bolivia, Ecuador, Panama, Sudan, Turkey, Malaysia, Iran, Senegal, El Salvador, Brazil, Philippines, New Hebrides, Bahamas, Korea Dem., Thailand	Nicaragua Zambia, Guatemala, Saudi Arabia, Syria	Ivory Coast, Brunei, Libya

Note: Countries in each group are listed in ascending order of the annual rate of change in their food production; MSA countries are underlined.

Source: Reference 4

TABLE 6. Estimated Number of Persons with Food Intake Below the Critical Minimum List: Developing Regions (Excluding Asian Centrally Planned Economies)

	Total Population		Percentage Below 1.2 x BMR		Total Number Below 1.2 x BRM	
	1969-71	1972-4	1969-71	1972-4	1969-71	1972-4
	Millions		%		Millions	
Africa	278	301	25	28	70	83
Far East	968	1042	25	29	256	297
Latin America	279	302	16	15	44	46
Near East	167	182	18	16	31	29
MSA	954	1027	27	30	255	307
Non-MSA	738	800	20	18	146	148
Developing countries	1692	1827	24	25	401	455

Source: Reference 7

TABLE 7. Population, Population Growth, Land Area and Population Density by Region

	Population Millions (1977)	Annual Rate of Growth 1965-1977	Population as Percentage of World Total %	Land Area as Percentage of World Total %	Population Density Number Per Sq Km
Asia	2355	2.2	57	20	85
Europe	478	0.6	12	5	97
Africa	424	2.7	10	23	15
Latin America	342	2.7	8	15	17
USSR	260	1.0	6	16	12
North America	242	1.0	6	15	11
Oceania	22	2.0	<1	7	3
Near East	318	2.8	8	14	20

Source: Reference 8
<u>Note</u>: Near East data were calculated from country values and are for 1979; values are not fully additive because the Near East Region is part of both Asia and Africa. Near East as here defined is larger than FAO region.

TABLE 8. Estimates of Infant and Early Childhood Mortality in Selected Regions of the World

	Infant Mortality (A) (per 1000 Live Births)	Early Childhood Mortality (1-4 Yrs) (B) per 1000 Population at Risk	Ratio A/B
More developed regions: Country range	8.3 - 40.3	0.4 - 2.0	20-21
Less developed regions			
North Africa	ca. 130	ca. 30	4-5
Sub-Sahara Africa	ca. 200	> 30	5-6
Asia	ca. 120-130	> 10	6-12
Latin America	ca. 85-90	ca. 6	ca. 15

Source: Reference 8
Note: Middle East overlaps North Africa and Asia in many WHO Tables.

TABLE 9. Comparison between National Maternal and Child Mortality Rates

	Highest Levels (A)	Lowest Levels (B)	Ratio A/B
Perinatal mortality[a]	120	12 - 15	8 - 10 : 1
Infant mortality[a]	200	8 - 10	20 - 25 : 1
Childhood mortality[b]	45	0.4 - 1.0	45 - 75 : 1
Maternal mortality[c]	1000	5 - 10	100 - 200 : 1

[a] per 1000 live births; [b] per 1000 population; [c] per 100,000 live births
Source: Reference 8

TABLE 10. Association between Infant Mortality and Socio-Economic Development

	IMR[a]	Food Energy Consumption (Kcal/capita/day)	GNP Per Capita U.S. $
Developed regions	22	3400	5200
Less developed regions	109	2200	470
of which least developed	156	2000	140

[a]IMR: Infant Mortality Rate, deaths (less than 1 year of age) per 1000 live births

Source: Reference 8

TABLE 11. Estimated Life Expectancy at Birth for World Regions

World	56-57
More developed regions	70
North America	73
Australia and New Zealand	73
Europe	70
Japan	74
USSR	70
Less developed regions	c. 54
North Africa	50-55
Sub-Sahara Africa	<50 (probably 40-45)
East Asia	50-60
South Asia	c. 50
Latin America	62

Source: Reference 8

TABLE 12. The Characteristics of Hunger and the Major Nutritional Disorders.

	Protein Energy Malnutrition (P-EM[b])						
	Hunger[a]	Nutritional Marasmus	Kwashiokor	Xerophthalmia	Goitre	Iron Deficiency Anaemia	Low Birth Weight Infants[c]
Causation/Precipitation Long Term	Poverty, poor agriculture		Low protein diet	Low intakes of carotene and/or retinol	Low intakes of iodine	Low intake/absorption of iron	Poor dietary intake since conception. Infections of Mother
Immediate	Poverty, crop failure, war	Early weaning; Infections	Infections	Early weaning; Infections		Blood loss from infestations	Low weight gain in pregnancy
Vulnerable groups and main age of incidence	All ages	Children less than 1 year	Children between 1-2 years	Children, preschool	Older children, females	Children (<3 yrs) and females of child bearing age	Mothers of poor socio-economic status
Major features	Growth failure, wasting, lethargy	Wasting	Oedema, fatty liver, reduced serum albumin	Night blindness, xerosis of conjunctiva and cornea, keratomalacia, low serum retinol	Enlarged thyroid	Low haemoglobin (microcytic hypochromic anaemia if severe)	Hypoglycemia, hypothermia, poor resistance to infection (low IgG)
Consequences	Reduced growth, reduced work capacity, high mortality	High mortality, impaired mental development	High mortality, impaired mental development	High mortality especially when associated with PEM. Blindness	Cretinism	Pallor, reduced work and learning efficiency	High mortality, suboptimal development. High incidence of infection
Areas of Incidence	All areas of poverty	Urban areas, large families with low incomes and poor education	Rural Africa, areas with low protein weaning foods	Rice staple: areas of poverty	Low soil iodine, Mountain areas and certain oases	Ubiquitous	Low socio-economic areas with high prevalence of infections
Prevalence	High	Widespread in poor areas	Increasingly rare in Middle East and North Africa	Not widespread in wheat staple areas of Middle East and North Africa	High in localized areas	High	Incidence highly correlated with socio-economic indicators, possibly 20% of all births in poor areas
Measures to Eliminate	Major socio-economic, agri-cultural and educational improvements	Major socio-economic and educational improvements, Control infections	Control infections Higher protein in weaning foods	Increased consumption of green vegetables. Fortification. Improved socio-economic conditions	Iodine enrichment	Iron enrichment Control of infestations	Maternal nutrition programs. Prevention of infections. Major socio-economic and educational improvements.

[a] There is a considerable degree of overlap with P-EM and LBW infants; [b] P-EM when early or of mild-moderate severity is usually sub-clinical and can only be diagnosed by anthropometric criteria (Wt/age, Ht/age and Wt/Ht); [c] Infants of birth weight below 2,500 g. In Developing Countries the majority of these are due to fetal growth retardation.

With acknowledgements to D.S. McLaren, Nutrition in the Community, First Edition, J. Wiley & Sons, Chichester, U.K. (1976).

TABLE 13. Estimated Numbers of Children Suffering from Severe or Moderate PEM in the Near East, North Africa, and Other Developing Regions

Region	Total Population[a] 1977 (m)	Number of Children[b] <5 Yrs (m)	Severe PEM[c] (m)	Moderate PEM[c] (m)	Total PEM[c] (m)
Near East[d]	318	50	1.4	9.5	10.9
Africa	424	67	2.0	16.8	18.8
S. Asia	1318	211	4.2	35.8	40.0
Latin America	342	54	1.0	8.9	9.9
Total developing regions	2973	469	10.3	93.8	104.1

[a] Source: Reference 8

[b] Proportion of children less than 5 years old in developing countries compared to total population is about 16%.

[c] Proportions of children less than 5 years old suffering from PEM in various regions from Bengoa and Donoso (Reference 17).

[d] Near East Region is not identical to FAO defined region. Values are not additive since Near East Region overlaps Africa and Asia and not all developing regions are shown.

TABLE 14. Criteria for Determining Whether Hypovitaminosis-A is a Significant Public Health Problem

Criteria	Percentage of Population
Bitot spots with conjunctival xerosis	$\geq$ 2.0
Corneal xerosis and corneal ulceration with xerosis and keratomalacia	$\geq$ 0.01
Corneal scars	$\geq$ 0.1
Plasma vitamin A 100 ug/litre	$\geq$ 5.0

Source: Reference 30 and Guidelines for the Eradication of Vitamin A Deficiency and Xerophthalmia (The Nutrition Foundation, Inc., New York, 1977.

TABLE 15. Estimated Number of Births of All Live Infants and of Low Birth-Weight Infants

Region	Live Births (Thousands)	Low Birth-Weight Infants %	(Thousands)
Africa	21,000	15	3,165
North America	3,684	7	269
Latin America	12,410	11	1,392
Asia	72,940	20	14,785
Europe	7,006	8	536
Oceania	506	12	62
USSR	4,752	8	380
World	122,300	17	20,600
Developed countries	17,400	7	1,290
Developing countries	104,900	18	19,310

Source: Reference 11

PROBLEMS IN THE ASSESSMENT OF HUMAN NUTRITIONAL NEEDS

NEVIN S. SCRIMSHAW

The previous paper has described the wide range of world nutritional problems, many of which are prevalent in the region. However, only the deficiencies of protein, calories, and vitamin A and possibly iron are significant for plant breeders. The other vitamin and mineral deficiencies occur sporadically, but not with a frequency, severity, or consistency that need to be taken into account in breeding programmes. Nevertheless, the avoidance of such deficiencies requires green and yellow vegetables and fruits in the diet, so that these cannot be neglected in either nutrition education or agricultural policy. Of course, animal proteins can also make a valuable contribution, not only to the protein content of the diet, but also to the vitamin and mineral content.

Interpretation of the nutritional significance of any given level of nutrient intake in a population depends on the nutritional criteria adopted. The principal criteria that have been used to identify a serious and persistent insufficiency of dietary calories or protein are:

(a) protein and calorie intakes relative to requirements for each, and for available protein calories as percent of total calories;

(b) growth performance compared with growth standards.

The value and significance of each are quite different, and they have been affected in diverse ways by changing expert judgments in recent years.

The adequacy of protein-energy intakes can also be judged from data on infant and preschool child mortality, measles mortality where immunization is not given, and when available, overall morbidity from infectious disease, especially among preschool children. The seriousness of these adverse functional consequences of such malnutrition should be a stimulus to agricultural efforts to assure adequate protein and energy supplies. While the prevention of protein-energy malnutrition depends ultimately on the ability to acquire food and on associated dietary practices, marginal improvements in the protein <u>value</u> of staple foods have important nutritional benefits.

Variations in the estimates of micronutrients are of less importance to agricultural planners and will not be discussed in this paper. Vitamin A and iron are partial exceptions. The biological requirement for vitamin A can be met either by preformed vitamin A from animal sources, in which case there is reasonable agreement on a daily intake of retinol from 65 ug (195 IU) per kg of body weight in children four months of age to 12 ug (36 IU) per kg in adults, or the same in retinol equivalents from vitamin A precursors in vegetable sources. In the latter case, the beta-carotene of carrots and other vegetables has half of the activity per mg of preformed vitamin A, and other carotenoid pigments have considerably less or none at all. For example, a pale yellow corn in which the pigment is mainly beta-carotene can have a higher vitamin A activity than a deep red or blue corn in which the pigments are carotenoids with little or no vitamin A activity. Similarly, although its beta-carotene content is high, most of the pigment in African palm oil has no vitamin A activity. The attempt to evaluate or breed vegetables for their vitamin A activity cannot rely on color as a reliable guide.

For iron the situation is equally complex. The requirement for iron is given as 14 mg per day for an adult male and 18 mg for adult women. However, this tells very little about how much iron is required in diets because both the source of iron and the presence of phytates, oxalates, tannins, and crude fibre greatly influences biological availability. The latter compounds severely reduce the availability of dietary iron. In general, iron of vegetable origin is poorly available (Figure 1), ranging from as low as 1 to 2 percent for spinach to only 3 to 5 percent for better leaf sources such as lettuce and cassava leaves, and 3 percent from *Phaseolus vulgaris* (1).

In contrast, the haem iron in red meat is at least 10 to 20 percent absorbed and also improves the absorption of vegetable iron in the diet. Iron absorption is enhanced by ascorbic acid in the diet and reduced by protein deficiency.

The adequacy of dietary iron intake is complicated still further by environmental factors. Hookworm, schistosomiasis, and malaria increase iron loss from the body, and enteric infections further decrease iron absorption. These effects of infection on iron requirements can generally be overcome by increased iron intake alone. Clearly, one can tell little about the adequacy of dietary iron intakes *per se* or the probability that they will be associated with the known functional consequences of iron deficiency. These adverse effects include reduced physical capacity and work performance, impaired resistance to infection resulting in increased morbidity and in absenteeism of workers, poorer cognitive performance, and lower cold tolerance. It is actualy more difficult to meet iron requirements than protein needs from vegetable sources alone.

Dietary Energy Requirements

Energy requirements in the 1973 FAO/WHO (2) and preceding reports (3, 4) have been expressed as average requirements with the implication that a population not consuming the average was to some extent calorie-deficient. While this may be true in one sense, it is quite wrong to assume that either individuals or populations whose average intakes are below estimated average requirements are actually in negative energy balance. As the new FAO/WHO/UNU report (5) and a previous UNU report emphasize (6), individuals adapt, within limits, to low energy intake level by decreasing their activity and to a small extent also their basal metabolic rate (BMR). This adaptation is at the cost of reduced discretionary activity and ultimately, lower work capacity. By these means, however, physiological needs for energy can be brought into balance with available food energy until a limit is reached.

A 1975 expert FAO/WHO consultation pointed out that very sedentary individuals could survive at levels averaging as low as 1.5 X their basal metabolic rate, although this did not allow for significant physical activity for work or recreation. It was intended to cover BMR plus the energy lost through the heat of metabolism of food, and minimal dietary energy necessary for dressing, eating, personal hygiene, and little more.

FAO statisticians reasoned that, if the coefficient of variation of BMR was 10 percent, as assumed in the expert committee reports, the absolute minimum for all but 2.5 percent of individuals would be 1.5 minus 20 percent (the mean minus 2 S.D.), or 1.2 X BMR. They then applied this figure to national food intake data to calculate the number of severely undernourished on the assumption that nearly all individuals below this figure would be beyond the limits of adaptation. However, this gives an underestimate of under-nutrition. One problem with this approach is that it assumes a distribution about the mean according to need that applies to *ad libitum* calorie intakes, but not necessarily to conditions of restriction. There will be a statistically predictable number of individuals with intakes above 1.2 X BMR who are also beyond the limits of their capacity to adapt. It should also be clear that even 1.5 times basal metabolic rate is not sufficient for either productive economic activities or long-term maintenance of health. Its application will fall far short of indicating the economic and social consequences of the reduced activity associated with low food intakes caused by poverty.

A re-examination of protein and energy requirements took place in Rome in October 1981 under the auspices of FAO, WHO, and UNU and the report will be published during 1984 (5). This new report notes that apparent paradox of the survival of populations consuming 90 or even 80 percent of their estimated energy requirements by international standards. Because these populations are not wasting away and dying, they are adapting to lower calorie intakes mainly at the cost of reduced physical activity. Viteri has documented the extent to which Guatemalan plantation workers are limited by their food intake in the amount of work they can do, and how they virtually collapse for the remainder of the day after working hours with little further activity (7). When additional food is provided to them, their consumption and activity both increase. This is true for children as well as adults and the reduced interaction of undernourished children with their environment, including parents and siblings, is probably a critical factor in the poorer cognitive performance of such children (8, 9).

Which criterion is used for arriving at estimates of numbers of malnourished makes considerable difference. This is illustrated in Table 1 for countries with four different population distributions and activity levels. The large differences in estimated numbers of malnourished individuals by FAO and the World Bank are easily understood on this basis. The FAO estimates shown in Table 2 are for individuals whose intakes are below 1.2 X basal and those of the World Bank below estimated requirements. In the former case the percentages range from 16 to 23 percent globally and in the latter from 61 to 73 percent. The actual figure thus varies from 436 million in the FAO *Agriculture Toward 2000* published in 1981 to 808 million in a 1980 paper of Reutlinger and Alderman for the World Bank (10). To either of these numbers WHO would add those children whose growth and development are significantly impaired by under-nutrition and those mothers whose pregnancies result in low birth-weight children.

Recently, Poleman (11) has claimed that both the FAO and World Bank figures are grossly inflated, but his own figure wholly ignores the problem of deficient calorie intakes of many populations and focuses only on preschool children. He acknowledges a possible range of 10 to 50 percent of this group malnourished in developing countries, or 82 to 309 million people, and proposes 100 million as a reasonable estimate without attempting to justify it further. His estimates of numbers of preschool children should be added to the FAO or World Bank figure and not substituted for it.

The new FAO/WHO/UNU report (5) also emphasizes for the first time the importance of adequate food for discretionary as well as work activities. It points out that there is no appropriate average figure for energy requirement unless the activity level is specified. Not only do individuals adapt, but also whole societies develop patterns that are compatible with low food intakes, although poorly adapted to the development goals to which they aspire. It should be recognized, therefore, that, as average intakes fall below average requirements, or as individuals consume less than their own requirements when food is freely available, the first consequence is a decrease in discretionary activity. As intakes drop, work activity will be progressively affected until a level is reached that will allow only for the energy necessary for basal maintenance, digestion of food, eating, hygiene, and a sedentary, dependent existence incompatible with long-term cardiovascular fitness. This is the 1.5 X BMR lower average or individual limit. At the mean minus two standard deviations, or 1.2 X BMR, nearly all individuals will be below the survival limit. Wasting and eventually death will occur.

In the future, countries will need to determine the caloric requirements for the pattern of work and of discretionary activities that they consider appropriate to their populations, whether or not the result implies the need for an increase or decrease in their observed intakes. Different segments of a country's population will have different mean energy requirements and these may vary seasonally or over time. Because energy requirements are likely to be higher in lower income segments of the population because of their work patterns, and food availability to them is usually less because of poverty, national averages are grossly misleading, especially when the increased wastage of food by upper income groups is taken into account. This kind of relationship between income and energy intake is illustrated in Figure 2, based on the 1970 national nutrition survey in Brazil (12). The high caloric intakes reported for the highest income groups are more indicative of food waste than overeating.

Safe Allowances for Protein

When, without elaborate rationale, the League of Nations in 1935 proposed 1 gram of protein per kg in a good mixed diet as the adult requirement, the figure was probably more correct than those recommended in the intervening years. Successive FAO/WHO committees proposed a figure for "reference protein" of 0.52 in 1955 and 0.71 per kg in 1963, in both cases with the optimistic assumption that in use this would be corrected for by the quality of usual diets to bring the figure up somewhat toward the old estimate by the League of Nations committee. The 1963 figure of 0.71 g/kg for adults resulted in evaluations of the diets of low-income populations of developing countries that frequently indicated protein to be the limiting factor, particularly for preschool children. During the 1960s, considerable emphasis was given to meeting the present and future protein needs of developing countries in national planning, agricultural research, economic policy, and nutrition education.

The situation changed dramatically when the 1971 FAO/WHO Expert Committee on Energy and Protein Requirements arrived at a figure that was 20 percent lower than the 1963 adult reference protein requirements and changed the estimated calorie requirements only slightly. Even before the publication of its report in 1973 (2), there was a rush to re-evaluate the relative deficiency of protein and energy in developing country diets, often without an appropriate adjustment for protein quality. This generally led to the conclusion that protein was less limiting than calories and that emphasis on additional protein in the diets of developing countries was misplaced.

With the publication of the 1973 FAO/WHO report, the pendulum shifted from a tendency to focus too narrowly on protein to the opposite extreme of neglecting protein to a dangerous degree. Four factors were responsible:

First, the estimates of the 1973 report were too low. This was not generally officially recognized and corrected until the October 1981 FAO/WHO/UNU consultation and the published report will not be available until 1984 (5).

Second, the discrepancies between the FAO/WHO estimates of the average energy requirements and observed energy intakes did not reflect physiological deficiency of energy, but rather adaptation to available dietary energy. Instead of indicating an absolute deficiency of energy, zero energy balance was achieved in most cases.

Third, it was generally assumed and frequently stated in dogmatic terms that, when the percentage of deficit protein intake compared with the "safe allowance" was less than the percent of energy intake compared with average energy requirement, additional protein in the diet is wasted because it is metabolized to meet energy, not protein, needs. Even if adaptation to lower energy intakes were not the rule, this statement is not supported by data from animal feeding studies nor by our own metabolic studies in human subjects (13). In fact, experience with so-called protein-sparing fasts for weight reduction of morbidly obese subjects indicates that 1 gm of protein per kg is sufficient to maintain nitrogen balance in individuals consuming a 500 calorie diet (14).

Fourth, there was a general failure to recognize that the same socio-economic circumstances that force physiological adaptation to low dietary energy intakes are frequently associated with increased protein requirements because they are conducive to frequent episodes of diarrheal, respiratory, and other infectious diseases. Unfortunately, unlike the situation for calories, there is no adaptation possible to protein intakes below either normal minimum requirements or those exacerbated by infectious disease.

The October 1981 Protein-Energy Consultation identified the reasons why the 1971/73 protein recommendations were too low. This had already been established beyond doubt by two kinds of experiments:

One approach was to feed the 0.57 gm of egg protein proposed as a safe allowance in 1971 to normal subjects, not for short periods as in the original studies, but for up to three months. When this was done in repeated studies, (15-17), many of the subjects fed this protein level with adequate or even excess calories showed significant loss of lean body mass, serum albumin and haemoglobin, and in some cases, serum enzyme changes indicative of altered liver function.

The other approach was to feed graded amounts of good-quality protein, such as egg, milk, meat, and soya in order to determine by linear regression the amount required for zero nitrogen balance. Repeated studies gave a mean intercept of 0.64 gm protein per kg with a coefficient of variation of 17.5 percent (18). In addition, the United Nations University sponsored a series of similar studies in 13 developing countries with the usual diets of these populations and, to the extent possible, under prevailing conditions (6, 18). They yielded mean intercepts ranging from 0.58 to 1.40 gm/kg. When corrected for the digestibility and protein value of the various diets, these values are similar to the 0.64 figure and much higher than the average values assumed in the 1973 FAO/WHO report.

The recognized shortcomings of the safe protein allowance of the 1973 publication were:

First, in order to be sure that calories were not limiting in studies of protein requirements, it was common practice in research studies to provide extra calories in metabolic balance studies (19). For example, in our work at MIT we routinely made the best estimate of the subjects' usual caloric intake and then added an additional 10 percent to be sure that protein needs were not exaggerated because of the need to use the dietary protein as an energy source.

Figure 3, taken from the work of Inoue et al. (20), indicates the consequences of such an experimental design. The additional calories tended to bring about an underestimate of the amount of protein required for zero nitrogen balance when dietary energy needs were only just being met.

Figure 4 shows the effect of caloric intake on the amount of protein required for nitrogen balance in our three-month studies at MIT. At the "safe level" proposed in the 1973 report, 0.57 g/kg of body weight, the three subjects illustrated were in strongly negative nitrogen balance when given a caloric intake appropriate to their needs. The addition of 250 calories made their nitrogen balance less negative, and 500 calories were sufficient to bring the individuals into nitrogen balance, but at the cost of a progressive gain in weight. Clearly, a "safe level" that is adequate for nitrogen balance only when an individual is consuming so high a dietary energy level as to be gaining weight is not acceptable.

Second, when nitrogen intake is carefully measured and compared with nitrogen losses in urine and faeces, the difference must be due to losses from the skin, hair, nails, saliva, and nitrogen in menses and semen. Isaksson and co-workers (21) have summarized data of their own and others to suggest that the difference is consistently in the range of 14 mg of N per kg; however, direct measurements by Calloway et al. (22) yield figures of 3 mg for sweat losses and 2 mg for miscellaneous losses for individuals consuming a minimum adequate protein intake. The 1984 report does not accept the value proposed by Isakkson et al. because of the possible effect of measurement errors, but it indicates that the losses at requirement levels are higher than the 5 mg of the 1973 report and proposes 8 mg per kg.

Third, the 1973 report allowed 30 percent for the difference between efficiency utilization of protein at zero nitrogen intakes and that at nitrogen equilibirum. More thorough review of available data suggests that the figure should have been in the range of 45 to 60 percent (5). Thus, the amount of nitrogen considered necessary for nitrogen balance on the basis of measured obligatory losses was not corrected sufficiently for inefficiency of utilization at requirement levels.

Fourth, there was a tendency for individuals using the 1973 report to fail to note that the 0.57 was expressed in terms of egg or milk protein, and hence to neglect the appropriate adjustment for the lower net protein utilization of ordinary proteins.

Fifth, in the case of children, it was assumed that they would grow at a daily rate of 1/365th of their annual growth rate. The trouble with this is that even normal children fail to grow for some periods of time and then grow at two or three times the average daily rate (8). This is important because the requirement of protein for growth is a much larger percentage of the total requirement than is the case for energy. For example, Table 3, based on the 1973 report, shows 2 percent of total calories for growth at 1/365th of the annual growth, while the corresponding figure for protein is 12 percent. Thus, normal growth would require 6 percent more calories and 36 percent more protein for peak periods than for the 1/365th of annual rate standard. This will be allowed for in the 1984 report. More significant, however, is the situation for catch-up growth after periods of acute infections and malnutrition. By the 1973 standards, a nine times average increment would require 16 percent more dietary calories and 96 percent more protein. I cannot re-calculate these percentages for the 1984 figures because they are not yet available, but the conclusion will not change.

This kind of analysis explains why protein is so important to the diet of the young child, especially in developing countries. It is lack of protein rather than calories that inhibits the peaks of catch-up growth and results in permanently reduced stature according to studies in both Peru (23) and Guatemala (24).

The net result of the October 1981 discussions, taking into account all of the above factors, was the recommendation that the new safe protein allowance for adults should be 0.75 gm of protein per kilo of body weight, expressed in terms of egg, milk, meat, fish, or soy. The group took into account both long-and short-term studies and decided to adopt 0.61 as the average adult protein requirement, and 12.5 percent as the coefficient of variation to arrive at the preceding figure. The "safe allowance" expressed for the protein of mixed diets will be in the range of 0.8 to 1.0 gm of protein per kilo, depending on whether it is predominantly animal protein or entirely vegetable protein of relatively high fibre content.

The practical significance of this can best be seen by comparing calculations for the requirements of a single country's population, based on the 1973 and 1985 reports, respectively (Appendices 1 and 2)[1/]. When calculations are based on the 1976 census in Egypt, and the age, sex, and physiological status distribution of that population, the differences are impressive -- 702,998 tons of protein of the quality of the usual Egyptian diet for calculations based on the 1973 report, and 932,881 tons per day based on the 1985 report.

Any estimate of protein-energy needs based on the 1984 compared with the 1973 report will indicate about one-third more protein, hence a need for a higher percentage of available protein calories than those estimates based on the 1973 report. The percentage of protein calories required by the elderly is generally higher than that for young adults both because of the reduced physical activity and poorer protein digestibility.

Percent of Available Protein Calories

Minimum acceptable protein calories as percent of total calories has been used as an indicator of dietary inadequacy. In 1961 Platt and co-workers (25) proposed a calculation of net dietary protein calories percent (ND_pCals %). This was calculated by taking the caloric equivalent of the average protein requirement corrected for Net Protein Utilization as percent of the total calorie requirement. The resulting figure was proposed as a reference point against which the percentage of available protein calories in usual diets could be evaluated. If the latter was less, it was judged inadequate to meet minimum protein needs even when the diet was consumed in amounts sufficient to meet calorie needs.

The concept was a good one, but the method of calculating the reference percentage and its application failed to take into account the individual variation in each of the three components of the calculation: calorie requirements, protein requirements, and protein quality. An individual can be at the upper end of the distribution for protein requirements and the lower end for energy requirements. In this case, the required percentage of available protein calories would not be appropriately described by reference to the average calorie requirement, but more properly to the average calorie requirement minus 2 S.D. The net result

---

[1/]Prepared by Dr. Aida El Asfahani, United Nations University Fellow from Egypt, in the MIT-Harvard International Food and Nutrition Program.

would mean that that individual would need a much higher percentage of available protein calories than the original ND_pCals % calculation.

Table 4 shows the percentages for the 1973 and anticipated 1984 publications utilizing average calorie requirements and safe protein allowances, and the same figures re-calculated to show the percentage of available protein calories calculated from the estimated variation at each of these expert meetings. The figures assume healthy individuals with _ad libitum_ dietary energy intake. They do not take into account the fact that many individuals in developing country populations are forced to consume lower energy intakes for lack of money, and may have higher protein requirements because of frequent episodes of acute infectious disease, the presence of intestinal parasites, and other chronic disease states.

It is noteworthy, however, that the ordinary diets consumed by the well-nourished populations of industrialized countries are not only well above the range of estimated adequacy of availability of protein calories for normal individuals, but that this is also true of most populations in developing countries as well.

When the diet is made up of a cereal staple and legumes, the available protein calories are generally sufficient if the caloric intake is adequate. In such a population, only individuals whose diets for reasons of poverty or other factors contain lesser amounts of legumes or other protein sources than the usual patterns, or whose dietary energy intakes are severely restricted, will run the risk of protein deficiency. Where the staple is cassava, however, or other roots and tubers, the complementary legume or other protein source in the diet becomes even more critical, and inadequate protein intakes may occur for some individuals consuming local diets even as adults. In any event, young children are always at risk when they do not receive sufficient legumes or other protein sources relative to either a cereal or a root or tuber staple such as cassava.

It should be clear that there are so many variables that it is very difficult to estimate the probability of deficiency from knowledge of dietary protein calories percentage alone. Nevertheless, this calculation can be used to identify diets so low in available total protein as to be likely to result in protein deficiency in most individuals consuming them.

Without going further into the matter, it can be stated that both direct observations on MIT students and the figures derived from the latest Protein-Energy Report indicate that about 10 percent of protein-calories of high value is needed. This figure increases to 11 to 12 percent with the predominantly vegetable protein diets of developing countries and 13 to 14 percent when roots and tubers are the staple. It will be higher when caloric intakes are restricted for any reason, and for recovery or catch-up growth after infections and other kinds of stress.

Growth

The growth of young children is a sensitive indicator of nutritional adequacy, and on a population basis, any improvement of inadequate nutrition is associated with increased growth. However, because most children in the lower socio-economic groups of developing countries are so much smaller than well-nourished children of comparable age in industrialized countries, there is chronic resistance to using the latter as a standard for comparison. On the other hand, adopting so-called local standards can lead to a gross underestimate of the influence of malnutrition.

Whenever it has been possible to obtain reliable data on the growth of sufficiently well-nourished and relatively privileged children in developing countries, they have not differed significantly from those of similar children in the U.S. and Europe. Many years ago the Institute of Nutrition of Central America and Panama (INCAP) found that the pre-pubertal growth of children of upper income groups in Guatemala, El Salvador, Honduras, Costa Rica, and Panama did not differ significantly from that of Iowa schoolchildren. The so-called Harvard Standards (26) have also been widely used in developing countries.

More recently, WHO examined comparable data from around the world and concluded that the most recent and extensive data from the United States, those of the National Center of Health Statistics (NCHS) (27), were appropriate to become the WHO reference standards. Nevertheless, the desire persists in many developing countries for local standards that are lower. The issue of what height and weight standards to use in calculating protein and energy requirements was thoroughly discussed during the October 1981 Protein-Energy Consultation, and the use of the U.S. NCHS-based WHO standards was endorsed. This is of critical importance in the use of weight and height for age to classify malnourished children and estimate percentages and total numbers of children in the various categories.

SUMMARY

In summary, the fluctuations in estimated protein requirements that have given low figures in 1975 and 1973 and much higher figures in 1965 and 1984, while estimates of energy requirements have changed very little, have caused great confusion. Diets that have been considered, since 1973, to be deficient in calories relative to protein may now once again be considered to be relatively deficient in protein. Renewed emphasis is also given to protein by the recognition that individuals adapt to low energy intake by reduced activity, but cannot adapt to correspondingly low protein intakes.

It is now apparent that added protein quantity or quality, when the protein value of a diet is inadequate, does bring about nutritional benefit whether or not calories are also inadequate. On the other hand, adequate caloric intake enhances protein utilization, and the adaptation to low calorie intakes is neither economically nor socially desirable. These changing estimates of energy requirements and safe protein allowances have profound implications for agricultural policy.

1. M. Layrisse, "Iron Absorption from Food," in Iron Metabolism and Anemia, Pan American Health Organization Publication No. 184 (PAHO, Washington, D.C., 1969).

2. Energy and Protein Requirements. Report of a Joint FAO/WHO Ad Hoc Expert Committee. Wld. Hlth. Org. Tech. Rep. Ser. No. 522 (WHO, Geneva, 1973).

3. Food and Agriculture Organization of the United Nations, Protein Requirements. Report of the FAO Committee, Rome, Italy 24-31 October, 1955. FAO Nutrition Studies No. 16 (FAO, Rome, 1957).

4. Protein Requirements. Report of a Joint FAO/WHO Expert Group, Geneva, 8-17 October, 1963. Wld. Hlth. Org. Tech. Rep. Ser. No. 301 (WHO, Geneva, 1965).

5. Energy and Protein Requirements. Report of a Joint FAO/WHO/UNU Expert Consultation,Rome 5-17 October, 1981 (WHO, Geneva, in press).

6. B. Torun, V.R. Young, and W.M. Rand, eds., Protein-Energy Requirements of Developing Countries: Evaluation of Data. The United Nations University World Hunger Programme Food and Nutrition Bulletin Supplement No. 5 (UNU Tokyo, 1981).

7. F.E. Viteri, "Definition of the Nutrition Problem in the Labor Force," in Nutrition and Agricultural Development - Significance and Potential for the Tropics, N.S. Scrimshaw and B. Behar, eds. (Plenum, New York, 1976).

8. F.E. Viteri, R.G. Whitehead, and V.R. Young, eds., Protein-Energy Requirements under Conditions Prevailing in Developing Countries: Current Knowledge and Research Needs. The United Nations University World Hunger Programme Food and Nutrition Bulletin Supplement No. 1 (UNU, Tokyo, 1979).

9. A. Chavez, C. Martinez, and T. Yaschine, "The Importance of Nutrition and Stimuli on Child Mental and Social Development," in Early Malnutrition and Mental Development, J. Cravioto, L. Hambraeus, and B. Vahlquist, eds. (Almquist and Wiksell, Uppsala, Sweden, 1974).

10. S. Reutlinger and H. Alderman, "The Prevalence of Calorie-Deficient Diets in Developing Countries," The World Bank Staff Working Paper No. 374 (World Bank, Washington, D.C., February 1980).

11. T. Poleman, "A Reappraisal of the Extent of World Hunger," Food Policy 6(4):236 (1981).

12. The Getulio Vargas Foundation, Brazilian Institute of Economics, Food Consumption in Brazil (The United States Department of Agriculture, Economic Research Service, and Israel Program for Scientific Translations, Washington, D.C., 1970).

13. N.S. Scrimshaw, Y. Taylor, and V.R. Young, "Lysine Supplementation of Wheat Gluten at Adequate and Restricted Energy Intakes in Young Men," Amer. J. Clin. Nutr. 26:965 (1973).

14. G.L. Blackburn, J.P. Flatt, G.H.A. Clowes, T.F. O'Donnell, and T.E. Hensle, "Protein-Sparing Therapy during Periods of Starvation with Sepsis or Trauma," Ann. Surg. 177:588 (1973).

15. C. Garza, N.S. Scrimshaw, and V.R. Young, "Human Protein Requirements: The Effect of Variations in Energy Intake within the Maintenance Range," Amer. J. Clin. Nutr. 29:280 (1976).

16. C. Garza, N.S. Scrimshaw, and V.R. Young, "Human Protein Requirements: A Long-Term Metabolic Nitrogen Balance Study in Young Men to Evaluate the 1973 FAO/WHO Safe Level of Egg Protein Intake," J. Nutr. 107:335 (1977).

17. C. Garza, N.S. Scrimshaw, and V.R. Young, "Human Protein Requirements: Evaluation of the 1973 FAO/WHO Safe Level of Protein Intake for Young Men at High Energy Intakes," Brit. J. Nutr. 37:403 (1977).

18. W.M. Rand, R. Uauy, and N.S. Scrimshaw, eds., Protein-Energy Requirement Studies in Developing Countries: Results of International Research, The United Nations University Food and Nutrition Bulletin Supplement No. 10 (UNU, Tokyo, Japan 1984).

19. N.S. Scrimshaw, Shattuck Lecture: "Strengths and Weaknesses of the Committee Approach. An Analysis of Past and Present Recommended Dietary Allowances for Protein in Health and Disease," New Engl. J. Med. 294:136,198 (1976).

20. G. Inoue, Y. Fujita, and Y. Niiyama, "Studies on Protein Requirements of Young Men Fed Egg Protein and Rice Protein with Excess and Maintenance Energy Intakes," J. Nutr. 103:1673 (1973).

21. B. Isaksson, B. Lindholm, and B. Sjogren, "Dermal Losses of Nutrients and Their Significance for Human Metabolic Studies," Acta Med. Scand. Suppl. 445:26 (1966).

22. D.H. Calloway, A.C.F. Odell, and S. Margen, "Sweat and Miscellaneous Nitrogen Losses in Human Balance Studies," J. Nutr. 101:775 (1971).

23. G.G. Graham, W.C. MacLean, Jr., C.H. Kallman, J. Rabold, and E.D. Mellits, "Growth Standards for Poor Urban Children in Nutrition Studies," Amer. J. Clin. Nutr. 32:703, 1979.

24. A.B. Wilson, "Longitudinal Analysis of Diet, Physical Growth, Verbal Development, and School Performance," in Malnourished Children of the Rural Poor, J.B. Balderston, A.B. Wilson, M.E. Freire, and M.S. Simonen, eds. (Auburn Publishing Company, Boston, Massachusetts, 1981).

25. B.S. Platt, D.S. Miller, and P.R. Payne, "Protein Values of Human Food," in Recent Advances in Human Nutrition, J.F. Brock, ed. (J. & A. Churchill, Ltds., London, U.K., 1961).

26. H.C. Stuart, "Growth Charts" in Textbook of Pediatrics, 8th ed., W.E. Nelson, ed. (W.B. Saunders, Philadelphia, 1964).

27. P.V. Hamill, National Center for Health Statistics, Growth Curves for Children, Vital and Health Statistics: Series 11, Data from National Health Survey, No. 165 (DHEW Publication; [PHS] 78-1650, Washington, D.C., 1977).

TABLE 1. Effect of Different Energy Requirement Criteria on Predicted Percentage of Individuals Below Own Protein Requirements[1]

Country	Ref. Req.	<100% Ref.	<90% Ref.	<80% Ref.	<1.5 X BMR
A	2210	(92)	23	53	41
B	2320	(99)	48	63	49
C	2330	(35)	13	22	14
D	2220	(49)	20	32	27

1 Calculated by S. Reutlinger, IBRD, Taking intake variation with income into account and assuming moderate activity + 10% household losses.

TABLE 2. Estimates of Numbers of Malnourished in World Population

Publication	Source	Data Year	Millions Undernourished	Criterion	Coverage	Percent
1963 World Food Survey	FAO	1958	300-500	3rd Perc.	World	10-17
1974 World Food Conference	FAO	1970	462	BMR x 1.2	World	16
1977 World Food Survey	FAO	1972-1974	455	BMR x 1.2	LDCs	25
1981 Agriculture towards 2000	FAO	1974-1976	436	BMR x 1.2	LDCs	23
1976 Malnutrition and Poverty	IBRD1/	1965	1,130	Requirement	LDCs	73
1980 Prevalence of Calorie-deficient diets	IBRD2/	1965 1973	704 808	Requirement Requirement	36 countries 36 countries	66 61

1/ S. Reutlinger and M. Selowsky, "Malnutrition and Povery: Magnitude and Policy Options". World Bank Staff Occasional Papers No. 23, World Bank, Washington D.C. (1976).
2/ S. Reutlinger and H. Alderman (Reference 10).

TABLE 3. Estimated Protein and Energy Requirements

Age (Yrs)	Wt (Kg)	Calories Total	Calories Growth	%	Protein (G) Total	Protein (G) Growth	%
2-3	13.6	1360	30	2	10.2	0.9	12
4-5	17.4	1720	35	2	10.7	1.0	10
9-10	31.3	2420	30	1	14.3	1.4	10

TABLE 4. Comparison of Available Percent Protein Calories for Adults, Calculated from 1971[1] and 1981[2] Protein-Energy Recommendations (Weight Men 65 kg, Women 55 kg)

	Based on Average Protein and Energy Requirement* Estimates		Based on Safe Allowance for Protein and Energy Requirements* Minus 2 SD	
	1971	1981	1971	1981
Men	3.7	6.1	6.2	9.9
Women	4.0	6.2	7.1	9.6

* Light Activity

(1) Energy and Protein Requirements. Report of a Joint FAO/WHO Ad Hoc Expert Committee. WHO Tech. Rep. Ser. 522, Geneva, 1973.

(2) Energy and Protein Requirements. Report of a Joint FAO/WHO/UNU Expert Consultation, Rome 5-17 October, 1981. WHO, Geneva, 1984.

APPENDIX 1

Calculation of Total Protein Requirements of the Egyptian Population According to the 1976 Census and FAO/WHO Energy and Protein Requirements (1973)

Age Group (Years)	Average Body Wt. (kg[1/])	Requirement per Kg Body Wt. per Day (g)	Requirement per Capita per Day (g)	Population	Total Requirements per Day (Metric Tons)
Infants					
0 - 1[2/]				698	
Children (Both Sexes)					
1 - 4	11.3	1.64	18.5	4,344	40,249
5 - 9	19.5	1.33	25.9	4,682	60,628
Adolescents (Male)					
10 - 14	32.8	1.1	36.1	2,582	46,579
15 - 19	53.0	.89	47.2	2,142	50,547
(Female)					
10 - 14	31.7	1.02	32.3	2,324	37,560
15 - 19	44.0	.59	26.0	1,850	24,012
Adults					
Men	59	.81	47.8	8,953	213,941
Women	46	.74	34.0	9,052	154,060
Allowance for					
Pregnancy[3/]			7.9	768	3,033
Lactation			24.3	698	8,480
					639,089[4/]
					702,998[5/]

1/ Body weight according to the 5th percentile of weight of NCHS Growth Curves (U.S.).
2/ No requirements are indicated for infants because they are combined with those for pregnancy and lactation.
3/ If the number of pregnant women in a population group is not known, it is assumed that there are 10% more pregnant women than infants aged 0 - 12 months, allowing for pregnancy wastage and perinatal mortality:
pregnant women = 697.938 x 1.1 = 767,732 (thousand).
4/ Per capita per day = 35 g (without wastage).
5/ With allowances for wastage = 35 x 1.1 = 38 g per capita per day.
6/ The safe level of protein is adjusted for the relative quality of the protein in the national diet relative to that of egg or milk by multiplying it by 100 divided by the score of the food protein, e.g., 100/70 = 1.43 and protein intake of a child 1-4 years = 1.15 x 1.43 = 1.64 g.

APPENDIX 2

Calculation of Total Protein Requirements of the Egyptian Population According to the 1976 Census and FAO/WHO Energy and Protein Requirements (1985)

Age Group (Years)	Average Body Wt. (kg[1/])	Requirement per Kg Body Wt. per Day (g)	Requirement per Capita per Day (g)	Population	Total Requirements per Day (Metric Tons)
Infants					
0 - 1[2/]				6,978	
Children (Both Sexes)					
1 - 4	11	2.00	22.6	4,344	49,090
5 - 9	20	1.62	31.6	4,682	73,971
Adolescents (Male)					
10 - 14	33	1.32	43.3	2,582	55,900
15 - 19	53	1.13	59.9	2,142	64,149
(Female)					
10 - 14	32	1.23	39	2,324	45,309
15 - 19	44.0	1.1	48.4	1,850	44,769
Adults					
Men	59	1.07	63.1	8,953	282,613
Women	46	1.07	49.2	9,052	222,763
Allowance for					
Pregnancy[3/]			7.9	758	3,019
Lactation			18.6	698	6,491
					848,074[4/]
					932,881.40[5/]

1/ Body weight according to the 5th percentile of weight of NCHS Growth Curves (U.S.).
2/ No requirements are indicated for infants because they are combined with those for pregnancy and lactation.
3/ See footnote No. 3 in Appendix 1.
4/ Per capita per day = 46 g (without wastage).
5/ With allowances for wastage = 35 x 1.1 = 38 g per capita per day.
6/ The safe level of protein is adjusted for the relative quality of the protein in the national diet relative to that of egg or milk by multiplying it by 100 divided by the score of the food protein, e.g., 100/70 = 1.43 and protein intake of a child 1-4 years = 1.15 x 1.43 = 1.64 g.

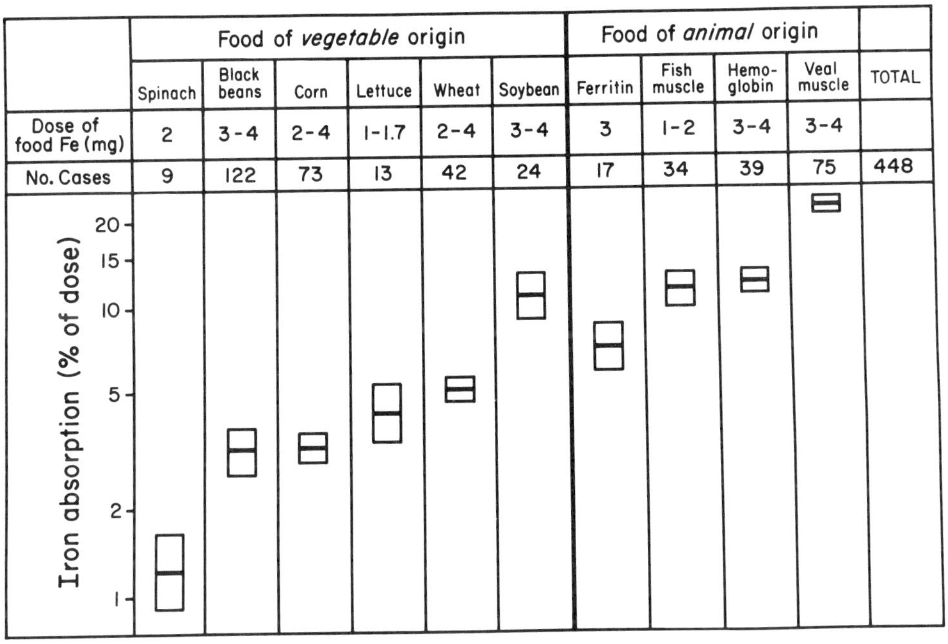

Figure 1. Iron absorption from foods; the result of a collaborative study conducted by the Department of Botany and Medicine at the University of Washington, Seattle, and the Department of Physiopathology IVIC, Caracas, Venezuela. The Mean absorption and standard error were calculated from the logarithms of the percentage of absorption.
Source: Reference 1

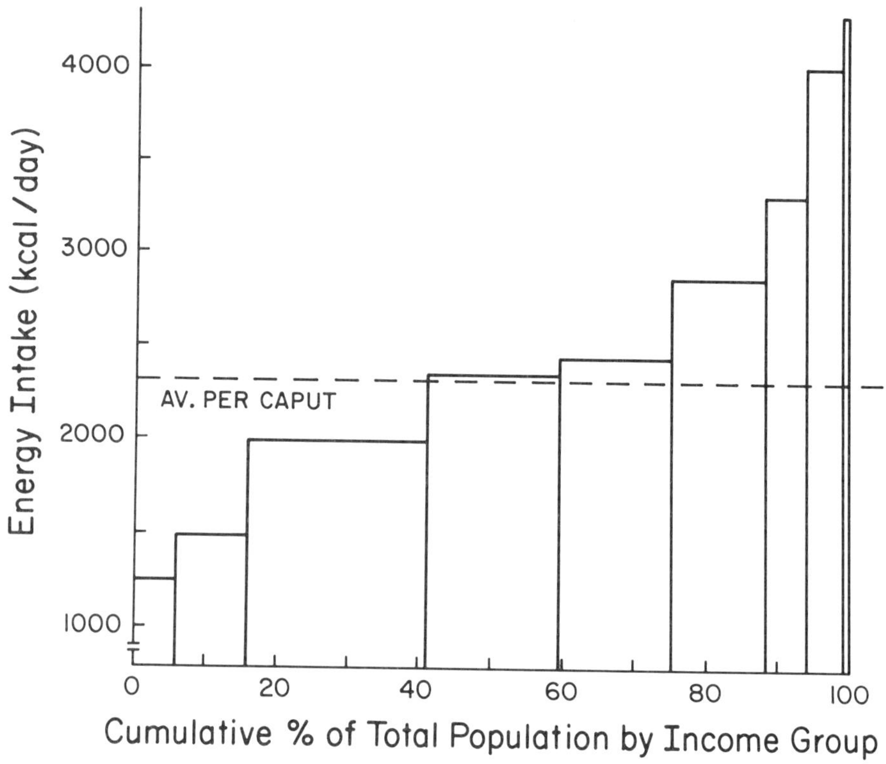

Figure 2. Effect of Income on Energy Intake in Northeastern Brazil (Requirement = 2450)

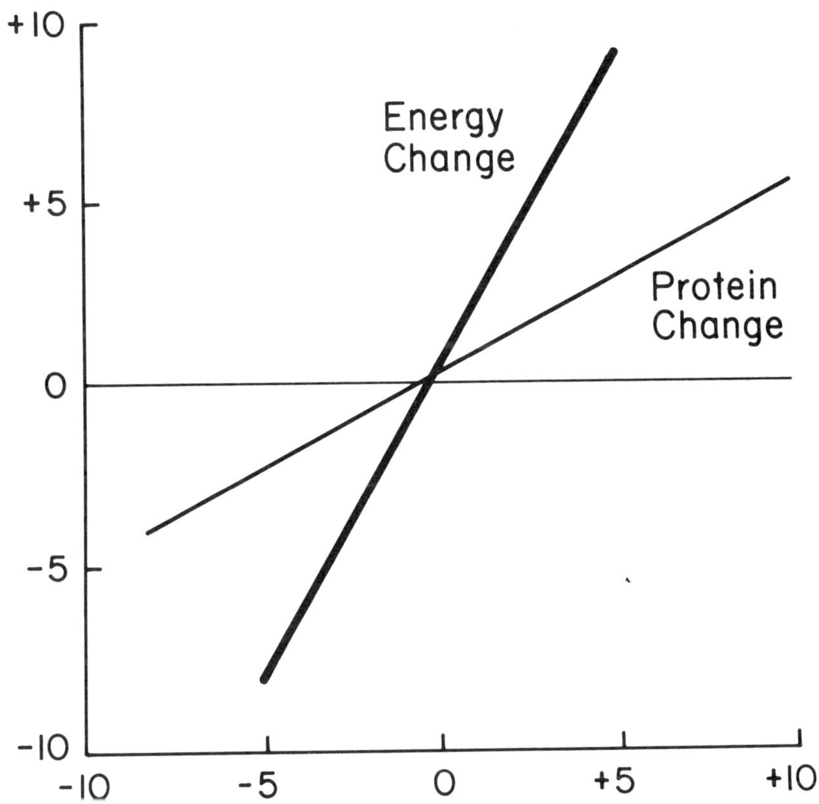

Figure 3. Change in efficiency of intake N with E and N intake varied barely above or below maintenance level.

Inoue et al., 1973 (Reference 20).

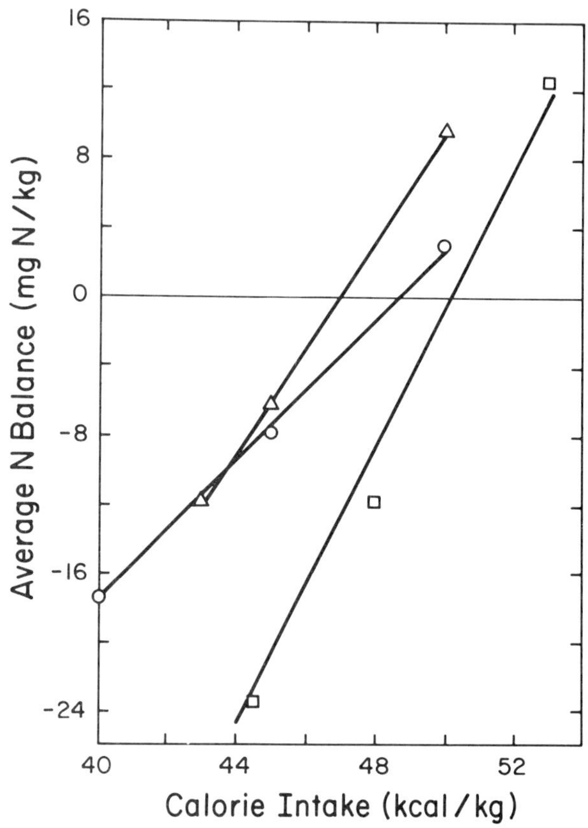

Average N balance (mg N / kg) vs. calorie intake (kcal / kg). Y = N balance, X = calorie intake. △ = T.C., $Y = -146.24 + 3.12X$, $S_b = 0.06$ $S_{YX} = 0.32$. ○ = D.K., $Y = -99.75 + 2.05X$, $S_b = 0.09$ $S_{YX} = 0.61$. □ = L.T., $Y = -203.26 + 4.05X$, $S_b = 0.56$ $S_{YX} = 3.56$.

Figure 4.

DISCUSSION

SESSION I - MALNUTRITION AND HUNGER

DAVID F. NYGAARD

It would be presumptuous of me to try to criticize two of the world's leading experts on human nutrition. What do I know about nutrition problems in the world? The only reason I am here at all is that the person we had invited to discuss this opening session was unable to attend. Therefore, I am going to play a rather devious trick and take the burden of discussing these two papers off my shoulders and put it on someone else.

Specifically, I would like to put it on the shoulders of the Minister of Economic Development, as well as his assistants, of a mythical country that I have created for use in this discussion. May I ask you to use your imagination for a moment? Imagine, if you will, that we are in a country called: well, you give it a name. It is a fairly small country in the Middle East of about 12 million people and has a fast-growing population. Its food production is stagnating, its food imports are rapidly increasing, and income distribution is becoming a serious source of social unrest. There is a rapid increase in urban population and consequently urban poverty. This is due, however, to rural unemployment and rural poverty. Thus, the Minister of Economic Development is under severe pressure from his President to sort out these problems.

As a first step, he has just appointed two new deputy ministers: a deputy in charge of nutrition and a second in charge of food production, an agriculturalist. He has called them into his office today, their first day on the job, to develop priorities for a plan of action. He opens the meeting with the following comments:

"Well, Gentlemen, welcome to your new posts. Let me warn you that you have no time for settling-in; the work begins now. The President has given us 25 million dinars to start a new development programme. If we get off to a good start, there will be more money in the future. What do you have to say? How should we spend the money?"

"Your Excellency, please permit me to begin", said the nutritionist, "I think we should put that money into determining where and what our nutrition problems are. I recently read an excellent article by a fellow named Pellett on hunger and malnutrition. He develops very clearly, and I believe with startling implications, the devastating impact of malnutrition on people's productivity and health. He also lists several of the more important nutrition problems. Clearly, we should use some of this money to identify these problems in our country".

Before continuing, the nutritionist paused to take a breath, and the agriculturalist cut in. "I also read that paper", said he, "and I think my friend the nutritionist misunderstood what Pellett was saying, although, as an agriculturalist I got a bit confused with his acronyms and I am still not sure of the difference between LBW and PEM or FEP and CHD. But I still think I understood his point. That is that many of the nutrition problems are very difficult to identify and measure, and he suggests that the causes of this malnutrition are many and very complex. The real solutions involve an improvement in the general standard of living - increasing real incomes, food availability, improving the environment, etc. I also read a paper by Nevin Scrimshaw of a few years ago that recognizes these same issues. He claims that the solutions to these problems lie in interdisciplinary research teams."

"Hold it", interrupted the Minister himself. "Now that is a fuzzy concept if I ever heard one. I have not had a chance to read these two papers you speak of by, what were their names, Pershaw and Scrimett, but I have read other articles coming out of the World Hunger Programme of the UNU: all stressing interdisciplinary research. Now I think that that is a nice idea but how does it work?"

"I recently accepted an invitation to visit ICARDA, this new International Center at Aleppo, Syria. They have a program there called the Farming Systems Program and those fellows keep talking about multidisciplinary research too, but they didn't convince me. Frankly, I can't see how such a team could work in our country. We can't waste money on that kind of thing. We have to get on with the objectives of economic development."

"I agree", said the agriculturalist, realizing that he had lost face on that last exchange, "What bothered me about Pellet's paper was that he said nothing about our country; in fact, he said very little about the Middle East. Perhaps the reason for this omission is that we do not have a nutrition problem in our region."

"All of Pellett's discussion on nutrition status is based on aggregate data at the regional level and we all know the problem of nutrition is not macro but micro. There is a parallel here in our experience in agricultural research. Problems identified at a macro level are of little relevancy to the farm level, and decisions based on aggregate data usually exacerbate the problem of income distribution".

"What really worries me", continued the agriculturalist, is Pellett's discussion of the causes of malnutrition. He cites a list of immediate causes, underlying causes, and finally basic causes, all from another article by Jonsson. The basic causes are obviously where the solutions lies. But the list includes things like: (i) political organization, (ii) historical cause, (iii) religion, and (iv) division of labour. Now, if we have to change these things before we can improve the nutrition status, we might as well give up".

"But", interjected the nutritionist, "there are things we can do even without changing these basic causes. A recent Scrimshaw article points out the progress made in the last decade on measuring nutrition requirements of human beings at different income levels and at different ages. If only we could apply these new standards in our own country...."

"Now that's the craziest notion I have ever heard", said the agriculturalist taking the offensive. "Progress -- you call that progress. All Scrimshaw's article points out is the lack of progress -- nutritionists themselves are still arguing about who is malnourished and who is not. You nutritionists can't agree about anything. Why you are worse than economists".

But the nutritionist was adamant. "That _is_ progress, only you are too stubborn to see it. It all boils down to a question of _priorities_. If we can identify the problem areas -- geographically, for example, in any of several fields, you can aim your research toward solving those problems and the solutions we would then come up with would have a higher probability of success."

"What I did like about both the Pellett and Scrimshaw articles", said the agriculturalist, trying to soften the mood of the discussion, "is that they are both alluding to the poverty trap in which poor people in developing countries find themselves. It seems to me, we are all searching for a way to spring the trap -- to break out. It may be with a nutrition solution, an agricultural solution, or something else. I have an idea that may work on the agricultural side and could solve nutritional problems as well. I believe we should use that 25 million dinars to develop a livestock project to get this agricultural sector off the ground. This would increase rural incomes, decrease our demand for meat imports, and solve, through meat and milk consumption, many of the protein deficiencies that exist in our country today."

And into the conversation charged the nutritionist, "Now that is a simple-minded idea if I ever heard one, Your Excellency." Turning to the agriculturalist, the nutritionist continued, "It is clear, my dear friend, that you may have looked at Scrimshaw's paper, but you didn't read it. You're just worried that agricultural projects are no longer the 'queen bee' of technical assistance money from abroad and you're afraid you won't get hold of this 25 million. Scrimshaw's message is this: We must have a far better impression of what the problems are and where are they prevalent. To suggest that a livestock project will solve our nutrition problems is naive and possibly erroneous. That project would have to be located in the east, while my guess is that the western part of our country is where the nutrition problem is. Who says that the poor in the western region could buy milk produced in the east?"

"And", broke in the agriculturalist, "to spend part of our development money identifying nutrition measures that even you cannot agree upon is certainly pouring money down the drain."

"So you see, Your Excellency", continued the agriculturalist now rising to the challenge, "what we drastically need is a major effort in food production. Perhaps an organization like ICARDA could help us. More food will solve the financial and social ills of the country. This would..."

But before he could continue, the nutritionist was on his feet interrupting the agriculturalist in mid-sentence. "Now, Your Excellency, that is a typical response of our narrow minded-colleagues in agriculture. As I have tried to explain, what we need is a clearly focused project, not only on nutrition, that will deal with poverty, malnutrition, and hunger. I recommend we use our development budget to feed the hungry and improve the lot of the poor, particularly in the cities."

"And what about the rural poor?" Again, it was the agriculturalist. It was turning into a shouting match.

"Gentlemen, Gentlemen, take it easy, take it easy", asserted the Minister, once again taking control of the meeting. "There must be other experts besides these people of whom you speak. What were the names again? These Messrs. Pellmell and Scrimage. The dilemma facing us is now clear to me and we need a joint effort. So, I am going immediately to call a workshop of experts on these issues and try to sort out, <u>not</u> a programme of nutrition and <u>not</u> a programme of agricultural development, <u>but</u> a programme of <u>this</u> both, and this is really what Messrs. Scrimshaw and Pellett, yes, that's it, what these two are saying. But you two are just not listening. Maybe an interdisciplinary approach is not so bad after all."

If I can bring you back to reality, Ladies and Gentlemen, to Aleppo, Syria, and the workshop on the interfaces between agriculture, food science and human nutrition in the Middle East, we are here to do just that! Sort out priorities for projects to solve these problems. Messrs. Pellett and Scrimshaw have done a nice job of defining the problem and helping us focus our efforts and we thank them. But now it is time to hear from you! I believe that we have some problems to work out.

A personal work to Drs. Pellett and Scrimshaw, if you disagree with some of the comments that the nutritionist and the agriculturalist made about your papers, would you please see them --not me! Thank you.

Nygaard: If I could take the discussion leader's prerogative and pose one question to Pellett. What do we know about nutrition in the Middle East, nothing?

Pellett: No, we know a great deal about nutrition in the Middle East, possibly less than about other regions, but I think we have a lot of country data, and we have information on morbidity and mortality. There are very wide ranging problems. This is a region with some of the richest countries and some of the poorest countries in the world. The message I would like to bring out as part of that answer is that there is not one grand solution with one grand answer. I think we have believed in the past that there is a single solution, but there is not: there are a thousand problems and a thousand different solutions that are going to differ not only from region to region but almost from family to family. We have to recognize that there are broad aspects, among which the elimination of poverty may be basic, but that is impossible in the foreseeable future. We thus have to look at things we can do and therefore, within one family it might be education on food use, in another it might be improvement in budgeting thereby increasing purchasing power.

Parpia: Mr. Chairman, I certainly enjoyed your method of introducing the subject, but you have opened a Pandora's box, and I intend to throw something more into it. First, when there is a Minister for Development, he cannot afford to look at only agriculture and nutrition. I do not intend to go into detail, but the nutrients you produce must be preserved, otherwise they won't be nutrients anymore. They must also be made available, and to make them available you have to have income. If a nutritionist said that the sole purpose of income generation only concerns nutrition, he or she would be making a serious mistake. Unless you can generate a surplus that can be reinvested, it will not be possible to bring about any development. If one follows the advice of some nutritionists and subsidizes all food, we will be distributing your total national income to the poorest and you will be holding back social and economic progress. This is very frequently done by nutritionists who look at only one part of the problem.

The next issue is that these developing countries need to have employment alternatives in rural areas. The field of post-harvest activities provides the largest single potential for this purpose, but the potential has not yet been developed. The reason for that is that more than 50 percent of all exports, according to the Brandt Report, is of agricultural raw materials and commodities worth 30 billion dollars. From this, 240 billion dollars worth of finished products are manufactured by the rich countries. This is how the poor developing countries, by exporting their raw materials, lose their income potential. If these products were processed at home it would increase and improve the food supply and generate employment. Therefore, Mr. Chairman, you need a third deputy for your Minister of Development who will look at certain other aspects besides nutrition and agriculture, and who will, in turn, stimulate both of them. May I suggest that we make our activity more interdisciplinary.

Nygaard: I certainly agree. However, I had trouble working on the dialogue with three people much less four. There probably should be 7 or 8 actors in my play.

Miladi: My first question is to Pellett. What can the International Centers do to avoid the problems and negative impacts of the Green Revolution? In this region, will the efforts of ICARDA to increase food production with new varieties, etc., improve the nutrition situation, or will we have another failure?

My second question is to Scrimshaw. Between 1935 and 1981, we have had five different recommendations on protein requirements. From 1935 to 1955 the world, which was apparently protein-deficient, became a world of protein excess because of changes in the requirement values. This is confusing and really affects agricultural policy and the whole exercise of development. This will affect the understanding between nutritionists and agriculturalists, if the nutritionists come up every 5 or 10 years with new protein requirements. Breeding programmes take many years to produce new varieties and cannot make changes this quickly.

Pellett: I do not have an immediate answer as to what the International Centers can do, but I hope that as the week progresses we will produce some answers. Your question to Scrimshaw, is I think, of much more immediate importance and I would like to pose a supplementary question to him and hope that he will answer both together. I agree that there is great confusion concerning protein requirements and what has happened with these recommendations. Is it really correct that the protein requirements for an adult were increased recently by 30 percent or, in fact, is it not true that the new (1984) values are almost unchanged from the 1973 values? The previous 1973 value for an adult was 0.57 g protein per kilogram body weight per day. This was for 'reference protein' -- a protein of high quality such as egg or milk -- with a net protein utilization (NPU) approaching 100 %. Thus, when corrected for protein quality (and incidentally, digestibility) by using a value of 70-75 percent for the NPU of an average western diet, the 0.57 g/kg/day was increased to about 0.80 g/kg/day. As I understand the situation, the new value for the adult will be 0.75 g/kg/day (yes an apparent increase of about 30 percent from the value of 0.57 g/kg/day) but no further correction for protein quality will be performed. The only correction will be for digestibility, which will be small, since for most diets it is above 85 percent and will be perhaps 90 to 95 percent in a good Western diet. Requirements for the adult in terms of dietary protein will therefore increase to 0.83.g/kg/day, an increase of less than 5 percent rather than the 30 percent you mentioned. Am I correct in this interpretation?

Scrimshaw: The reason I told you more than most of you wanted to know about the origin of protein requirements was precisely to be able to give a reasonable answer to these kinds of questions. I think it is safe to say that there will not be another drastic revision of protein requirements. I was involved in each of the past international meetings that established them, except for the first one at the League of Nations in 1935. In the 1957 meeting, there were only two data points: the amount of protein that a breast-fed infant obtained from breast milk, and the metabolic balance study that gave an anchor point for young adults. There was simply no knowledge to supply the points between. People assumed that there had to be a decrease from the high requirement of the infant to the relatively low requirement of the adult but the shape of that curve was a subject of debate for two years; it vibrated like a violin string and finally came to rest, but was based on very inadequate data. The next meeting (1965) introduced a new approach, which was that the requirements must be capable of being calculated from the nitrogen losses from the body under conditions of maximum adaptation. Again, there were no good data available. This was the factorial approach, and to determine urinary nitrogen losses, they used an equation that seemed true for animals from the shrew to the elephant, based on the relationship between the basal metabolic rate (BMR) and nitrogen excretion, forgetting that most of those animals do not lose nitrogen from sweat as man does. Thus, the figure that they adopted was clearly inappropriate. Subsequent studies by Mohamed Hussein Amir, who is at this meeting, used human subjects. One hundred MIT students were given a nitrogen-free diet for twenty-one days. Their obligatory urinary and faecal losses were measured. A small group from California was studied in the same way. These studies provided the data base for the next meeting and the 1973 recommendations. The problem was that, with the best of intentions, we were giving extra calories at the time with the results that I showed earlier. For the 1984 figure, we have data on the amount of protein required for zero nitrogen balance and its coefficient of variation from Korea, Thailand, the Philippines, Mexico, Guatemala, Chile, Brazil, Nigeria, Egypt, Bangladesh and India, with very good agreement. Whether the exact safe allowance should be .75, .78 or.8, is not important; it is now in the right order of magnitude.

Concerning Pellett's question. The net effect of the increase will not be quite as much as one-third for two reasons. One is that the correction for children is much smaller because the 1971 allowance was much more generous to them than to adults. Second, the data from the multi-country study suggest that, at requirement levels, protein quality, judged by the amino acid pattern and the amino acid score, is generally not the main determining factor but rather it is digestibility. There must be a correction factor for digestibility that increases the safe allowance upwards from .75. That correction factor is much smaller for mixed diets containing animal protein than had been previously assumed. Since the average figure in the new recommendation is definitely higher, however, than the safe allowance of the 1971, there is a considerable increase in the amount of protein considered to be required.

Hussein: I would like to comment on one of the slides presented by Pellett on the energy intake of Egyptians in 1976, which is a quotation from FAO This is around 108 percent of the minimum requirement. We had the impression that it is not the total energy intake per se that is important for a population but rather the percentage of energy derived from fat -- in other words, the nutrient density. In growth studies in Egypt with school children we were able to produce improved growth with both protein and fat supplements. The poor growth was related to high bulk of the food.

Pellett: Two brief comments. The food balance sheet data are only averages. Second, it is clear that uneaten food has no nutritional value. If the food bulk is large because of high water-holding capacity then a stomach-full of food is not the same as a stomach-full of nutrients, and thus the child is not getting the nutients he needs. Food bulk is of paramount importance in child-feeding.

To return to Miladi's question on the activities of the International Centers. You are asking about the potential impact of plant breeding programmes on the overall improvement of nutritional status of populations. I think several things have happened in recent years that are extremely important and ICARDA recognizes these. There was a time not so long ago when merely improving the yield of a product was the be-all and end-all of a breeding programme. It is now fully recognized that unless a wheat makes good bread or a legume makes good hommus there is not necessarily an improvement. This is recognition of the importance of the acceptability and edibility of a product. That is a tremendous step forward for breeding programmes. ICARDA and other centers are now looking at the overall impact of changes on people's consumption habits, on families' economic status, and on the environment. Until relatively recently this was not even considered in agricultural research efforts, but it is now an integral part of ICARDA's research. I think this is indicative of a change in thought and a much more realistic recognition of what breeding programmes can do, and I assume that is what we will be addressing during the rest of this meeting.

Nour: When the Centro Internacional de Mejoramiento de Maiz Y Trigo (CIMMYT) was formally established in 1966, the main issue was a question of producing enough food in a similar climate to prevent the Indo-Pakistani sub-continent from entering a phase of mass starvation. In the late 1950s and early 1960s the sub-continent had enormous food problems and was forced to import food to alleviate starvation. Therefore, within this context, I think CIMMYT did an admirable job. It reversed the trend of imports and these countries are now approaching self-sufficiency in food. In general, I think we can safely say the International Agricultural Research Centers have addressed themselves to issues of socio-economic importance and also toward nutritional as well as agricultural problem-solving .

After the problem of low production was successfully addressed, second generation problems arose. It is these problems that spawned questions about not the quantity but the quality of what the breeders are producing. ICARDA has learned many lessons from the "green revolution", particularly in India and Pakistan. As a local example, Turkey was a cereal-importing country, but the trend was completely reversed when some of the better varieties were introduced with help from multi-national agencies like the Rockefeller and Ford Foundations, USAID and others to encourage farmers to adopt them. It would, however, be an error to say that, if a country is not self-sufficient in its basic food requirements, there is a breeding programme available to reverse the trend of food importation. This may be the wrong issue since we must often worry about other problems such as the how the new production is distributed, how it affects the resource-poor farmers, and how we protect them from the richer farmers who sometimes reap many more of the benefits?

These are second-generation problems that need to be looked at and to do so is one of the main objectives of the Farming Systems Research Programme. It is for this reason that we have a model at ICARDA that is different from earlier models; we have introduced into our commodity programmes an approach whereby we look at the farming systems as a whole, consider the farmers' income, income distribution, and how the package of technology that we are trying to develop will address itself directly to the poorer sectors of the community. It is in this context, that I think ICARDA has learned some of the lessons about problems that Miladi raised.

It is still necessary to boost breeding programmes so that we are able to produce greater quantities in order to reverse a trend. In the Middle East region, I think we are right on the mark. As will be seen, this region needs to look very carefully into its food production, and to assess carefully its requirement for increased imports of food. We are the highest per capita food-importing region in the world; a trend of that nature will have to be addressed by increasing production, and to achieve that we must breed higher-yielding varieties.

Scrimshaw: As nutritionists many of us were concerned with the initial preoccupation of the international agricultural research centers with cereal yields. Then, as high-yielding varieties were developed and governments subsidized them in various ways, legumes, which are necessary to supplement the protein in predominantly vegetable diets, suffered. Legume production per capita went down, and sometimes even absolute legume production decreased. Prices soared and people suffered, but the lower protein recommendations of the 1970s drew some of the attention away from the fact. The data that I presented re-emphasize the importance of a balanced programme that will include legumes such as beans, and lentils, as well as cereals.

The second conclusion from the information I presented is that small improvements or small losses in the protein value of the cereal staples could be of real nutritional significance. A third conclusion, is that, by and large, preocccupation with amino acid balance or protein quality will be less useful than emphasis on protein quantity for human diets. This is because the human is less demanding of amino acid balance at requirement levels than is the rapidly growing animal that has been used for most protein quality tests. But even more important is that, because of complementary patterns among various food proteins, sometimes small increases in consumption of something like green leaves can contribute significantly to the overall quality of the diet.

Hussein: In comparing nutritional status or agricultural production figures among countries there should be standardization. The table on weight-for-height shown by Pellett of figures available from various countries is an example. There are very high figures in some countries and low ones in others, but we cannot compare these figures unless these surveys have been done on a standardized basis. If we look at these figures for Egypt, we find that one to two percent of the population is under-nourished, which gives an impression that we do not have a big problem. But as a matter of fact if we use the figures of height-for-age, it shows that 20 percent of the population is affected by malnutrition. I just want to call your attention to the problem of data sources and I think we should find some standardization from the figures.

Salameh: I commend Pellett for his presentation, but I would like to summarize the subject to my own way of thinking and answer some questions he raised. Opinions on the world's food problem today is divided into two groups, pessimists and optimists. However, both groups agree scientifically about the solutions to hunger and malnutrition. I believe there are five things that must be done. First, we must fully use land and natural resources that are available to produce food. Second, farmers must be better trained to be decision-makers, and development should not be forced upon them. They should be allowed to create and control their own internal infrastructure, but rural areas need to be stabilized by small industry and services provided by the government. Third, food should be fairly distributed among family members, families, villages, provinces and countries. Fourth, the nutritionist must be recognized as a scientist with rights and duties. He/she must be treated equally with respect to salary and research support in comparison to other officials in the government. He/she should be allowed to work in his own field and control his own destiny. The fifth requirement I suggest is the better use of food itself. It must be available in adequate quantities and reasonably priced and we must be careful that it is not contaminated chemically or biologically. These should be the cornerstones of government nutrition plans.

Pellett: I think you have summarized the situation in an excellent manner. There is only one major concern that I would add, and that is the availability of health services and a clean water supply so as to allow for the full metabolic utilization of food.

Singh: The goals and objectives of plant breeding have been mentioned several times. In most of the developed world, plant breeders give attention to improving grain quality as well as increasing yields, but in most of the developing world, the breeding goal continues to be only for high yield. At ICARDA we are breeding cultivars that give higher yield and we are trying to monitor quality, particularly protein and cooking quality, to avoid releasing a cultivar that may give a high yield but be low in protein or have some other poor-quality characteristics. Nour pointed out that this region is a food-importer so the main and immediate goal is to make the region self-sufficient. Perhaps once that is achieved, the goal of improved quality may be looked at in greater detail.

Pellett: In relation to the large amount of food imports in the Middle East, I think it is worth mentioning that it is the only area in the developing world that, within the last decade, has shown a decrease in the proportion designated as malnourished. Of course, countries within the region differ enormously, but the region as a whole has shown a net improvement. This, of course, is not unrelated to the general increase in wealth.

Nygaard: One of the very interesting things we have found at ICARDA is that there is a nice balance in the sheep-crop system in Syria in which almost every component plays a complementary role in determining total production, income, and income stability. Intervention on the cropping side is going to have large repercussions on the animal side. We are trying to understand the system well enough to maintain this balance and, therefore, to avoid some of the negative consequences that changing the cropping side will have on the animals. I would like to ask Scrimshaw if one can automatically assume that animals in the system will improve the diets of rural people, or is that too simplistic?

Scrimshaw: First, the attention to cropping systems, which again were not characteristic of the International Centers in the beginning, is very important. It has been the emphasis on monoculture, whether of a food crop or a cash crop, and neglect of the farmer's interest in producing complementary foods, at least for his family, that has led to some of the increases in malnutrition. In some regions, anything that promotes a greater variety in the diet of the farmer and his family will contribute to improved nutrition. Whether increased animal production results in increased protein consumption or simply in more cash and less poverty, it will still likely result in an improvement in the family diet, and therefore is desirable.

Bressani: We have conducted a similar seminar on the interfaces between agriculture, food science, and nutrition in Latin America. It was developed in a way similar to this one, except that after three days of discussing the problems, we spent two extra days and tried to put what we had learned into practice in a case study. Unfortunately, we were not very successful. The point of Pellett's talk was that malnutrition is a problem caused by many factors, and he also emphasized that to solve this problem we need many solutions. The solutions will come from the interactions among agriculturalists, nutritionists, economists, and government officials. We had several government officials in our seminar in Latin America because we felt that the final action had to be taken by them. I would like to know how we can be more successful at developing the interactions among different disciplines.

Scrimshaw gave a figure for protein requirement of 0.75 g/kg/day. The way I interpret that is to determine what this means in terms of protein production for a country. Should we just limit ourselves to producing cereal grains and legumes, or should we incorporate animal production into our farming systems? My own feeling is that animal production is important because this is the way of life for people in these countries. There are always animals in their farming systems. I would like to hear more discussion on this point.

Khattab: The two papers we have heard have demonstrated beyond any doubt the multidisciplinary nature of food and nutrition problems. Therefore, I think that the first practical step in solving such problems is to understand them. In order to do so it is necessary that the various disciplines and various specialists should have some basic knowledge of food and nutrition so that they can appreciate how nutrition affects their own speciality. In the Faculty of Agriculture at the University of Khartoum, for example, we are moving toward including a course on food and nutrition as part of the curriculum for B.Sc. agricultural students. I think this should be followed in other disciplines as well, so that the people who are in charge of education, research, and administration of agriculture will have a good idea of what food and nutrition problems are. Without this kind of exposure it will be very difficult to use the interdisciplinary approach and make it work.

Nygaard: One point of confusion is the way one defines multidisciplinary or interdisciplinary. Interdisciplinary is often assumed to mean a person who has studied several different areas and is thus an interdisciplinarian. I disagree with this definition. It seems to me instead that it is important to have different people in the process and that each should have his own expertise and not necessarily be broadly trained. I think that, early in the development of the farming systems programme at ICARDA, we were looking for people with two or three areas of specialization and that we wasted too much time trying to find people who did not exist. I agree with Khattab that in undergraduate training institutions one needs to have, if it is a nutrition programme, exposure to agriculture, and in an agricultural programme, exposure to food science and nutrition. However, this idea should not be taken too far. We still need highly trained agriculturalists, nutritionists, economists, etc. -- all working together.

It is not easy to put together a multidisciplinary team. I would like to give you an example of the difficulty of applying this in practice. ICARDA has an economics component in a faba bean research project in Egypt. This was in a government administrative structure where the economists are separate from the food production scientists and it was very difficult to develop collaboration between them. We tried to get an economist assigned to the food legumes group and failed. We set up these strong, strict disciplines and now we are suggesting that they should be changed, and there is much resistance to this by administrators. Perhaps this is a subject we can discuss later in the workshop?

Karrar: I would like to mention our experience in the University of Gezira. It is a very new university, and one of its objectives is to be community-oriented. We have studied many methods for assesssing nutritional status in the community, and one of those used, as explained by Pellett, was the food balance sheet. I know that in most of the agricultural institutes they use these food balance sheets, and, as we have seen in FAO Yearbooks, they tend to over-use these figures. An example is in the prediction of how many people are suffering from P-EM. We train our students on how to assess nutritional status by using the food balance sheet. In Sudan the average figures from the food balance sheets show that the country has enough protein and energy. However, at the micro-level, 50 percent of the children are malnourished. One has to be careful of this sort of contradiction.

We have four faculties in the University, and we have designed a summer course whereby all the disciplines will come together and participate in a rural development project. One objective of the course is to get the students to realize that there is interaction between these disciplines that is neglected in most of our other training. For example, in classical nutrition training, one concentrates only on food intake by human beings and the important interacting factors. Agriculturalists, however, look at nutrition only as food availability. Therefore, I think if we include interdisciplinary research within our formal training we can help scientists realize that there are many factors that interfere with nutrient utilization. When they go to the field and find an agricultualist, a doctor, and an economist, they will realize that they can cooperate and together improve the nutritional status of the population.

Thomson: During the last twenty years there have been many controversies about dietary fibre, high-fibre diets being better than low-fibre diets or animal products being detrimental to health. Do the speakers feel that the pendulum is slowly moving towards the center on these issues? Also, in the future will revisions of requirements, say for protein, remain close to this latest figure you have recommended?

Scrimshaw: I think it very unlikely that we will have any further large swings that would significantly affect policy in estimated protein requirement for adults. The data for pregnant and lactating women are, however, still quite inadequate. The energy requirements have not changed for the past three decades, and they are not going to change much except as the activity levels of populations change.

The controversy over animal fat in relation to cardiovascular disease and cancer is by no means over. I think the result is going to be a considerable emphasis on leaner grades of cattle and of breeds that will provide less animal fat. We are already seeing in the industrialized countries a decrease in saturated fat intakes that will certainly affect markets and agricultural goals. The question of crude fibre still is a matter of controversy, but I doubt if it is a very important one. As there is some decrease in animal protein intake in the industrialized countries and an increase in animal protein intake in the developing countries, I think probably the fibre content of diets will take care of itself.

Pellett: I would like to add one thing to what Scrimshaw has said concerning activity levels. These, particularly in relation to requirements in industrialized countries and possibly as time goes on in the developing countries, are very important. What is happening is that, as activity levels are reduced and as the energy needs fall as a result, there is a need for higher nutrient concentrations within the remaining part of the diet. If one were eating 3,500 calories per day all nutrient needs would probably be met. If one only eats 2,500 calories and is still meeting energy requirements, the original need for the various micro-nutrients still exists, but the diet no longer provides it. This has become a very important consideration in making the recommended dietary allowances (RDA) for developed countries.

Scrimshaw: The FAO/WHO meeting actually concluded that the levels of energy requirements for some populations in the U.S. were below the levels adequate for cardiovascular fitness and prolonged good health. Instead of countenancing any further reduction in the estimated requirements for the U.S. population, there needed to be an increase in the activity of the U.S. population. A corollary of that, as Pellett pointed out, is that as energy intakes decrease, the concentration of protein and other nutrients in the diet must be higher. This is particularly a problem with aging populations because the elderly tend to be less active and it is much harder to get sufficient protein and other nutrients in their diets.

Gerhart: We heard that FAO solved the protein problem by reducing the recommendation by 50 percent and now has adjusted it back to a more realistic level. I would like to ask Scrimshaw what the main functional results were of this reduction in the estimates. In other words, how important is the accuracy of estimates for actual behaviour either on the part of national governments with their own investment policies, on the part of donors with their investment policies, or on the part of research agencies? Is it clear that there is a relationship between estimates and the behaviour of these specific actors?

Scrimshaw: This is not an easy question to answer. In countries with chronic underemployment, if you give additional calories the people want more work and there is not more work available. Or, if you give them more work according to their increased capacity, then you have to discharge others, thus adding to the unemployment. It is clear that many societies have undergone social adaptation to low levels of energy intake. These include the long siesta or the assignment by <u>terrare</u>, by unit of work, whereby they can take a short time or a long time to finish work rather than being paid by the hour. A sudden increase in the availability of dietary energy may not have constructive work outlets. On the other hand, we do see that the adaptation to low dietary energy intakes virtually rules out some of the kinds of discretionary activity, for example, community organization, which is essential for community development. On balance, I think it is important in planning to provide for increased dietary energy availability for populations now consuming energy intakes well below the requirement level, but this should be gradual and not by a sudden readjustment to the requirement levels.

<u>Mansour</u>: I would like to return to the 1971 FAO-WHO recommendations in order to stress the policy implications of these requirements on food and agricultural production. In Tunisia, we have been conducting a national food consumption survey for five years that serves as a basis for the elaboration of a five-year development plan. The analysis of this national food consumption survey was based on the FAO-WHO nutritional requirements, especially for energy, protein, and other nutrients. FAO advisors suggested we use what they called minimum requirements. These are about 1.5 BMR and half of the usual requirements for micro-nutrients, vitamins and other minerals. The results gave a false sense of achievement to planners and implementers, because the proportion of the population malnourished apparently decreased when the recommendations were lowered.

<u>Nygaard</u>: I would like to thank Drs. Pellett and Scrimshaw for starting the workshop off in the way they have. I look forward to another two and a half days of discussion of this nature, and I hope that this does not conclude discussion on this subject. At some point, if nobody else does, I would like to ask: What happens to nutrition when people have rapidly increasing incomes but are not fully aware of the implications for nutrition when their diets are changing? Is this an important factor that we should be looking at in the Middle East - one that is perhaps not so important in other parts of the world?

SECTION II

FOOD POLICY AND AGRICULTURAL DEVELOPMENT

FOOD POLICY AND HUMAN NUTRITION

PER PINSTRUP-ANDERSEN

The nutritional status of an individual is determined primarily by his or her food intake and health. Thus, policies and programs affecting food intake and health of the undernourished and those at risk of becoming malnourished are likely to have nutritional effects irrespective of whether such effects are intended. This paper addresses food-related policies and programs only. The exclusion of explicit discussion of health policies and programs should not be interpreted to mean that they are considered unimportant. The interaction between nutritional status and health is of great importance and must not be ignored in efforts to deal with nutritional problems.

This paper is divided into three sections. An overview of the causal links between food policy and nutrition is presented first, followed by an analysis of the nutritional effects of selected food policies, and ending with a discussion of how nutritional considerations may be more closely integrated with other goals in the design of food policies.

An Overview

The nutritional status of an individual is affected by: (i) the amount and kinds of food available in the market or on the farm at a given time and place; (ii) the ability of the household of which the individual is a member to obtain available food; (iii) the desire of the head of the household to obtain food to which he/she has access; (iv) allocation of the acquired food among household members, and (v) the physiological utilization of ingested food by a malnourished individual (Figure 1).

Malnutrition may be the result of deficiencies in any one or more of these five factors. Thus, efforts to orient food policies toward the alleviation of existing malnutrition or avoiding its future occurrence should include an analysis to determine which of the five is or are the immediate reasons for malnutrition. Is it a general shortage of food? Is it lack of access to available food on the part of the malnourished? Is it a lack of desire to obtain food to which households with malnourished members have access? Is it a problem of misallocation within the household? Or is it a problem of poor physiological utilization of the food obtained by the malnourished? The five factors are interrelated. Changes in one may be ineffective unless others are changed simultaneously. Efforts to expand food availability will have no nutritional effect if malnourished people do not get access to more food. Similarly, efforts to improve the ability to obtain food may be of little use if food availability is strictly limited, or if households with malnourished members do not desire to take advantage of such improved ability to obtain food but instead translate it into the purchase of non-food commodities.

DRA-F

Many past and current efforts to improve human nutrition focus on one of the factors while ignoring their interactions. Policies aimed at the promotion of food production tend to pay little attention to the fact that the additional food may be inaccessible for malnourished people because they do not possess the necessary purchasing power. Direct nutrition intervention programs such as direct feeding schemes or other food transfers to malnourished groups frequently fail to realize that households may not desire net additions in food consumption of the magnitude provided by the programme, but instead make opposing adjustments in food purchases. Nutrition education programmes may neglect the fact that better nutritional knowledge *per se* need not improve access to food.

The point to be made here is not that all past and ongoing food and nutrition programs and policies are ineffective, because obviously they are not. Rather, the point is that many food and nutritional programs are based on a very narrow perception of the problem. The lessons to be learned from the failures of many of these programs are that food and nutrition policies should be integrated, or at least closely related, and not kept separate, and that efforts to assess the nutritional consequences of food policies should incorporate the effects of all five factors and their interactions.

Food policy measures influence human nutrition through a number of intermediate steps. These must be identified and the process within which they operate must be understood in order to predict effectively how alternative policy formulations will affect nutrition. Figure 2 presents a schematic overview of the principal intermediate steps and causal links between food policy and nutrition.

Human nutrition is affected by food policy through changes in: (i) incomes of households with malnourished members; (ii) the quantity and quality of food available to those households and the prices they have to pay; (iii) fluctuations in incomes, food availability, and food prices; (iv) household income composition; (v) intra-household income and budget control; (vi) women's time allocation, and (vii) access to nonfood items and their prices.

Although the reasons for existing calorie-protein deficiencies differ among countries and population groups, low household incomes, insufficient food availability, and high food prices are likely to be primary ones. Changes in any of the three are likely to influence food consumption. From a nutritional point of view, only changes in food consumption by households within which some or all members are currently malnourished, or where the risk of malnutrition is significant, are of interest. Thus, changes in food supplies affect the nutritional status of individuals only to the extent that the food consumption of malnourished or at-risk individuals is affected. Estimates of total per capita food availability for a given country or region are of little or no use as indicators of the magnitude of protein-calorie undernutrition. Protein-calorie undernutrition frequently coexists with a more or less plentiful food supply, but plentiful food supply is irrelevant to households without access to adequate food.

Changes in the incomes of households with malnourished members and the food prices facing these households influence the ability of these households to obtain food and may also change the cost of food relative to other goods competing for the household budget.

Additional income obtained by households with malnourished members is unlikely to be spent entirely for the purpose of improving nutrition. It may be spent on food for well-nourished members of the households, it may be spent on foods with low nutritional value, or it may be spent on non-foods. Furthermore, increasing household incomes may cause commodity substitution towards more expensive nutrients. Two points are important in this regard. First, household spending and consumption patterns, while rational to the head of the household, may not be optimal from a nutritional point of view. Nutrition is only one of a series of considerations entering into decisions on spending and consumption patterns. Needs other than nutritional ones may carry considerable weight and there is no reason to expect that the fulfillment of all other needs is subordinate to the fulfillment of nutritional needs. Lack of knowledge regarding food and nutritional needs by household members is another reason why the ability to obtain food is not fully exploited. Nutrition education may help, but wrong information imposed from outside the household and promotion of non-foods or non-nutritious foods add to the problem.

Second, spending and consumption patterns may depend on who within the household controls incomes and decides on spending and consumption. Thus, although knowledge on the subject is extremely deficient, there is reason to believe that, as a rule, the nutritional effect of real income expansions, whether in money, in kind, or through price decreases, will depend on who in the household controls such income expansions and who decides what should be the appropriate adjustments in household consumption patterns. Wipper (1), Kumar (2), Tinker (3), and Guyer (4) provide empirical support for this argument. In a study in Kerala, India, Kumar (2) found evidence that the marginal propensity to consume food varied among women's incomes, men's incomes, and incomes from home gardens. Referring to the rural poor of Asia and Africa, Tinker concludes that ...."greater income-producing activities for women will have a more immediate impact on providing basic food and health to the poor than similar activities aimed only at men" (3, p.8).

The importance of this point has been grossly underestimated in past economic analyses. Traditional economic analysis tends to overlook the point by assuming that the household operates as a single decision-making unit and that no conflict exists between the utility functions used for decision-making and the utility function of individual household members. On the basis of research in rural areas of Africa, Guyer (4, p.1) found that ...."the classical assumption of the household as an undifferentiated decision-making unit applies poorly to many African kinship systems." Thus, the assumption may cause considerable error in estimations of nutritional effect and may result in faulty policy guidelines. This is an area where additional research is likely to be very useful.

The proportion of additional incomes spent on expanding calorie consumption (the marginal propensity to consume calories) has been found to vary widely among groups of households with similar levels of apparent calorie deficits. In some cases even severely deficient groups appear to spend very little additional income on increasing calorie intakes, while a considerable portion is spent on upgrading the diet in the sense of substituting toward more expensive calories. Thus, Williamson (5) found that the urban poor in Brazil would spend only about 25 cents of each additional dollar on expanding calorie consumption and spend about as much on shifting their diet towards higher-priced calories and considerably more (36 cents) on improved housing. While these households were deficient in calories they were also deprived of many other basic material goods. Thus, expanded incomes would be divided among the most pressing needs according to the preferences of the head of the household. Improved calorie intake was only one of these needs.

In other cases, the proportion of additional income spent on more calories is high. The large variation in the marginal propensity to consume calories among deficient households is a puzzle for which existing empirical explanation is insufficient for policy guidance. For the purpose of policy design it is important to know the approximate amount of income that will be spent on food by the population group of interest and the factors and processes by which spending is affected.

While severe calorie deficiencies are obvious, although they may not be identified as such by the household members, they are not widespread. Mild and moderate deficiencies are widespread but may not be recognized because they may be counteracted by adjustments in the level of activity. Furthermore, calorie requirements are influenced by a series of factors, and food intake data may not provide a good indicator of actual deficiency. Thus, some households that appear to be deficient may not be perceived to be so by the household decision-makers. Part of the explanation of the large variation in the marginal propensity to consume calories among calorie-deficient households may be found in these factors:

Incomes of malnourished households may be affected by food policy through: 1) income generation, e.g., policies related to technological change in agriculture and food-for-work programs, 2) income transfers in cash or redeemable coupons (e.g., food-stamp programs), or food distribution (e.g., food supplementation schemes of various types), and 3) food price policies. Food price policies may also change the price of one or more foods relative to other foods and non-foods. Thus, in addition to the effect of the real incomes embodied in price changes, these policies may -- but need not -- influence household budget allocation through changes in relative prices, and, thus, food consumption and nutrition. This is further discussed in the section on price policies.

A large part of existing calorie/protein deficiency, particularly among the rural poor, appears to be a result of fluctuations -- seasonal or irregular ones --in food prices, in incomes of the malnourished, and food availability. Thus, policies affecting these fluctuations, e.g. storage, transportation, foreign trade, and crop insurance policies, may have significant nutritional implications. In addition, changes in the income flow, including frequency and regularity, may be important.

The composition of household income may also be important for nutrition. According to neoclassical demand theory, the effect of changes in household real incomes on food consumption is independent of income type and source; i.e., it does not matter whether additional incomes are received in the form of food, cash, or from some other source as long as the receipt is infra-marginal (less than the amount that the household would acquire in the absence of the additional income). Many nutritionists, on the other hand, assume that infra-marginal food transfers to malnourished households result in a larger addition to household food consumption than effected by transfer of an equal amount of cash income. In fact, this assumption seems to underlie a great many past and ongoing food supplementation schemes that, as further discussed elsewhere, tend to be infra-marginal. Furthermore, there is some evidence that real incomes in the form of food from home production contributes more to food consumption than an equal amount of cash income.

The apparent conflict between actual food acquisition behavior and what would be expected on the basis of demand theory may be a result of erroneous calculations of the real cost of food to the household. Another possible explanation is that different types of income are controlled by different household members, and that the proportion of additional incomes (the marginal propensity to spend on food -- MPF) that each member wishes to spend on food differs. As discussed earlier, there is some empirical evidence to support the argument that MPF differs between heads of households and spouses in parts of Africa and possibly elsewhere. However, this is an area where additional research is urgently needed to sort out the relevant causal links.

The nutritional impact of changes in the demand for women's time is another area where additional research is urgently needed. It is likely that policies and programs that increase the demand for women's time influence food preparation, child care, and other nurturing activities and cause dietary shifts towards higher-priced calories. However, existing empirical evidence is very limited.

Having briefly discussed the principal ways in which food policy may affect nutrition, I shall turn, in the next section, to an analysis of the nutritional effects of selected kinds of policies according to available empirical evidence.

Nutritional Effect of Selected Policy Types

Existing food policies are many and varied. Four of the most common policy types discussed below are: (i) food supply policies and programs; (ii) consumer-oriented food price policies; (iii) food-linked income transfer, and (iv) food transfer programs.

Food Production Policies

Production-oriented policies may affect urban as well as rural malnutrition. The impact on urban households depends on the extent to which food prices are affected and on food/price/wage linkages.

Food consumption by the poor -- particularly the urban poor and those rural poor who do not produce part or all of the food they consume -- is very sensitive to changes in food prices. Thus, policies that affect food prices and their fluctuation over time are of particular interest from a nutritional point of view. High price levels and severe price fluctuations are much more harmful to the poor than to the better-off consumers. On the other hand, low price levels may have severe negative nutritional effects among the rural poor who depend on food production for their incomes whether they are producers or farm labourers. Furthermore, the long-run nutritional effects of low food prices on urban as well as rural poor may be severe because the low prices depress food production.

The effect of expansions in food production on food prices, and, thus, on urban and some rural malnutrition depends on a number of factors, particularly foreign trade and price policies. If free trade is maintained and domestic food prices reflect international ones, local production expansions of tradable commodities are unlikely to result in significant price reductions except perhaps for short-term local price decreases caused by ineffective marketing and transportation facilities. In those cases, the nutritional effect on the urban poor may be negligible. On the other hand, if foreign trade is controlled and domestic prices are permitted to adjust to reflect the additional domestic supply, then the nutritional status of the urban poor may be significantly improved because their real incomes increase and food becomes less expensive relative to other goods. Thus, household food acquisition will be affected by income as well as by substitution effect.1/

1/ For additional analysis and discussion of the distributional effects of production expansions, see references 6 and 7.

The impact of food supply policies on food acquisition and nutrition of rural households is more complex and poorly understood. Clearly, food acquisition by producers of the commodities influenced by the policies may be affected through income as well as price changes. Agricultural labourers deriving incomes from the production or marketing of such commodities will be affected by price changes and may -- but need not -- experience any income change.

There is considerable evidence to show that the introduction or expansion of the production of cash crops among subsistence or semi-subsistence farmers may cause negative nutritional effects (see 3,7,8 for a review of the findings in this area). Since overall incomes are expected to increase and semi-subsistence farmers would be expected to have positive income elasticities for food, it is not clear why the nutritional effects could be negative.

The explanation obviously differs among cases. However, it appears that factors other than income that influence household food acquisition behavior may play an important role in many instances. Foremost among these are the impact on intra-household income and budget control and the resulting effect on food consumption. Policies and programs that transfer budget control from household members with high propensities to household members with low marginal propensities to consume food (MPCF) would result in reduced food consumption that might offset the positive impact of increased household income.

One of the principal underlying factors appears to be that the responsibility for the production of food for use in the household in many African and some Asian countries rests with women, while incomes generated by cash-cropping frequently are controlled by men. Expanded cash-cropping reduces the availability of land and household labour for food production and, thus, women's control over household real incomes decreases. But because women have traditionally been responsible for assuring the necessary food supply for the family, and since a strong separation may exist between men's and women's incomes and their uses, the loss in food consumption from their own production may not be matched by increased food purchases.

Transformation from semi-subsistence to a cash economy frequently expands the spending opportunities by making more goods and services available in a region. This would be expected to exercise pressures towards more emphasis on non-foods and higher-priced food at the expense of low-priced staples. Farm gate-retail price spreads for food as well as local food price increases caused by local supply reduction and failure to compensate through food imports into the region would also push the farmer in the direction of non-foods as he ceases to produce his own food.

Inability of the existing marketing system to cope with a situation of rapidly increasing demand and reduced supply of basic food staples in rural areas is a major problem that may contribute to sharp food price increases in local markets.

Household reactions to changes in the frequency and fluctuations of incomes may also be responsible for a reduced emphasis on food. While semi-subsistence farming may produce a constant flow of income in the form of food and some cash, income from cash-cropping frequently comes in large lumps and may be spent quite differently.

Introduction or expansion of cash cropping may alter the demand for women's time. This, in turn, is likely to affect nutrition through changes in child care, breast-feeding, food preparation, and food acquisition. Finally, cash crop policies and programs may alter existing resource ownership patterns and thus make some households economically and nutritionally worse off.

Much of the evidence on the nutritional effects of rural change is anecdotal and there is an urgent need for additional research to assist in the design of policies that will assure success of otherwise appropriate rural transformations from a nutritional point of view. It is possible that observed negative effects on nutrition are of a short-term nature and exceptions to a general rule of positive long-term effects of such transformation. Even if this is the case, the exceptions are sufficiently widespread and the short-term effects sufficiently alarming to warrant research and policy attention. In addition, research is needed to assist in the design and implementation of other food supply policies, including the choice of commodities to be promoted and the design of production technology that takes nutritional and distributional effects into account.

Consumer-Oriented Food Price Policies

Consumer-oriented food price policies are widespread and may take many forms. In most cases they are aimed at maintaining low food prices to urban consumers and are frequently linked to government desires for low urban wages. Explicit and implicit subsidies are usually included in such policies.

Although nutritional concerns are sometimes used as arguments in support of government intervention in food pricing, the principal goals are usually of a broader socioeconomic and political nature. But whether improved nutrition is part of the principal objectives or not, nutritional status may be significantly affected by price policies.

Studies of food subsidy programs in Kerala, India, (9); Sri Lanka (10); Bangladesh (11); and Pakistan (12) conclude that such programs may provide an effective means of reducing protein-calorie deficiencies among low-income households, although the cost-effectiveness tends to be low and the costs high.

The fiscal costs of food subsidy programs depend on the price wedge that must be introduced between the government purchasing and selling price. The size of the wedge, in turn, depends on the source and prices of the food available to government and the desired consumer price level. Sometimes the wedge may be quite large, whereas at other times governments may sell low-cost food aid commodities at a profit.

In Sri Lanka food price subsidies accounted for 18 percent of total government expenditures in 1975 (10). These subsidies have since been replaced by a less expensive food stamp program. In Bangladesh, the costs of food subsidy programs were estimated at 14.7 percent of total government expenditures for 1979 (11). In Egypt an even larger share of government expenditure is spent on food subsidies. Egypt reportedly spent about $1.5 billion, or about 20 percent of government expenditures in 1980 and the cost is increasing (13).

These high government costs together with the implications for foreign exchange spending is one reason why goverments in some countries are forced to reduce the size of existing food subsidy programs. Such reductions have occurred recently in Peru, Sudan, Sri Lanka, Jamaica, and other developing countries.

Food price subsidy programs may be implemented in various ways. In some cases such as India and Egypt, public ration shops or publicly licensed private shops distribute the food. If attempts are made to identify target households, these households may be issued ration cards (e.g., Egypt) or food stamps (e.g, Sri Lanka) that may be exchanged for subsidized foods. Such measures both identify the target household and ration the amount of food that can be obtained under subsidy.

Although food price subsidy policies have been implemented with reasonable success in many urban areas, their success in rural areas has been very limited. Such an urban bias is exemplified by the public food distribution system in Bangladesh (11). Relatively few attempts have been made even to try to reach the rural poor with these programs. Food price subsidies programs in Sri Lanka, India, and Egypt are exceptions to this general rule. Results from research undertaken by IFPRI indicate that the rural populations in these countries obtain significant benefits (9, 10, 13).

The impact of price subsidies on the food acquisition of a particular household is influenced by the size of the subsidy and household food acquisition behavior. It is important whether the subsidized quantity is infra-marginal. In many cases, food price subsidies are limited to specified rations that are less than the quantity that would be acquired without subsidy; it is infra-marginal. This implies that the nutritional effect would be expected to be no different from that of a transfer of cash income equal to the real income embodied in the price subsidy. Except for such income effect and possible effects of changes in intra-household income control discussed earlier, there is no apparent reason why the household should allocate more of its real income to food because the marginal cost does not change. If the marginal propensity to consume calories is around 0.5 -- a reasonable magnitude for many households with malnourished members -- then it would be expected that only one-half of any income transfer would be spent on increasing the quantity of calories consumed irrespective of whether the income transfer is in the form of food or cash as long as the transfer is infra-marginal.

In other cases food subsidies are available in quantities exceeding those that would be purchased in the absence of the subsidy. This includes those cases where subsidized quantities are unlimited to the individual household, such as bread and wheat flour in Egypt. Here the marginal cost of food or particular food commodities is lowered relative to a situation without the subsidy. Thus, the quantity demanded would increase not only because of a transfer of real income embodied in the subsidy, but also because the food is cheaper relative to other goods. Of course, rationing reduces the cost of a subsidy program, but it also reduces the effect on food consumption by the target household per unit of subsidy cost, i.e., the cost effectiveness. The cost may also be reduced by targeting more effectively on those households where malnutrition is most prevalent. This would increase the cost-effectiveness. Thus, if the goal of a particular food price subsidy is to maximize the increase in food intakes among households with malnourished members per dollar of subsidy, effective household targeting should be pursued and rationing to target households avoided. Unfortunately, to be effective, targeting may depend on some kind of rationing.

While consumer-oriented food price policies may interact with household food acquisition behavior in a number of ways, one aspect, the non-price costs to participating households of obtaining subsidized food, deserves special attention, partly because it may play an important role in determining the nutritional effects of such policies, and partly because it is frequently ignored in policy design. One of the principal elements of the non-price costs is the time required to obtain the food. The waiting time in food lines and the disutility of standing in line may be considerable. Such time requirements may make it unattractive for some households to participate because of high alternative cost of time, perceived loss of status, or high marginal utility of money. The first two reasons are likely to reduce participation by better-off population groups and thus bias the program in favor of the most needy. When low wages are linked with extremely scarce leisure time, the bias may be in the opposite direction. Malnutrition is frequently found in households where both income and time are extremely scarce. Thus, the use of queuing as a targeting device may not be effective in reaching the most needy.

The impact of food price subsidies on real increases and food consumption by the poor is also influenced by the price-wage linkages. In many countries, attempts to keep food prices low originate at least in part from a desire to keep wages low and thus promote economic growth. In those cases, the immediate benefits captured by poor consumers from food price subsidies are lower than those indicated by the difference between the free market and the subsidized prices, because existing wages are lower than they would have been in the absence of the price subsidies.

Food-Linked Income Transfers

Food-linked income transfer programs may take many forms, with food stamp programs probably being the most common. These programs attempt to transfer incomes to target households in such a way as to assure that the income is spent on food. Frequently, the quantities of food covered by these programs are infra-marginal. Thus, as discussed above, the effects on household food acquisition would not be expected to differ from those of an equal cash transfer. However, there is some evidence that the marginal propensity to consume food is higher for food-linked income transfer than for other incomes (2, 14). One possible explanation is that the intra-household budget control is a function of the income source and that the marginal propensity to consume food varies among household members.

However, food-linked income transfers need not be infra-marginal. One way to design transfer programs to have an effect on food acquisition beyond the income effect is to require the household to pay some amount close to what it is currently spending on food in order to obtain food stamps covering a larger quantity. Such a puchase requirement was included in the U.S. food stamp program up until 1979. Programs designed in this fashion are likely to have a greater impact on household food acquisition because in addition to the income effect, they make food relatively cheaper at the margin, at least by the transaction costs or discount associated with resale of the food stamps.

Purchase requirements are difficult to implement in a socially just manner. If the amount to be paid for the food stamps is based on the average food expenditures by the target group, then the program would tend to be regressive among target households and may exclude the most needy from participating because the amount may exceed what they are able to pay. On the other hand, in most societies it is impossible to extract a different amount from each household on the basis of ability to pay.

Even if food-linked income transfers do not influence nutrition in a manner different from cash transfers of the same magnitudes, the former may be politically feasible where the latter is not. Better-off population groups generally derive more utility from income transfers aimed at the alleviation of overt human misery such as extreme and highly visible malnutrition than from general income transfers where the spending decisions related to the transfers are left in the hands of the recipient households. For this reason, income transfers to the absolute poor may be politically desirable or feasible only if earmarked for alleviation of extreme human misery even though the final result is not different from non-earmarked transfers. Further discussion of this matter is presented by Harberger (15) and Scandizzo and Knudsen (16).

Food Transfer Programs

Food transfer programs may be targeted on households or individual household members. A variety of food supplementation programs fall into this category. Most such programs are targeted on individual household members such as infants, preschoolers, and pregnant or lactating women. The "leakage" in such programs, i.e., the difference between the amount of food transferred and the net addition to the quantity consumed by the target groups, is usually large. Such leakage is a result of the sharing of transferred food among household members and a reduction in the quantity of food acquired by the household through other channels. From a review of about 200 food supplementation programs for infants, Beaton and Ghassemi (17) found that the net addition to food intakes of intended beneficiaries was 20 to 70 percent of the food transfers.

When food transfer programs are targeted on households but not on particular household members, one of the sources of "leakage" mentioned above --the sharing with non-target household members -- disappears and a lower magnitude of leakage would be expected. However, even in those cases the leakages may be high. Thus, a food supplementation program transferring 850 calories to each of the participating households in Bogota resulted in an average net increase of only 155 calories per person, i.e., a leakage of 82 percent (18).

The prevalence of leakage is not surprising because the quantity of food transferred is usually less than the quantity consumed prior to the program. While the magnitude of leakage in many programs may conform to expectations, the large variation among programs and population groups is a puzzle for which there is little empirical or conceptual explanation. One possible explanation is that some programs transfer more food than what was previously consumed, thus lowering food prices at the margin. However, such programs are rare. Differences in program design that make substitution more difficult in some programs than in others, e.g., direct feeding versus take-home rations, may assist in explaining these variations, particularly if direct feeding exceeds food intakes of the particular individual without the program. Other program design matters such as entry/exit criteria, program duration, and timing of supplement assist in explaining differences in the degree of substitution. Differential impact of the various program types on intra-household budget control linked with differential marginal propensities to consume food among individual household members, as well as differential impact on the demand for women's time, may also be hypothesized to play a role in explaining the large variations. (See Knudsen [19] for additional discussion of factors influencing the benefits of food supplementation programs).

Improving the Nutrition Impact of Food Programs

Food policies are frequently designed to achieve a number of objectives. While improved nutrition may be an expected outcome, it is frequently not one of the explicit policy objectives. It is even more rare to find cases -- outside the highly targeted nutrition program -- where nutrition goals and considerations have influenced policy design. However, it is essential to pay explicit attention to nutritional effects of food policies if the achievement of nutritional goals is of high priority. Modifications in policy design or introduction of complementary measures may have significant nutritional effects without causing unacceptable changes in the achievement of other policy goals. Which trade-offs related to the achievement of conflicting goals are acceptable is, of course, a political question. But to deal effectively with this question, the trade-offs must be explicitly considered. Merely assuming that increasing food production, higher incomes, and/or lower food prices will result in improved nutrition, or that increasing production of non-food crops and/or higher food prices will have adverse nutritional effects is to avoid the issue.

Successful efforts to improve the nutritional impact of food policy measures must be based on: (i) A political desire to improve the lot of the poor, (ii) effective institutional and analytical capacities to deal with the issue, and (iii) a thorough understanding of the relevant processes and access to the necessary information. Deficiencies in one or more of these areas currently prohibit effective incorporation of nutritional consideratons into policy design in most countries. Each of these three areas is further discussed below with emphasis on ways to remove existing deficiencies and, thus, improve the impact of food policy on nutrition.

Political Desire

Political desire to do something about existing malnutrition is essential. The political power structure that explicitly or implicitly contributed to past and current malnutrition may show no greater desire to improve the nutrition situation now than before. However, in some countries increasing urbanization, the related accumulations of the absolute poor, and increasing awareness among the latter regarding the power embodied in threats of urban social unrest, have brought more government attention to the issue of absolute poverty and the need to deal with it. Furthermore, it is possible that recent evidence of high payoff to society from investment in human capital may begin to have an impact on government policy towards the poor.

Efforts to improve nutrition could and frequently do play an important role in the broader attempts to raise the living standards of the poor for a number of reasons. First, better-off population groups (who are usually the ones possessing the political power) generally derive more benefit from income transfers aimed at the alleviation of overt human misery, such as extreme and highly visible malnutrition, than from general income transfers where the spending decisions related to the transfers are left in the hands of the recipient households. For this reason, income transfers to the absolute poor may be politically desirable or feasible only if the transfers are earmarked, even though, as discussed above, the transferred income is fungible. Second, malnutrition is a reasonable although not perfect indicator of poverty. Thus, government policies benefiting the malnourished would generally be expected to benefit the absolute poor. Third, identification of the target group (the absolute poor) and minimization of leakage to non-target population groups from government transfer programs may be more effectively achieved within a food and nutrition-related program than within other government policies.

Thus, even though the political desire for improving the lot of the poor may not be strong, there are reasons why governments may wish to improve the nutritional benefits of public policies (20).

Institutional and Analytical Capacities

Institutional changes are needed in many countries to facilitate closer interactions among agriculture, food policy, and nutrition. A number of countries have recently established nutrition monitoring units, food policy units, and similar agencies focused on various aspects of these interactions (21). Such efforts should be strengthened. Their success is critical to sustained incorporation of nutritional goals into food policy. A number of factors tend to oppose success. The elements of an integrated approach to agricultural policy and nutrition are usually found among a number of existing institutions, and attempts to integrate the appropriate activities run counter to vested interests and traditions. Furthermore, shortage of funds and of well-trained manpower and analytical capacity is common. The international assistance community has promoted the establishment of analytical units in a few countries, but the support has usually been of a short-term nature, and while the institutional problems may have been at least partially overcome, support to develop appropriate analytical approaches and capabilities has been deficient. Yet, without it those units will not succeed.

Improved Knowledge and Access to Information

Efforts to guide the choice and design of food policies to meet nutritional goals better must be based on a solid understanding of the underlying processes and empirical estimates of the likely impact of alternative policy choices and designs. This is an area where additional research is urgently needed. While the specific research needs vary among countries, particularly insofar as the empirical estimates are concerned, there is a need for research that will produce generalizable results capable of improving existing understanding of the most important processes and relationships and, thus, provide the framework for location-specific empirical analyses. In particular, there is a need for further research on: (i) food acquisition behavior among households with malnourished members; (ii) food policy design and implementation procedures, including more cost-effective ways of reaching the target population without excessive leakage to non-target groups; (iii) economy-wide implications of alternative food policies, including effects on foreign exchange, domestic food production, income distribution, growth, and fiscal costs, and the most appropriate role of external food aid, and (iv) food market-related matters.

In order to assure a high degree of policy relevance, such research should be undertaken within a policy framework. Emphasis should be placed on four policy areas: (i) agricultural and rural development programs and policies, (ii) food price policies, (iii) income and food transfer programs, and (iv) integrated health and nutrition programs.

In addition, more information is needed at the national and local level to identify the malnourished and to estimate their responsiveness to changes in food prices, incomes, and other variables, as discussed earlier. Traditional aggregate demand analysis is of only limited value because no attempts are made to separate demand characteristics for well- and malnourished. Price, income, and other relevant factors must be estimated specifically for the malnourished or the absolute poor. At present, such estimates are extremely scarce.

Last but not least, there is an urgent need for research to improve current understanding of the decision-making process as it relates to the choice and design of food policy. A better understanding of the behavior of governments and how this is influenced by the various interest groups and changes in the power structure is likely to enhance the effect of other policy analysis by making it more relevant to the decision-making process.

1. A. Wipper, "African Women, Fashion, and Scapegoating," Canad. J. Afr. Studies 6(2):329 (1972).

2. S. Kumar, "Role of the Household Economy in Determining Child Nutrition at Low Income Levels: A Case Study in Kerala," Occasional Paper No. 95, Department of Agricultural Economics, Cornell University (November 1977).

3. I. Tinker, "New Technologies for Food Chain Activities: The Imperative Equity for Women," Office of Women in Development, US/AID, Washington, DC (1979).

4. J.I. Guyer, "Household Budgets and Women's Incomes," Working Paper No. 28, African Studies Center, Boston University (1980).

5. C. Williamson, "Food Consumption Parameters for Brazil and Their Application to Food Policy," Research Report No. 32, International Food Policy Research Institute (IFPRI, Washington, DC, 1982).

6. P. Pinstrup-Andersen, Agricultural Research and Modern Technology in Economic Develoment (Longman, London, 1982).

7. P. Fleuret and A. Fleuret, "Nutrition, Consumption and Agricultural Change," Human Organization 39(3):250 (1980).

8. K.G. Dewey, "Agricultural Development, Diet and Nutrition," Ecol. Food Nutr. 8:265 (1979).

9. S. Kumar, "Impact of Subsidized Rice and Food Consumption and Nutrition in Kerala," Research Report No. 5, (International Food Policy Research Institute IFPRI, Washington, DC, 1979).

10. J.D. Gavan and I.S. Chandrasekera, "The Impact of Public Foodgrain Distribution on Food Consumption and Welfare in Sri Lanka," Research Report No. 13, International Food Policy Research Institute (IFPRI, Washington, DC, 1979).

11. R. Ahmed, "Foodgrain Supply, Distribution and Consumption Policies within a Dual Pricing Mechanism. A Case Study of Bangladesh," Research Report No. 8, International Food Policy Research Institute (IFPRI, Washington, DC,1979).

12. B.L. Rogers, Consumer Food Price Subsidies and Subsidized Food Distribution Systems in Pakistan, Ph.D. Dissertation, Brandeis University, Waltham, Massachusetts, 1978.

13. H. Alderman, J. von Braun, and S.A. Sakr, "Egypt's Food Subsidy and Rationing System: A Description," Research Report No. 34, International Food Policy Research Institute (IFPRI, Washington, DC, 1982).

14. R.B. Reese, J.G. Feaster, and G.B. Perkins, "Bonus Food Stamps and Cash Income Supplements," U.S. Department of Agriculture, Economic Research Service, Marketing Research Report No. 1034 (USDA, Washington, DC, 1974).

15. A.C. Harberger, "Basic Needs Versus Distributional Weights in Social Cost-Benefit Analysis," Background Notes for a Seminar, World Bank, Washington, DC, 1979.

16. P.L. Scandizzo and O.K. Knudsen, "The Evaluation of the Benefits of Basic Need Policies," Amer. J. Agric. Econ. February, 1980.

17. G.H. Beaton and H. Ghassemi, "Supplementary Feeding Programs for Young Children in Developing Countries," Amer. J. Clin. Nutr. 35:(4, Supplement):864 (1982).

18. J.O. Mora, B. de Paredes, M. Wagner, L. de Navarro, J. Suescun, N. Christiansen, and M.G. Herrera, "Nutritional Supplementation and the Outcome of Pregnancy," Amer. J. Clin. Nutr. 32:455 (1979).

19. O.K. Knudsen, "Economics of Supplemental Feeding of Malnourished Children: Leakages, Cost, and Benefits," World Bank Staff Working Paper No. 451 (World Bank, Washington, DC, April 1981).

20. P. Pinstrup-Andersen, "Food Policy, Household Behavior, and Nutrition," paper presented at the Fourth Biennial Meeting of the Agricultural Economics Society of Southeast Asia, Singapore, Nov. 3-7, 1981.

21. P. Pinstrup-Andersen, "Nutritional Consequences of Agricultural Projects: Conceptual Relationships and Assessment Approaches," World Bank Staff Working Paper No. 456 (World Bank, Washington, DC, 1981).

Figure 1. Schematic Overview of the Principal Policy-Related Factors Affecting Nutritional Status

Food availability
(time and place)

↓

Ability of household
to obtain available food
(household food acquisition power)

↓

Desire to obtain available food
(household food acquisiton behavior)

↓

Allocation of acquired food
among household members
(household food allocation behavior)

↓

Physiological utilization of
ingested food
(health status and household nurturing behavior)

↓

Nutritional status
of individual

Figure 2. Schematic Overview of the Principal Causal Links Between Food Policy and Nutrition

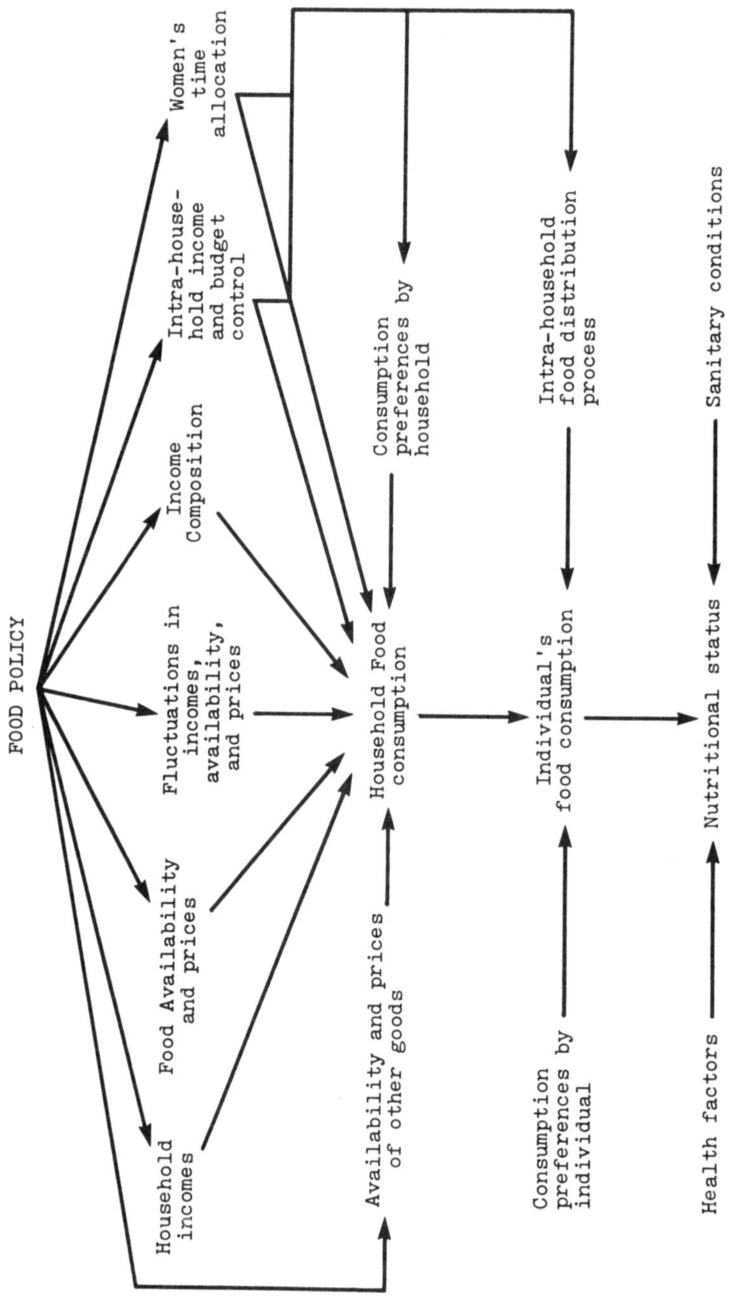

NUTRITIONAL CONSEQUENCES OF AGRICULTURAL AND RURAL DEVELOPMENT PROJECTS*

PAUL LUNVEN**

INTRODUCTION

Traditional nutritional solutions - by direct interventions - give generally short-term effects, and indeed have only had a marginal impact in the past; they cannot be expected to be effective in combating the problem of hunger and malnutrition as a whole. The only way a sustained impact can be made is through the main-stream of development efforts, so that the resources invested in development by governments and donors have the maximum effect on nutrition -- within the constraints imposed by economic and other considerations. However, these resources do not invariably have a beneficial effect on nutrition; and often any effect they do have is more by chance than by intention. It is evident, from available statistical data, that they have not had sufficient impact in the past to reverse the rising trend of malnutrition. More resources and better use of them will both be needed to reduce malnutrition.

While it can reasonably be expected that, in the long-term, hunger and malnutrition will be solved effectively through general economic and social development, and especially through national food and nutrition strategies, it is clear that actions targeted at the rural poor need to be implemented in the short- and medium-term in order to provide an effective benefit to the community and to the family.

This is why, for reasons of efficiency and speedy action, it is necessary to work _also_ at the level of projects - or ecological areas - to make sure that agricultural and rural development projects, well-intentioned as they may be, actually improve the level of living and the socio-economic conditions of the rural poor.

Evaluation of a number of projects has revealed that improved nutrition is not automatically a benefit of development. The economic and social conditions of a region can change with no real impact on nutrition. Or, even worse, the most well-intentioned development plans can have a negative effect on the nutrition of those at risk.

Why is there this discrepancy between the logical, reasoned theory of the relationship between nutrition and rural development and the actual nutritional impact of the projects? Perhaps there is more involved in integrating nutrition objectives in rural development and in achieving nutrition benefits than just providing inputs and services necessary for increased production, improved employment, and better incomes.

* An earlier version of this paper has already been published in the UNU _Food and Nutrition Bulletin_ Vol. 4, No. 3:17 (1982).

** Dr. Lunven was not present at the meeting, but the paper was read for him by a member of ICARDA staff.

DRA-8

There is a need therefore, within the planning undertaken at area level, to take nutrition considerations into account. Most planners will be familiar with making decisions based on trade-offs between the social and economic factors involved, but they are likely to find the nutritional context unfamiliar, and the techniques of analysis and computation of nutritional benefits much less proven and definitive than those of standard economic analysis.

In addition, data on nutrition and food consumption are usually poor or non-existent for the specific population groups likely to be affected by projects in developing countries, and national statistical systems are frequently not sufficiently well-organized to make effective use of such data.

Although the assessment of potential nutrition effects should be a normal routine exercise of project appraisal, achieving that objective in a given country will require initial concentration on a limited number of carefully chosen projects, and gradual extension and strengthening of data and information services.

In an attempt to analyse the failure of projects to provide nutrition benefits, and to ensure that future development efforts will live up to their potential to improve nutrition, we offer details from case studies of six rural projects (1).

ASSESSMENT OF PROJECT IMPACT

Case History I

Large areas of a developing country in Africa are arid or semi-arid. The climate is severe, the terrain is rugged, the people are poor, and malnutrition is widespread. The inhabitants of these regions raise livestock (cattle, goats, sheep, shoats), slaughtering the animals to feed their families, selling any surplus animal products to earn income that can be used to purchase other food supplies. Because the land is rough and vegetation scarce, the herds must be constantly on the move to sources of food and water, making the work highly labour-intensive.

Over a period of about ten years these arid and forbidding regions have been hit hard by droughts and animal diseases. An already tenuous existence became even more vulnerable and the risk and incidence of malnutrition increased. More and more households began to turn to crops to supplement food supplies, to provide another source of income, and to produce the fodder needed for the livestock.

The government of the country realized that something had to be done to improve life for those living in these arid regions, and developed a programme, tested in one region of the country, designed to increase productivity and incomes.

The pilot project, consistent with the overall plan, provided for transportation infrastructures, social services, livestock development, rural industries, afforestation, soil conservation, dryland agriculture, and small-scale irrigation. From the plans it appeared more than likely that the project would achieve its objectives, that people in the region would be better off, and the risk of malnutrition would decrease.

An analysis of the project indicated that certain components were successful. The new rural industries, developed under the auspices of the project, created a market for local products (honey, fish, etc.) and provided alternate sources of income for people who otherwise would have been forced to go outside the region to find work.

The agricultural components of the project were less successful. To reinforce the shift from livestock to farming, which was already occurring in the region, the project introduced a number of small-scale irrigation and dryland crop schemes. The water provided by irrigation was to help compensate for the months of low rainfall, make the crops less vulnerable to drought, and make the arid region more productive. The irrigation systems were designed to be labour-intensive, bringing to the region not only water but jobs.

An evaluation of the irrigation/crop schemes revealed a number of problems hindering the project. First, the irrigation schemes were concentrated in the sub-regions of the project area that had the best soil, the closest access to water, the most innovative people, and a lower risk of poverty and malnutrition. The poorer sub-regions that were the areas most in need and most likely to provide the technical results and information that could be applied in other arid parts of the country were the areas least likely to benefit from the project.

Second, the kind of seeds provided to the farmers were not as drought- or pest-resistant as they should have been, given the conditions and growing/storage problems in the region. The crops encouraged by the project were not as nutritious as others that might have been recommended, though the late introduction of cowpeas promised to benefit local diets.

Third -- the most serious problem with the scheme -- the demands for heavy amounts of labour for field preparation, clearing, burning, fencing, weeding, etc. coincided and conflicted with the time at which the livestock herds also demanded intensive amounts of human labour. As a result, those who could have benefited from the income earned working on the irrigation/crop schemes could not spare the time from their herds to do the work. Those who were trying to raise livestock and produce crops had to divide their time between the two to the detriment of both. Only those wealthier farmers who could afford to hire others to do some of their labour could hope to achieve good yields in livestock and in crops and increase their incomes and food supplies. With the kind of labour conflict created by this project, poverty and malnutrition will continue to be a problem for a majority of the people in the region.

Case History II

In a region of an African country, population was increasing at an alarming rate while the land struggled to support it. Problems of poor soil quality were being complicated by frequent droughts and damaging agricultural techniques. Soil erosion, overgrazing, soil depletion, and deforestation were threatening to turn the area into a wasteland, making it even more difficult for the people to eke out a marginal subsistence living. With the growing population there was less and less land available and more and more pressure on the available food supplies. Those most at risk of poverty and malnutrition were the landless and those holding very small tracts of land - who were unable to produce or buy enough food to feed themselves.

To counter these problems and provide more opportunities for production and employment, the government started a five-year integrated development programme. The strategy of the programme was to deal with the constraints facing the small farmers: inadequate extension services, lack of training, inadequate inputs and marketing facilities, and lack of available credit.

Through the project much progress was made in soil conservation and in providing water to households. But most of this work was concentrated in the central part of the region -- the area least affected by severe climatic conditions, poverty and malnutrition -- and has not yet been extended to the most seriously affected areas. Those most in need are not yet feeling any benefits.

To encourage the small farmers to increase production, and therefore increase their incomes, the project included a credit programme. Farmers who agreed to plant two acres of cash crops - usually cotton - were eligible for a loan. The credit cooperative that administered the programme urged the farmers to plant, in addition to the two acres of cotton, one acre of staple crops and one acre of "rescue" crops in case the staple crop failed. Credit was supplied in seeds and agricultural inputs. There was also a guaranteed market for the cash crop once it was harvested.

The expected income increases from the sale of the cash crop might have had positive nutritional effects, but a closer analysis of the programme showed that the shift from food crops to cash crops put even more pressure on the food supplies produced and available in the region. An increase in income can only have a positive effect on nutrition if there is food available to buy. Not only did growing cotton take up land that had been used to grow food, but cotton depleted the soil and added to the problems of soil conservation in the region.

The main disadvantage of the credit scheme, in terms of those most at risk of poverty and malnutrition, was the land requirement. Two acres of cash crops, plus one acre of staple crops plus one acre of "rescue" crops means a minimum land requirement of four acres. That excluded all the landless and over half of the small farmers. Those most vulnerable were least able to participate. If the credit programme continues as it was designed, the larger farmers will get larger and richer, food supplies in the region will be more scarce, and the landless and the small farmers will suffer more.

Case History III

In a highland region of a developing country, tea-growing was a profitable business for those who owned large tracts of land or estates. On the other hand, small farmers managed to earn only a subsistence living. A high rate of stunting and wasting was reported in the children of households owning only small tracts of land, and the standard of living was low.

In an effort to alleviate the poverty of the small land-owner, the government introduced a tea-growing project. By providing training in tea cultivation, materials, transportation and marketing facilities, the project was to help the small farmer produce tea that could then be sold to bring a steady cash income into the household.

Researchers studying the project after it had been operating for a number of years discovered that those small farming households involved in the project did have higher incomes and exhibited other signs of affluence, such as better cattle. But there was no improvement in nutrition. In fact, the children of the tea-growers had a higher risk of stunting and wasting than the children of those not growing tea.

The main reason for this situation is that, during the transition period between subsistence farming and cash cropping, farmers and their families are faced with a drastic change in their community life and environment. They also have to adopt new cultivation practices, and consumption patterns that affect their traditional cultural patterns and -- as in this case of tea-growers --decrease the amount of food available for home consumption. Owing to lack of assistance from social workers, home economists and nutritionists, whose role had not been foreseen in the plan of operations, those with the money to spend in the market place did not know how to buy food to ensure the proper nutrition of their children.

In addition, the project had a negative effect on the buying power and nutrition of those outside the project. With the shift in the region to tea-growing and a cash economy, land and food prices increased drastically. Those not growing tea were finding it more and more difficult to feed their families, but did not have the cash to purchase in the market place. It seems likely that the incidence and severity of malnutrition will continue to increase.

Case History IV

A developing country in Africa wanted to encourage agriculture in the high potential regions of the country and improve rural conditions. Most of the land is held and worked by subsistence and small farmers. Although land potential is high, agricultural techniques are poor and poverty and malnutrition are widespread.

The development programme offered loans as an incentive to small farmers. Loans in kind (seed, fertilizer, extension services, marketing assistance) were available to farmers willing to grow cotton or maize, which were in short supply in the country. The cotton loans were managed by the cotton marketing company, the maize loans by the farmers' cooperative. The loan of seeds along with technical assistance and a guaranteed market for the crops was to increase productivity and crop quality and give the farmers a source of cash income.

An evaluation of the project indicated that there were a number of problems. First, the poor farmers owning the smallest tracts of land, who were most at risk of malnutrition, did not qualify for the loans; and any loans they did manage to get were seasonal and had to be repaid within the year.

The second problem was administrative. The cotton marketing company ran a much more efficient, businesss-like credit system than did the farmers' cooperative. Cotton loans were based on the suitability of the farmer's land for growing cotton. Seeds and other inputs arrived in time for planting, and were delivered right to the farm. Cotton extension workers paid regular visits to the farmers and supervised them from ground preparation through harvesting, ensuring large and profitable crops. The farmers' cooperative maize programme, on the other hand, ran much less smoothly. The system for approving farmers' loans seemed to be highly influenced by local politics and had little to do with the farm land being used. Seeds and other inputs often arrived late, and the farmer was responsible for getting the seeds from the local stores to the farm. (This regularly involved great distances. Cart delivery service was expensive and had to be paid in cash that the subsistence farmer did not have). Extension services were uneven: most of the help was given to the farmers who held the largest tracts of land. Marketing practices were such that farmers were encouraged to sell their entire maize crop and buy back the maize meal (at a higher cost) to feed their families.

In addition, the price for cotton was much higher than the price for maize. Given the smooth administration of the cotton programme, and the higher price for cotton, most farmers preferred to apply for the cotton loans.

The situation that rapidly developed in the region is that the poorest farmers have received no benefit from the credit programme: their farms are no more productive, their incomes have not increased. Those farmers holding slightly larger tracts of land are putting as much land as possible into growing cotton and they are earning good incomes from it. Because of the failure of the maize programme, less and less maize is being grown in the region and food supplies are threatened. With food supplies down and food prices up, the potential is for increased poverty and malnutrition among those who cannot produce enough food to feed themselves and cannot afford to buy it.

Case History V

In rural Asia, problems of poverty and malnutrition exist beside great wealth and affluence. The society is structured rigidly and it is difficult to improve life for the poor without threatening the wealthy and the powerful within the communities. As in most developing countries, the landless and those who own only very small tracts of land are the most vulnerable. There are severe problems of protein-energy malnutrition.

A few years ago the government of one Asian country initiated a cooperative dairy development project designed to increase the incomes of the smaller, subsistence farmers and supply wholesome, unadulterated milk to the urban poor. Because the dairy industry was to be run through a cooperative rather than the middlemen, profits were to be reinvested in the communities to the greater benefit of the rural poor.

Over the short term, the project was, in fact, quite successful. Several milk processing plants were built, creating a larger, more profitable market for milk. More and more farmers attempted to take advantage of the opportunity for a higher income by buying cows. Any of the deficit farmers (less than 2.5 acres of land) and the subsistence farmers (2.5 to 5 acres of land) who owned cows were able to use the profits from milk sales and the bonuses from the cooperative to buy rice, vegetables, and fruit to feed their families. The project also created some limited opportunities for employment in the processing plants and in the milk delivery system in the cities.

A closer look at the social and economic situation in the region showed that there were potential problems with the industry. The landless, who make up a large proportion of the population and suffer most from poverty and malnutrition, cannot benefit from the project. These people, with no land on which to graze a cow, could not take advantage of the dairy project except through membership in a cooperative. An investigation of the cooperatives showed that the number of landless members is very small (10%) and dropping.

Although shares in the cooperatives are divided evenly, bonus payments are related to the quantity of milk sold. Therefore, the rich farmers, with more land and more cows, earn more from the cash sale of their milk and receive a disproportionately large amount of the bonus payments. The richer farmers invested no more in the industry than the deficit or subsistence farmers but, in fact, made much more profit.

Any landless members of the cooperatives are eligible only for the dividend on the share, not for any of the bonus payments, so they gain little from the cooperatives. The rich become richer, and though some of the poorer farmers are slightly better off, the gap between rich and poor grows steadily wider.

Within the cooperative themselves, the wealthier farmers tend to dominate, as in most community structures. This means that the cooperatives' investments in the communities do not necessarily serve the interests of the people the project is trying to help.

In addition, the rich and powerful are prone to manipulate and victimize the poor through nefarious money-lending practices. With more money available from the milk profits to lend, and growing pressure on the poor from rising prices and the importance of belonging to the cooperatives, the project may unwittingly have accelerated the pauperization of the small farmer.

It is also interesting to note that the price of the processed milk is so high as to be beyond the means of the urban poor, so there are not direct benefits to these people from the project. What began as a well-intentioned development effort for the needy has become a vehicle to maintain the wealth and influence of the powerful.

Case History VI

Social structures can be a major stumbling block in efforts to improve life for the rural poor. For example, in a country in Asia, the rural population lives in family groups that are strictly hierarchical. (A young brother must not speak before the elder and must defer to his opinion). The position of anyone within the family hierarchy determines his position in any social group. The old and the wealthy dominate, the young and the poor are subservient. Outside the family groups there are other relationships that also make it difficult for the poor to make any progress. The poor labourer is bound by almost semi-feudal ties to the landowner for whom he works. These social structures maintain the position and the influence of the rich; they keep the landless and the deficit farmers struggling for a subsistence living. Poverty and malnutrition are widespread and are accepted as a way of life.

The government of this country recognized that the poor needed to be educated out of their poverty and initiated a development programme for small farmers and landless labourers. Workers for the project were to go into rural communities and encourage the farmers and labourers to form groups and work together in activities such as potato farming, pond and river fishing, animal husbandry, rice husking, rick-shaw service, netmaking, and silk production. Through this kind of a cooperative the project hoped to give the poor alternative sources of income, and the confidence to break out of the subservient relationship with the wealthy in the community.

Some groups were successful. Where the project provided access to credit along with social and economic support for the changes, the poor in some groups reported a standard of living that had improved by 30 to 40 percent in only two years. Food consumption increased in aggregate terms, but there was still a great demand for food among the most deprived families. (This was indicated by the fact that, according to group records, some business loans were "misapplied" for food by some of the poorer members).

Other groups ran into serious problems. The traditional elite in some communities saw the groups as a direct threat to their position and influence. They feared they would lose their cheap labour and that the present system of production and profits would be destroyed, so they did everything they could to prevent people from joining, to the point of threatening their employees. Because of the hierarchical and semi-feudal relationships at work in these communities, these threats were effective.

In other communities, the wealthy saw potential for profit in the groups. They would join, take control, attempt to exclude the landless from membership in order to increase the size of the loans available to the groups, and use their position to borrow money from the project and then default with immunity.

On the whole, it is clear that the members were more concerned about accumulating wealth than encouraging total participation of the poor. To date, the project has improved life for only a very small percentage of the rural poor. Most of the benefits have accrued to the wealthy. Poverty and malnutrition continue to be serious problems in these communities.

IMPROVING NUTRITION THROUGH PROJECT ASSESSMENT: PROPOSED METHODOLOGY

The experience of the nutritional effects of projects is hardly sufficient to put forward procedures for an automatic selection of suitable projects based on typology or a scoring system. However, a series of fairly liberal criteria can be applied as a first filter: the size of the population likely to be directly affected by the project, the vulnerability (i.e., the poverty) of the region (or sometimes of the country) in question, the intensity of the direct changes in the way of life resulting from the project; the strength of the link between the project and the local food system; the government's awareness of the importance of poverty and malnutrition; and the existing level of food and nutritional information in the country. This list of criteria makes it abundantly clear that, for example, any rural development project is a candidate for the introduction of nutritional considerations.

In the case of the projects we have examined, all six were well thought-out, well-intentioned efforts to improve life for the rural poor. The problems they encountered with their credit schemes, their cooperatives, and their choice of crops limited their effectiveness. Often the problems were targeting ones: the projects were not reaching the people most in need, or the regions most in need. In many cases it was simply a case of not understanding the social and economic situation in given areas.

Sometimes the fact that the project affected people outside as well as inside the project area was not sufficiently taken into account during the planning process and, generally speaking, not enough attention was paid to assessing the indirect effects of development.

The attempt we have made to assess the nutritional impact of development projects without explicit nutritional objectives should not be interpreted as a discredit of development efforts. On the contrary, we still believe that rural and agricultural development is the most efficient way to create the social and economic changes that will eventually ease world problems of malnutrition. But, if better nutrition is going to be a legacy of development projects, we have to do more than just sit back and wait for it to happen. We have to contribute to the process in order to avoid the kinds of problems and disappointments just described above.

For nutrition to be either an implicit or explicit objective of development, nutritionists must be involved in the early stages of development planning. To that end, FAO has developed a methodology that makes it possible to integrate nutrition considerations into rural and agricultural development projects (2).

In summary, the methodology applies to projects that involve substantial investment, development and management of resources, and area development.

Among investment projects selected are those that provide resources to agriculture, forestry, and fisheries. Resource development and management projects provide direct support to land and water management, crop or animal production, and development of forestry resources. Area development projects have many aspects and include rural development.

The seven stages commonly used by United Nations agencies and others for the planning of a project have been adopted as the basic sequence to which the four major steps of the nutrition planning process correspond. These steps are a desk review, an initial assessment, an in-depth study, and monitoring and evaluation.

1. Review of the project proposal:

   The desk review, which corresponds to the pre-identification stage, involves an examination of all reference materials and staff knowledge related to nutritional and the potential project area. From the desk review it may be possible to derive valid information on the extent and causes of malnutrition and existing efforts to combat it. Tentative project ideas are screened for relevance to nutrition problems in the area. Project objectives and flexibility for altering the design are reviewed to ascertain potential contributions to improvements in the nutrition of the most disadvantaged people. Available evidence of government interest in nutrition is sought because of its critical importance. The time taken to complete this stage generally involves one to two weeks.

2. Initial assessment of the potential nutrition impact of the project:

   This step corresponds to the project identification stage. The nutrition planner travels to the project area with the project identification team whose task is to develop a broadly described proposal that will include justification for the project, its objectives, participants, activities, management, inputs-outputs, and priorities. Further information is gathered on the food and nutrition situation in the area. A preliminary appraisal must be made of the potential impact of the project on food supplies and demand of the population groups worst-off nutritionally, and suggestions made for including nutritional considerations in various aspects of project design. Discussions are held with government officials and those financing the project. The need for continuing the nutrition investigations into the third phase (in-depth study) must be assessed. Consideration must be given to the availability of country experts for all these tasks and to the necessary efforts to obtain community involvement in deciding on the activities of priority for the project. A visit to the project area for discussions with potential beneficiaries is essential. The initial assessment would normally require three to four weeks.

3. The in-depth study is based on a more detailed analysis of the information used in the initial assessment, or if necessary, based on new survey data. During the intensive project formulation work, the nutrition planner may have to carry out an independent feasibility study on food consumption and nutrition to get new information specific to the needs of the project. It may involve a survey or re-analysis of existing data. The scope and activities of this study evolve from initial assessment supplemented by questions raised with government officials and local beneficiaries as the project design is formulated. Data will be required for use in making decisions on project objectives, participants, inputs, activities, and outputs. The groundwork for monitoring and evaluation is laid. It should lend objective evidence to the subjective impressions derived in the initial assessment, and indicate the impending impact on food consumption and nutrition. During this phase, discussion between the nutrition investigators and the project planners must deal with how to balance projected nutrition and social benefits with possible economic and political costs. If this is achieved at a very early stage in the feasibility studies for the project and continued during subsequent design work, nutritional considerations can be included successfully. An in-depth study (which usually lasts for six to nine months) is not essential and should be carried out only when available data are inadequate for this project stage.

4. Monitoring and evaluation of the effect of the project on nutrition in the area:

   An important output of this planning methodology is to provide guidance on any monitoring and evaluation (M & E) of the project that may be carried out. If the data base is good, as indicated particularly by the desk review, information collection by the nutrition planner can provide an adequate base for future M & E. As a matter of fact, the planning process so far followed will have generated interest in food consumption and nutrition and alerted those implementing the project to the importance of using nutrition data in its monitoring. It will have uncovered all the relevant data relating to food consumption and nutrition and, in the process, a great deal more relating to poverty and resources allocation among target groups between and within families. The latter include women and children who are not always considered by planners insofar as the family is regarded as the unit to be benefited by the project. In addition, the initial assessment and in-depth study will have collected new data, or re-analysed existing data, and it is this that may provide a basis for future M & E. If a national nutrition, food consumption, or household expenditure survey has been carried out in the project area within the last five years, this will probably have been re-analysed during the in-depth study. As such, it will provide an ideal baseline to monitor changes in food consumption or nutritional status.

   In a general sense, the nutrition planning methodology will have provided valuable experience in order to decide what data to collect for M & E, how much and when. It will have provided insights into how much time is required to reach isolated groups, to collect information with acceptable sample sizes, and how to interpret data provided by respondents. Much of the formulation of M & E activities will be dictated, therefore, by common sense.

   This process allows the nutritionist to determine that the project is truly intended to help the rural poor and has the potential to improve nutrition. The initial assessment helps identify the groups within the regions who suffer most from malnutrition and why. That information can be fed back into project planning so that project components can be designed with specific target groups and specific target areas in mind. Through the in-depth study, the nutritionist can predict the potential effect of the project on the nutrition of those both within and outside of the project areas. That kind of analysis will help development projects avoid the mistakes that were described in the case histories. Monitoring and evaluation ensure that the project is achieving its objectives. The project team then has an opportunity to adjust for any weakness or problems before any irrevocable harm is done.

   It is to the benefit of everyone involved -- governments, funding agencies, those working with rural and agricultural development projects -- to integrate nutrition into the early stages of project planning and use nutrition throughout the project as a measure of project effectiveness. The methodology described very briefly here and in greater detail in one of our other publications (3) can help ensure that rural and agricultural development projects bring about the kinds of social and economic changes that will begin the end of poverty and malnutrition.

As a result of a request for technical assistance received in 1982, FAO was entrusted with the task of appraising the nutritional and food entitlement aspects of an Integrated Agricultural Development Project (IADP) already in operation in a West African country. In particular, it was an objective of the mission to ascertain whether single project components and measures chosen were expected to have any relevant influence on the nutritional condition of the project's target groups and to determine the expected effect and results.

It is now clear that food shortage problems in the world, and especially in Africa, will be solved only through production of basic foods by small farmers. In such cases food production and consumption cannot be separated, and the systematic introduction of nutrition considerations in agricultural projects will not prove incompatible with other national level considerations, such as saving foreign exchange, increasing rural employment, etc. It is therefore important to draw the attention of all concerned in project planning to nutrition issues and to enable the trade-offs between different project components to be fully examined and discussed. We think the FAO methodology is a structure by which this may be achieved.

DRY AREA AGRICULTURE AND NUTRITION

1. Food and Agriculture Organization, Integrating Nutrition into Agricultural and Rural Development Projects: Six Case Studies. Nutrition in Agriculture Series No. 2 (FAO, Rome, 1984).

2. Food and Agriculture Organization, Integrating Nutrition into Agricultural and Rural Development Projects: A Manual. Nutrition in Agriculture Series No. 1 (FAO), Rome, 1984).

3. P. Lunven and Z.I. Sabry, "Nutrition and Rural Development," Food and Nutrition (FAO) 7(1):13, 1981.

DISCUSSION

SESSION II - FOOD POLICY AND AGRICULTURAL DEVELOPMENT

PETER R. GOLDSWORTHY

Goldsworthy: I am going to disappoint those of you who may be expecting Act 2 of the drama of where to put your dinars. I could not equal Nygaard's animated introduction to the last session and, therefore, I do not propose to try. In my role as Chairman, I would like to say that I am new to ICARDA. Also I am an agronomist and I have nominated another agronomist, Alister Allan, to assist me in taking notes during the discussion. Should this bias come through in my comments, the nutritionists among you will have a chance to correct that during the discussion.

I propose to recap some of the principal points that have been covered in this session as they have appeared to me.

It is clear from what has been said that malnutrition is but one manifestation of hunger, but as pointed out by Pellett in the first session, the two words are not synonymous. Also, it is clear that one of the first causes of hunger is poverty. Pellett and Scrimshaw have summarized the principal causes of malnutrition, but most of them are poverty-related. As agriculturists we are aware that poverty restricts the effective demand for food and it also restricts the production of food. This is a relationship we have been exposed to by the economists.

Nevertheless, the most direct way for production scientists to combat hunger is to increase the supply of food and decrease its cost. The assumption is that this will increase food intake and thus improve the nutrition of people. However, many examples have been given in the two papers in this session to show that nutrition is not automatically improved by such development. The speakers emphasized these points in many different ways. We have heard an analysis of the causes of failure of some principal food policies and also some examples of poor development projects.

Pinstrup-Andersen has outlined for us links between different policies and nutrition and highlighted five main factors: (i) the availability of food, (ii) the ability of the household to acquire that food, (iii) the desire on the part of the household to obtain the food that is available, (iv) its allocation within the household, and (v) the efficiency with which it is used by the individual. A deficiency in any one of these fields can result in malnutrition. Malnutrition occurs commonly alongside ample supplies of food, and therefore to alleviate malnutrition, we have to consider all of these factors. Pinstrup-Andersen gave us a clear and very interesting account of the strengths, and perhaps the limitations, of four principal common food policies. Lunven's paper analyzed the causes of failure in six case studies of development projects. The main cause of the failure was that the projects failed to reach the sectors of the population most in need of assistance.

Many of us are aware of the limitations of agricultural policies based solely on the aim to increase production. The objectives of maximum yield or outputs, which are so dear to the hearts of agronomists and breeders, obviously have their limitations. In response to a question in the first session, Nour noted the circumstances CIMMYT faced ten years ago, of the urgent need to increase the amount of food in countries like India where there were huge food deficits. At that time the response of CIMMYT was the right one. However, the message of papers in this session is that, if there is to be a nutritional benefit as a legacy of development, we need to plan for it. Both speakers emphasized that it was not their aim to discredit past development efforts, and I think we must be cautious that we do not appear to be doing so. Many of the projects in the past did not have explicit nutritional objectives. Nor do we want to conclude that, because it is often difficult to forecast the results of change, it is better not to try to induce change. That clearly is not what we want.

Examples have been given of projects that have fallen short of their goals and the reasons for this have been clearly stated. It might also be helpful to ask whether there are examples of projects that have attained their goals and what such projects can teach us.

In the past ten years, we have learned some valuable lessons. At the same time we should accept that if we are to progress, we must also be prepared to make some mistakes in the future. We need to avoid the inference that the breeder or agronomist should do less of what he is doing, but perhaps ask should he be doing it differently, and by corollary should economists, social scientists, nutritionists, and health specialists be making their own contribution in a rather different fashion? A development project calls for many people of different disciplines and it is a simplification to think in terms only of the agriculturalist and the nutritionist. We have to remember that in a less than perfect world an individual may be working in a remote situation where he is unable to consult frequently with people in other disciplines.

Another thing that has emerged from the papers and discussion so far is that the situations in the developing world are extremely diverse and there are no simple solutions. Many of the solutions need to be location-specific. They will involve a knowledge of the environment and a fairly complete understanding of life systems as a whole. That knowledge certainly extends beyond the fields of the breeder and the agronomist or perhaps any other single discipline. Pinstrup-Andersen notes that much of the evidence on nutritional effects of rural change is anecdotal, and he highlights the need for additional research on existing life systems and the whole management of rural change, including what governs the form that it takes and the rate at which it proceeds.

It was noted in the discussion in the first session that there is increasing participation by the international centres, among them ICARDA, to look more comprehensively at the problems of these life systems; their aim is to design more productive systems that are more appropriate for the environments in which they are supposed to function. More attention to cropping systems and promoting new crops within those systems, as Scrimshaw mentioned, are likely to benefit nutrition by introducing a greater variety of foods.

It is important for the farmer to help make the decisions about what is appropriate, and here I would like to pay tribute to the work done at ICARDA. I can do so without fear of appearing to claim credit for myself since I only arrived here about two months ago. At ICARDA, natural scientists are working with social scientists, looking at many of the different aspects of development, and I look forward to participating in this work.

I have discussed with Alderman the project he is working on in Egypt. He seems to be trying to avoid previous mistakes and is certainly taking nutritional issues into account. I would like to ask him if he would tell us something about that project. It is too early to say that this approach is successful, but it is addressing some of the issues we are discussing in this workshop.

Alderman: I am working with IFPRI on a two year study of the food subsidy system in Egypt, along with Von Brawn and Sakr in Egypt and Pinstrup-Andersen as the Director in Washington, D.C. We are at the halfway point of the study, so many of the things that I will say are based on tentative conclusions and may be changed at a later date. I would like to mention that the nutritional impact of the subsidy system in Egypt falls much more into the domain of food policy than of agricultural policy. A system of subsidies puts a wedge between the agricultural prices and the market prices and there is a fair amount of separation of food policy, marketing policy, and agricultural production prices.

I would like to give a brief description of the salient features of the project and then try and tie these in with a few points that have been made in the workshop. Egypt subsidizes wheat flour or bread well below the market price --about one-fourth of the world price -- and these subsidies are available without ration to the entire population. It also makes sugar, tea, oil, and rice available to anyone with a ration card, and this includes approximately 90 percent of the population. These items are also available at prices well below the market price. They are also usually available outside the ration system at a second tier of prices, higher than the ration prices, yet lower than the open market price. A monthly quota of beans and lentils is available to all individuals, but the supply is slightly less regular than for sugar, tea, oil, and rice. Meat and chicken are available mostly to the urban population.

Our study indicates that wheat flour or bread is fairly well distributed among the entire population. The benefits of this subsidy seem to show no strong urban bias and no strong regional bias when you take into account other variables. Most of the population receive their ration of sugar, tea, oil, and rice. Again, this is true in both rural areas and urban areas, except for sugar, where the rations are slightly smaller in rural areas. There is more disparity for beans and lentils, but they are still fairly well distributed among the population. Meat, including chicken, is the most inequitably distributed commodity.

This brings up a point that relates to something mentioned earlier. The amount of meat and chicken available has increased in the last few years. One of the policy arguments for this is the need for "animal protein". Meat is inequitably distributed, most is consumed in the urban areas, but it may not be distributed to all the income groups even in the cities. We are studying the reasons for this. The situation provides a warning on what may happen to a nutritional goal (here, to provide more animal protein) when it is translated into a nutrition policy or a price policy. In this instance it did not benefit those most needing help.

The widespread subsidy system in Egypt may be a major reason why, as Pellett observed in his presentation, there is apparently much less malnutrition in Egypt than would be expected in a country in its economic bracket. Food is cheaper than it is in almost any other country. This has been achieved with a very low level of food security; only 25 percent of the wheat consumed in the country is locally produced, the other 75 percent is imported. About 50 percent of the vegetable cooking oil consumed is locally produced, the rest is imported, and similar figures apply to lentils and beans, depending on the crop yields in any one year.

In the short run, Egypt seems to have maintained high food consumption with low food security. This is perhaps a caveat to the expected relationship between food self-sufficiency or food security and food consumption. It seems now to be a somewhat vague concept that, without refinement, may not be a useful guideline for nutrition policy. The food policy in Sri Lanka at the beginning of the 1970s, or in Brazil today, are two opposite cases, and they do not show a strong correlation between equitable food distribution, high standards of nutrition, and food security, at least not in the short run. The long-run issue of Egypt's food policy is perhaps more controversial.

Agriculture has stagnated during the last decade in Egypt, and the low food prices are a significant cause of this. Whether policy makers correlate low producer prices with low consumer prices is not known, but it seems likely. In Zimbabwe there are high producer prices and low consumer prices, but in Egypt the two prices are linked in the planning. The long-run implications of readily available cheap food to the poor has some impact on the agricultural sector if farm prices are also low. Furthermore, the effect on the entire economy of the approximately $2 billion a year that is spent mostly on scarce foreign exchange has long-term implications for the country's ability to pay, and the ability to substitute current consumption for investment. This is an area that needs further study.

Egypt's problem is that its system is unnecessarily expensive because there is very little targeting. The ability to target a food-subsidy system takes both a developed bureaucracy and a rather strong government that can risk alienating groups who are used to existing food subsidies. This is, of course, very dangerous. Egypt had food riots in 1977; these are recalled in all discussions of food policy today. Targeting involves political questions as well as technological and administrative questions.

Parpia: I would like to comment in some detail on the paper by Lunven, but before I do I would like to make a brief comment on the valuable paper presented by Pinstrup-Andersen. I congratulate him and I agree with a large proportion of what he said. The only point I want to raise here is that there is need for a greater emphasis on the capability of a government to formulate a food policy and on those factors that determine this capability. In my view these would be: (i) what is the political and economic strength of the government? For example, a government that has a mixed and balanced economy will have to formulate a type of policy different from that for a subsistence economy or for a country where agriculture is responsible for 50 to 90 percent of the GNP. The government must have that power to prevent the negative effects to which Pinstrup-Andersen referred. For example, a transnational corporation or a national monopoly can very easily distort the entire policy. The moment people have more money someone will succeed in selling them toothpaste and junk food. (ii) What is the ability of a government to manage and administer the structure of food policy? How would it be implemented? What is the information system for decision-making? It is not infrequent to find decisions made on very inadequate information and as a result failures occur. (iii) What is the scientific and technological capability of the government? India would not have been able to implement the policy of the green revolution without scientific and technological competence. Therefore, food policy has a direct relationship with the scientific and technological policy of the government. Also, the credibility of the scientific community and the degree to which it is involved in the corridors of power and decision-making is important, because if scientists are not involved in decision-making they may keep on talking as most of us are doing here without any decision being made or implemented.

To go to Lunven's paper, I am grateful for the presentation of case study number 5. First of all, the case studies seem to raise problems but offer no alternative solutions. I think this can have a rather demoralizing, negative effect. A second point is that there is only one vague reference to a paper by himself and Sabry and no documentation for that reference.

In case 5, the study to which he is referring was a large cooperative in Asia. This programme was evaluated during its initial period by Prof. Mogens Jul of Denmark, and I think it is one of the best studies I have come across in which positive and negative aspects were carefully analyzed in order to have a positive effect on the development of the project. The second evaluation was carried out by a team of 12 in which each of the team members represented a single advanced country, so they were looking at the project not only from a very different point of view, but one diametrically opposed to the viewpoint of the members in the cooperative and the national government.

I wish to analyze this briefly. The objective of the dairy project was not simply milk production, because it was realized that poor people cannot afford to buy milk. (It is absurd to think so when an animal needs 6-7 kgs of feed in order to produce 1 kg of dry material) Thus, it is necessary to discern what impact the project had on social and economic development, and I should like to point out some of the benefits that were not listed in Lunven's paper.

The project resulted in doubling the income of the entire district, and today it accounts for over 40 percent of the income for these people. It has generated employment in many peripheral areas and has encouraged greater investment in agricultural inputs and related fields as a result of the dairy industry. The district constructed the so-called "milk roads" for milk collection and distribbution and this provided quite a large amount of employment. Clinics, maternity homes, and schools have also been built. The organization works closely with research institutions to develop weaning foods and, in fact, foods that save the country $50 million of foreign exchange. It has contributed to building capabilities in science and technology and today it runs the Institute of Rural Management. It has stimulated creation of cooperatives for oil seed processing and rice milling, and even for earning money through the manufacture of chocolate and confectionary goods.

Jul, in his evaluation, pointed out how the income generated from milk production is providing food for low-income people, which has contributed to better nutrition. Obviously, as pointed out by Pinstrup-Andersen, all the income generated is not spent for additional food, but this district today has become the leading one for manufacture of machinery and equipment -- a new type of capability that is leading to a new form of industrial revolution in the district.

Therefore, if one were to say that the poor still do not get the milk, I would call this "nutritionist determinism" rather than objectivity. Instead, we should look to those factors that, in the longrun, will raise the standard of living and eliminate poverty. This is the reason why the United Nations University's new programme is entitled "Food, Nutrition, and Poverty".

My idea in this intervention is to show the interdisciplinary approach used in this project. This represents, in my view, one of the best integrated production, conservation, processing, and distribution systems and it has generated much employment. I think it might turn out to be a scheme from which we can learn quite a lot. In case, by any chance, Lunven has referrred to another scheme and not to this one, may I suggest that he include this as a case study of positive accomplishment rather than of negative criticism.

DRY AREA AGRICULTURE AND NUTRITION

Lunven:[1/] I am grateful to Parpia for having taken as a positive example of successful agricultural projects a dairy project that is under operation in Asia. I am well aware of this project; I have carefully studied the evaluation reports prepared by Jul. I find myself perfectly in agreement with Parpia's view about the efficiency of this project and, in addition, I fully agree with him on the exaggerated prestige of milk, especially when discussing adults' diets.

I am therefore not biased by any "nutritionist determinism" in looking a little more closely at the consequences of this project for the people living in the project area. Although I would not be satisfied myself with broad statements based on aggregate data, it is probably correct to say that income and employment increased in the project area, that the impulse given by the dairy scheme to social and economic development has had positive consequences for people (probably the best off) and trade. Therefore, the project can be considered successful with regard to its stated objectives, and agricultural planners, food technologists, and economists have good reasons to be proud of these achievements.

The point I have been trying to make, however, regarding the importance of nutritional impact assessment, carried out by the method that FAO has developed recently, is illustrated by Parpia's own statement. He says a poor man cannot afford to buy milk. In terms of a meaningful food and nutrition policy I would argue that milk should be accessible also to the poor among whom, it is well known, the highest PEM rate is found, especially in children. Parpia goes further in saying that it would be "...absurd (that a poor man can afford to drink milk) when animals need 6-7 kg of feed to produce 1 kg of dry material". I would simply ask, at this stage, why it is not absurd to say the same for the rich man as well? Because he can afford to pay? I would not question this if it is clearly stated and the consequences of such an approach for the poor are frankly admitted. After all, development cannot start from nil, and in the dairy project the minimum asset requested from the participants is one cow. Those who have no cow are excluded from the benefits. It happens that in the project area this amounted to 60 percent of the total rural population. If it cannot be denied that some direct or indirect benefits accrued to them from the dairy project, I personally think -- because it is my job to look after the poor man's nutrition and welfare -- that a close association of modern nutrition planners with the project planning team would have permitted them to take informed decisions with regard to all groups of people (beneficiaries and non-beneficiaries) instead of hoping the best from a problematic "trickle-down" effect of the project.

However, nutrition should not become an obsession in development planning and the main FAO objective is to attack under-nourishment and malnutrition in developing countries through its combined support of expanding food-crop production on small farms and in improving food distribution.

The only point I wanted to make in illustrating some of the negative effects of rural development projects aimed at the small farmer was that improving nutrition is not just a matter of increased production, employment and income, but also of better distribution and access to food. To do this, special knowledge and methods are required that, I hope, we have contributed by improving them and making them acceptable to development planners.

1/ As Lunven was not present at the workshop these written comments were submitted subsequently.

Goldsworthy: I think Parpia has illustrated one of the things I was looking for. It also reinforces the point that Scrimshaw mentioned in the first session on how the increase in variation or diversity within the farming system can itself bring benefits.

Parpia: But agriculture would not develop without a system.

Scrimshaw: We should not fall into the trap of condemning programmes simply because they do not reach the poorest of the poor or do not benefit the poorest segment of the population. This may be so difficult as to be impossible to achieve immediately in a given situation. But we should not withhold benefits to other needy people simply because we cannnot reach the poorest ones.

Incaparina represents a product that has been repeatedly criticized because it does not solve the problem of severe protein-calorie malnutrition in Guatemala or Central America. As a processed food, even though much less expensive than milk, it is still too expensive for those who do not have a cash income and do not have the money. This was recognized when it was developed. There was a large segment of the population asking for help for malnourished children, and at the time all one could say was to give them milk. Yet, it was recognized that they could only afford a teaspoonful of milk in a glass of water, which would have made matters even worse. Or one could recommend feeding eggs. But one egg cost as much as enough rice to feed the whole family. In Guatemala and also in Costa Rica, when Incaparina was made available (and now other substitutes are available) this did and still does represent a product many poor people can buy, and the project did benefit some people in low-income groups.

Incaparina is also criticized because it benefits the middle class and even the upper class, and this is true, too. But it is not a subsidized product and to the extent that it is used by people in the middle class and increases market volume and helps maintain a minimum price, it is also good for the poor. We hear over and over again that Incaparina does not reach the poorest of the poor, and only middle and upper income people consume it, which I think, on analysis, is unjustified. This kind of thinking seems to have been involved in some of the case studies presented by Lunven.

Myntti: I would like to reiterate some of Pinstrup-Andersen's points. When talking about how policies affect populations and the nutritional status of these populations, we tend to oversimplify and exaggerate the differences between rural and urban areas. In terms of production and consumption, "the rural" is becoming more like "the urban" every day. In many parts of the Middle East we can no longer talk of agricultural production as being the major source of rural incomes, for most rural households have incredibly diversified sources of income. Thus, if we are concerned with policies affecting rural incomes, we must not simply concentrate on those affecting crop production, but also those affecting meat and dairy production, or even urban wages and international migration.

The differences between the levels and styles of consumption in urban and rural areas are also lessening. In many parts of the rural Middle East, for example, imported foods of little nutritional value are more readily available than local produce. Surely this affects the nutritional status of rural populations. Certainly government policies on food imports and the pricing of local agricultural goods affect what villagers eat.

Miladi: I would like to comment first on Lunven's paper. Actually, as Parpia said, the paper discussed the projects that have failed and then gave us methodology on how nutrition can be involved in development projects. Let us take the case of Cyprus, which is one country in the region. Six or seven years ago, Cyprus lost about 40 percent of its agricultural land, 80 percent of it to tourist hotels, and about 50 percent of it to schools. I went there to give them assistance in nutrition, but I could not find any nutritional problem in the country. Infant mortality is the lowest in the Middle East -- 17 per thousand compared to a country like Saudi Arabia with 50 per thousand, and I did not see children with low weight for height. In addition, I did not see any nutritionists. Therefore, it seems that Cyprus did not need a nutrition project to solve its nutrition problems. Were there nutrition problems in the first place? Good nutrition requires participation and the political involvement of people in decisions about social and economic factors that are important, and it shows how people can cooperate in hard times to make things work. I think the case of Cyprus is a very good illustration of the involvement of people in improving the whole social and economic environment along with improved nutrition.

I would like to tie food policy with another factor. Years ago in the Sudan, people were unacquainted with wheat. Wheat was introduced to Sudan through food aid, and as a result the largest food import in the country today is wheat. Food aid can change the consumption patterns of a population. Previously, the Sudanese lived on sorghum and millet, and now they have become wheat consumers even though the country cannot produce wheat economically. Food aid can thus contribute to changing consumer patterns in the long-term, with possible detrimental effects. This should also be taken into consideration.

A further aspect of food policy is improving the rural infrastructure. Roads per se can contribute much in terms of stimulating production and making food more accessible. In Somalia, the people were able to create some kind of stability in the prices of sorghum and millet by the creation of cooperative storage places. Food policy is made by governments, and I cannot see how women's time allocation is related to policy. Is this a government decision?

My final comment is on Egypt and the question of subsidies. Actually, it is a good example of subsidies going directly to nutrition. The rural population in Egypt 30 to 40 years ago was consuming corn, and pellagra was predominant in this region. The subsidy of wheat enabled the peasants to mix corn with wheat, an improvement that helped eradicate pellagra.

Naturally, one has to be careful with these subsidies. Egypt is currently importing five million tons of wheat that costs $1 billion a year. One cannot say this will improve nutrition because bread quality is poor, and much bread is fed to animals, not to people.

Goldsworthy: I would ask Pinstrup-Andersen if he would like to respond to those comments and also whether he wants to refer back to an earlier question on policy that was posed by Parpia. I did not give him a chance to respond to that.

Pinstrup-Andersen: I have no disagreement with Parpia's suggestion that generating a nation's capacity to deal with food policy and planning is extremely important. I split it up into two parts -- the institutional capacity and the analytical capacity -- but nevertheless, I think we are saying basically the same thing.

On the comment of Myntti, I completely agree with her on research priorities. I think the focus should be at the household level in order to understand better household behaviour in food consumption as well as production. In a recent document that IFPRI prepared for the UN Sub-Committee on Nutrition, that was precisely what we said. It is not the only research priority, but it is certainly one of the most important ones. We are interested in household food acquisition behaviour and related questions.

Regarding food aid, I completely agree that this is an extremely important problem in a number of countries. It has a number of negative and presumably also positive sides. We are currently collaborating with the Ministry of Planning in the Sudan, as part of a PL 480 study with the United States, to look at the extent to which one could promote the expansion of sorghum consumption as a replacement for wheat. We do not have any results from this work, but it is similar to recent efforts in a number of countries to introduce composite flours. The objective of this research is to withdraw from dependence on imported wheat in countries that cannot produce it. This is an extremely important issue.

There was a question on the role of women in inter-household distribution of income and the demand for their time. How is that related to policy? I think it is very closely related and it has been grossly ignored in the past. To give an example: When we promote rural development projects, we must take into account what effect it will have on the demand for women's time, because if we do not we ignore the impact this will have on nurturing behaviour in the home, including cooking, child care, breast-feeding, and so forth. I cannot tell you that it is <u>always</u> important, but in a number of cases it has been very important, and we know virtually nothing about it.

The same is true for food transfers versus income transfers of cash or food stamps. We have a number of studies available now. Half of them argue that a food transfer is more effective nutritionally than an income transfer. The other half argue that there is no difference. One way of trying to explain these apparent inconsistencies may well be to look at who, within the household, controls the food transfers or cash incomes, or food stamp transfers.

<u>Williams:</u> I would like to ask Pinstrup-Andersen if the study in Egypt considered wastage, specifically the impact of subsidies on wastage? I understand there is some evidence that there is more wastage of cereals because of the subsidy than there would have been otherwise. Is that true?

<u>Pinstrup-Andersen:</u> As far as I know we do not have any evidence one way or the other. We are going to try to look at the extent to which wheat is being fed to livestock, but I do not believe we have any answers to that question as yet. Alderman may want to add something about this.

<u>Alderman:</u> We are in the process of doing a household survey in the rural areas, and we hope to do a second visit in a few months. In the first visit, one of the questions we asked was "Do you buy bread or do you use your wheat flour for animal feed?" Virtually nobody admitted to feeding the wheat to animals. Thus, we are rephrasing this question for the second visit to ask what portion of the bread is fed to animals. The difference is that the type of bread used in Egypt, which is the same type of bread you see in the market in Syria, cannot really be stored. It is not like a loaf of bread in the U.S. or Europe, and a fair amount of leftover bread is fed to chickens. This is fairly certain, but not something we have been able to confirm. You certainly see bread being fed to animals, but you cannot tell whether it is purchased for that reason. I am certain that no one feeds flour to animals, since there are cheaper sources than that.

<u>Williams:</u> I believe bread is very cheap -- one piaster a piece.

Miladi: Actually, the subsidy is not for the household, it is through the baker who profits by selling it to the people.

Williams: Of course, this would be limited mainly to cities anyway; village areas do not make or eat that type of bread.

Alderman: They usually make their own bread with subsidized flour rather than buying it baked.

Nygaard: Let me address the issue of household micro-level data collection and highlight the difficulty of getting food data from certain types of questions. Two issues come to mind. One is a question of nutritional data and the other is a question of women and household allocation of women's time. The Farming Systems Programme in ICARDA is starting to become confident enough to ask a farmer how much phosphate he puts on his barley field. We have less confidence in our ability to find out what the yield is from his lentil crop, and it is very difficult to find out what he does with those lentils. Yet these are easy questions compared to those about how much wheat a family consumes in a day or a week and who consumes it. A study that I am aware of on this issue is being done by Rafiq Hamdan in Jordan. He is having much trouble with how to approach these questions on utilization of production. Ali has done a questionnaire on faba bean consumption in Sudan, but he is not satisfied with the answers he has received on utilization. In Syria, in the lower rainfall areas where poorer families live, women play a larger role in family labour, but if you try to find out where income goes you run into some major problems with data collection. Does any one have any ideas on how to get answers to these more difficult questions?

Somel: I have two comments. The first one aims at eliminating some of the delusions that may have been created by Pinstrup-Andersen's classification of policy types. This classification does not mean that these policies can exist individually. Usually, we find mixtures of them. The most standard set, as indicated by Alderman, consists of existing agricultural or food production support policies and consumer-oriented food price subsidy policies. In fact, support policies invariably involve input subsidies, which compounds the whole issue of determining the effects of these policies. The effective protection rates, as calculated by various researchers for the developing countries, are really quite high. This indicates that input subsidies are sometimes more important than the subsidies for the final commodities. They also usually cover such things as meat and sugar. In other words, these policies are not discriminative enough to target subsidies toward those who need the food or have nutritional problems. In the final analysis, subsidies can only go so far and somebody has to pay for them. Invariably, in developing countries subsidies are financed through inflationary measures, and hence costs are regressively reflected back on the poor more than on the rich.

My second comment requires a preamble. I am amazed at the atmosphere of agreement that exists in this workshop, even among economists. Pinstrup-Andersen commented on the justification for consumer-oriented food policy subsidy policies. One justification is claimed to be that low food prices imply low wages. Nowhere have I seen an empirical substantiation of this claim, and I think it is a myth. Causality in the opposite direction, i.e., low wages that barely cover food requirements is based on totally different factors. Man does not live by food alone, he has to purchase transistor radios and TV sets, and I do not see why we should discriminate against the peoples of the developing countries when we find such expenditures to be totally justifiable for people in the developed countries. The theory shows that a family at the micro-level allocates its expenditures to maximize the satisfaction it gets from these expenditures. If politically minded governments and policy makers wish to alter these expenditures in such a way as to achieve nutritional benefits, then policies should be adjusted to promote these ends. I do not think that subsidizing food prices is the solution, let alone the only solution.

Pinstrup-Andersen: I have to follow up the challenge since now I know two economists who disagree. Except I am not sure we do disagree, because I never suggested that low food prices were the solution to all evils. What I said was that there is a clear link between government efforts to keep food prices low and government efforts to keep wages low. I think that link is very well established. It is particularly clear in countries where the public sector employs a large proportion of the labour force. For example, this has been brought home to me on several occasions in discussions with high-level officials in the Egyptian government. Whether this is scientifically proven or not, it is very obvious that it is in the minds of the decision-makers in the Egyptian government. If food prices are permitted to increase, then eventually there will be a need to increase wages in the public sector. How that is reflected in the private sector depends on the labour market and I am not prepared to go deeply into it here, although I am sure there is a linkage. I am not saying that this should be promoted. I am totally open on the question because I think it depends on the country, the set of circumstances, and the time. The cost of food subsidies is often reported as being so high as to justify eliminating food price subsidies. It is not nearly as expensive as it looks if we take into account that there is, in fact, a wage subsidy embodied in food prices.

Gerhart: I would just like to say a word about the point Pinstrup-Andersen made. We tend to focus on food subsidies and the costs of carrying them, and this is particularly true in Egypt. Yet the same governments often have enormous subsidies for other goods, particularly energy subsidies. In Egypt, the energy subsidy is greater in terms of total cost to the government than the food subsidies and this has a much more regressive impact on income distribution. It is also much more damaging in terms of long-run competitiveness, because energy is an input for all manufacturing and production enterprises. These become increasingly noncompetitive as this factor is increasingly subsidized. In some respects, Egypt can take pride in its food subsidy and relatively low levels of malnutrition compared to its low per capita income. Of course, Egypt can improve its food subsidy programme by reducing the target costs and increasing efficiency. But before one would encourage the Egyptians to give up these food subsidies, one would certainly want to look at the extent and cost of energy subsidies in that country. I think this is true in many Middle Eastern countries as well.

Khattab: As a general comment on Pinstrup-Andersen's paper, I would like to congratulate him on his clarification of such a diverse and complicated issue. I fully agree with him that when we are launching rural development programmes we should not be content to remove the constraints to better nutrition, but rather emphasize the need to develop programmes that will enhance good nutrition. These are very important points because in most cases economists and planners tend to believe that if you increase the income of people, this automatically means better nutrition, although this point has been much debated and it is very difficult to convince them otherwise.

Pellett: I have a comment relevant to the last point and I am glad it was raised. I would like to summarize briefly the results of a survey we did a few years ago in Libya, as it demonstrates this very point that increased wealth does not necessarily mean better nutrition. A study was performed in the paediatric hospital, Tripoli, Libya, where the familial backgrounds of 50 marasmic infants were compared with those of a group of 50 essentially healthy infants of similar age. Families with marasmic infants had more children but lived in smaller homes than the comparison families. Total income, however, was similar in both sets of families, and major consumer items such as TV sets, cars and refrigerators were widely present in both groups. Families with marasmic infants, however, had less literate mothers who tended to breast-feed for shorter periods and to feed purchased pureed baby foods more frequently. The causation of marasmus in these circumstances was probably unhygienic infant feeding despite the availability of clean water and modern kitchen facilities. All three factors, i.e., adequate housing, adequate income, and an adequately educated mother, appear to be necessary simultaneously before infantile marasmus can be prevented. Certainly there are special circumstances in Libya but I think we still so often look at changes and do studies by the traditional 19th century scientific approach, i.e., vary or look at one factor at a time. In the real world for nutritional improvement to occur, several changes may have to be made at the same time before any real result can be seen.

Goldsworthy: It seems to me we are giving the food policy part of the discussion fairly good airing. The second subject was on the nutritional consequences of agricultural and rural development, and I would like to begin to exercise my bias as a chairman and an agriculturalist and ask a question in this area. The examples of rural agricultural development given here have usually involved the introduction of a new component into the system, whether it was a cash crop or some fairly radical revision of the traditional cropping systems. I would like to draw some comment from economists and nutritionists on some of the less dramatic changes that the biological scientist is trying to introduce when he is working only with crops. Often the biological scientist is faced with a situation in which he is looking at the capacity for increasing the productivity of traditional crops. Usually there is a technical margin that is comparatively easy to achieve and yields can be increased, but in rural areas communications and markets or access to markets are limited.

For example, in Central America or many parts of Africa with which I am familiar, agriculture is based on a cereal crop, and legumes are a staple part of the diet. The yields of many of the legume crops are extremely low, maybe two or three hundred kilos per hectare, and the possibility of doubling those yields is well within the technical capabilities of most production programmes. the agriculturalist often does not know the inelasticity of the market for that crop in these villages. In many situations the farmer is not going to take advantage of the opportunities that are available to him because there is little incentive to produce more than his family's immediate needs. It seems to me that these are important parts of the interface between agriculture and nutrition, and they may govern how the agriculturalist should respond to some of the circumstances in which he finds himself. We have not heard much about this in this session and I invite comments.

Nygaard: I would like to pick-up on the subject raised by Goldsworthy and play the devil's advocate by asking a question. We have several plant breeders and soil scientists and at least one agronomist in the room. We have talked about agricultural policy, agricultural projects, and nutrition. Is there anything that you have learned today that would encourage you to go out tomorrow and do your job differently, or are we whistling in the wind, as it were?

Williams: I will answer your question with a "no". I have not heard anything today that would change anything that I am likely to do. I think you will probably find the soil scientist in exactly the same category. Nutrition is really not my job per se -- I am a chemist. A soil scientist is a soil scientist. Certainly we are conscious of nutrition; there is no question about that at all. You have developed a number of aspects that deal with nutrition, but with all due respect to the speakers, I did not need to come today to learn how to do my job. I think you will find that the lack of response to your question is because of this basic reason.

Scrimshaw: In one sense this indicates that the ICARDA agriculturalists are far ahead of those in most of the other international agricultural centres and in the national institutes, because if you visit other centres you find them talking about yield of cereals while they often have a total disinterest in legumes. Some of them lack interest in farming systems and crop rotations. This is beginning to change, but it is very refreshing to come here and find a balanced emphasis that includes legumes. That is point one.

We need not discuss my second point now, because we will get into it when we discuss goals for plant breeders. However, it should have come out of the discussion in the first session that there certainly should be attention paid to the protein content of the staple crops. This is necessary to ensure that protein nutritional status does not deteriorate. Therefore even a marginal improvement in the protein content could be of some use. This is by no means as important as maintaining the role of legumes as a protein complement of predominantly cereal diets.

Finally, I would like to mention that it would be unfortunate if the renewed emphasis on protein were interpreted as meaning that more animal protein is required. There is no requirement for animal protein. There is only a requirement for protein. From a policy point of view, the incorporation of animal protein in the diet may be desirable for both nutritional and economic reasons, but it is not required.

Goldsworthy: In your account in the first session, Scrimshaw, of how the assessment of protein needs or requirements in diets has changed, Gerhart questioned you about the impact of those changes on the policies of governments and particularly on institutes like ICARDA. In the early seventies, I was working at CIMMYT in the maize programme in which there was a very large effort for production of high-lysine maize. (Many people said yield was being sacrificed). There were in addition many technical difficulties in trying to pursue that line of research. It came under attack because of the revaluation favouring the need for more calories in the diet as opposed to more protein. That answers Gerhart's question, I believe. These sorts of things can change the assessment of research priorities and did have an impact on the maize breeding objectives.

I subsequently worked at another international institute, IITA in Nigeria, where I was involved with legume crops. This was also during a period when the question of the priority given to the protein content of the diet was open to debate. These tropical legumes are low-yielding, and due to budget constraints at the center we were asked about possible returns from such research. Did food legumes really warrant the effort? There was a period when all of these research projects were at risk of being dropped. Fortunately they were not. I think it would have been disastrous had this occured, because legumes are vital parts of the diet in many parts of the world and their productivity can be improved.

The Technical Advisory Committee to the International Agricultural Research Centers has been deliberating on the issue of plant breeder rights. How are results of breeding tabulated, and how can we encourage the further development of plant breeding material? Ten years ago, there was almost no work on many of these basic legume crops, and work on them began long after work on cereals. In this discussion on plant breeders rights one of the things that emerged quite clearly was that the collection of cultivars of various legume crops has been carried out, and now plant breeders working in the developing world have access to much greater genetic diversity than they otherwise would have had, and they are using the collection much more actively. I hope this is something that will be amplified in the discussion on legumes in Session IV.

Bressani: I think that the international centres during the last five or ten years have become very much interested in nutritional standards for food crops. For example, CIMMYT still continues with work on improving the performance of high lysine corn; CIAT is involved in the acceptability characteristics of beans; ICRISAT is interested in improving the protein digestibility of sorghum; and IRRI is doing a beautiful job in improving the cooking qualities of rice. The biggest problem we find in one area of the world, Latin America, is that the national breeders and the national agronomists are not close to this research, and they are still not giving nutrition much emphasis.

Cooper: To go back to Nygaard's question -- do we feel, as a result of these discussions, that any of us should do our jobs differently? I think that is a rather important challenge because as he said, if not, what are the discussions for? I think this meeting could very well have focused on the interfaces between agriculture and social science. Had it been, many case histories and many examples could have been quoted in which agricultural projects failed because researchers did not take into account the social or economic context of the environment in which the projects were introduced. In this session, we are talking about nutrition and I think the question Nygaard should have asked was: "As a result of the discussion does ICARDA feel that it is paying enough attention to nutrition aspects?" We certainly realize that without a social science aspect or without an economics aspect to temper or guide our agricultural research, we will go up the wrong street more often than not. Now let us rephrase the question: Should we have a greater input or greater guidance from nutritionists?

Goldsworthy: Let us see if Pinstrup-Andersen has an answer.

Pinstrup-Andersen: No, I do not have the answer to the question that Cooper posed, but I would like to emphasize the need to look at the nutrition effects of agricultural research in a much broader perspective. I have worked for a number of years on technological change and related economic analysis, and it has become obvious to me that we are asking much too much of agricultural research and technological change. We frequently sit back and say that, irrespective of quasi-government policies in all other aspects, agricultural researchers should produce a technology that will solve not only production problems and consumption problems, but also income distribution and a number of other problems as well. It must be extremely frustrating for a plant breeder to be faced with this kind of challenge that he has no way of meeting. What we should talk about is what agricultural research and technology can do, and what do we ask governments to do to supplement or to complement technological change? If governments are determined to have confused policies, which is what we are talking about today, there is very little we can do through agricultural research except expand food production.

Parpia: We have been talking of nutrition and Pinstrup-Andersen correctly raised the question of making the discussion broadly based. We have talked of lysine and methionine and we have talked of increasing protein content. I do not think this is adequate and we have to go beyond that. There is a serious effect of insect infestation on protein quality in the case of wheat that has reduced the PER in four weeks from 1.8 to 1.4. Are we going to have insect-resistant varieties in the future?

Second, there is the question of the husk to grain ratio. Take the case of grain legumes. In Egypt and the Indian subcontinent legumes are consumed after dehusking and splitting, and this is a very difficult, time- and energy-consuming process. Is it possible to produce, instead of the 10 to 15 percent husk, a crop with 5 percent husk/grain ratio? Is it possible that the pericarp and testa can be separated from the endosperm more easily? Is it possible that crops could be more resistant to toxins that pose threats to health and nutrition in the developing countries? Already some thought is being given to eliminating the toxicity of the lathyrus pea, but I do not think enough attention is given to all the other aspects.

At a Joint Symposium on Grain Legumes, ICRISAT scientists were surprised to find that grain/legume milling and processing present so many problems. For example, if you dehusk legumes, it cuts down the processing time from three hours to one. These are factors that must enter future agricultural research priorities and should interact with post-harvest/processing and conservation to make a valuable contribution to nutrition.

Karrar: Pinstrup-Andersen has raised two interesting points about food subsidies. Actually, food subsidies in the Sudan have created problems for the nutrition of the population. Two food items that are subsidized are wheat flour and sugar, without any consideration of nutritional needs or whether the people affected have low protein or low calorie diets. As a result, sugar consumption is much too high. We did a survey in a suburban area near Khartoum and found that the average intake of sugar was about 200 gms/day/person, which can lead to dental caries. Nobody knows the basis for beginning these subsidies, but it appears to have been a haphazard sort of thing.

Consider the wheat subsidy. We are a sorghum-producing country and now, because wheat flour is subsidized, many people have given up eating sorghum. Thus, the government is obliged to import more wheat. When the Sudan tried to withdraw the sugar subsidy, it triggered a political crisis -- one that is still going on. I think we need to orient policy-makers such as agricultural economists and other economists to nutritional issues. They should have an idea about what type of nutrients are available in the country, which ones people need and why, and then they would be able to provide useful advice on what sector or commodity should be subsidized and what the effects would be.

Hayani: Although this conference is taking place in Aleppo, we have not said much so far about Syria. We have talked about food subsidy policies in Egypt and other countries, and I would like to say that in Syria the government is undertaking a very comprehensive food subsidy programme. There are two aspects to this that I would like to raise. The subsidy programme encourages waste, especially the waste of bread. In addition, this subsidy, as Somel mentioned, is not without cost, the brunt of which is really borne by the rural sector. Lentils, wheat, and cereals are bought by the government at fixed prices -- prices that sometimes do not even cover the producers' costs -- and thus the rural sector is subsidizing urban consumers.

A second comment concerns the impact of trade policy on nutrition. The impact of milk formulas for infant feeding in place of breast-feeding is making the nutrition situation for babies worse than before because these milk formulas are not used properly. Milk is improperly prepared or stored and when used, of course, it creates problems for the children. The rate of infant mortality is actually increasing rather than decreasing.

Scrimshaw: You have just heard the negative influence of the trend away from breast-feeding associated with the economic and social changes and the introduction of commercial formulas. This is occurring in all of the countries of the area. You would be interested in some figures that came from a UNICEF study in Bahrain. In 1977, the proportion of mothers breast-feeding children three months of age was down to approximately 9 percent, and the infant and preschool mortality was up in the range of 70 to 80 per thousand. A programme was introduced that barred the use of uniformed company nurses from the hospitals, barred the direct advertising of formulas to the mothers, and included an intensive educational campaign to promote breast-feeding. By 1981, the proportion of infants breast-fed was up to nearly 50 percent and, more important, there had been a surprisingly large decrease in infant mortality. It had gone down to about 30 per thousand. Policy trends can work both ways, and they can work much more rapidly than we had hitherto believed.

Ali: From what I have heard so far about the nutrition situation in most of the countries within the region, it has been concluded that neither food availability nor income will improve nutrition. Also, there seems to be a complete lack of nutrition education. Therefore, my suggestion is to start with a comprehensive nutritional education programme that would benefit the whole region.

Pinstrup-Andersen: I would certainly not like to see this session closed on the note that all that is needed is nutritional education. I have not said at any point that improved food availability does not have nutrition impact - obviously it does. Neither have I said that increased incomes for the poorest will not result in improved nutrition -- it will. I think the point I was trying to make was that expanding food supply by itself, if it does not have a price effect, may have very limited nutritional effect, if any. A second point was that not all additional income available to malnourished people will be spent on improving their diets.

SECTION III

FOOD PRODUCTION AND NUTRITION IN THE MIDDLE EAST

PERSPECTIVES FOR FOOD PRODUCTION - THE MIDDLE EAST AND NORTH AFRICA

MOHAMED A. NOUR AND DAVID F. NYGAARD

INTRODUCTION

Many of the chronic problems limiting agricultural production in developing economies throughout the world are also prevalent in the Middle East. But there are also differences -- differences between recent trends of agricultural development in the Middle East and other regions. The common problems are familiar to most of us and listing them here would have little value (1). Therefore, this paper concentrates on these differences: specifically, the special characteristics and problems of Middle Eastern agriculture are pointed out and the problems associated with these characteristics are described. Thus, new solutions to new problems are required and several strategies are considered.

The development of this paper is based on three assumptions with respect to the current status of agriculture in the region, and these should be stated at the outset. First, there is great potential to increase agricultural productivity and consequently, agricultural production in all countries in the region. Second, while recognizing that there has been agricultural growth in the region in the past 20 years, the current and expected future demand requires substantially higher rates of growth. Third, there is wide recognition of both of these factors by responsible leaders of the countries in the region and an apparent willingness on their part to take the necessary steps to realize the agricultural potential and meet the urgent requirements for food. Yet little has been done in the face of the pending crisis.

Certainly, ICARDA's research thrust is based on the assumptions in this chapter. We feel that the region needs, and is ready to accept, new and creative approaches to solving agricultural development problems. Thus, we are undertaking a sincere effort to find solutions and are optimistic that the results of efforts by ICARDA and many other organizations that are active in the region will make a significant contribution towards increasing agricultural production and improving the livelihoods of the rural families. In doing so, we must keep in mind that production of more food at lower prices will benefit consumers in general, perhaps more than producers.

Several questions need to be addressed. What are these differences? Where is this potential? What are the problems or constraints, and what are the priorities for alleviating them? The subsequent discussion is organized in four sections. First, some of the major trends in the region's agriculture, population, and food trade are reviewed. Examples of the indications of physical production potentials are given in the second section. The third examines the stumbling blocks in the way of realizing these potentials, while the final section focuses on priorities for dealing with these constraints.

DRY AREA AGRICULTURE AND NUTRITION

FOOD PRODUCTION AND TRADE PERSPECTIVE[1/]

Changes in total and per capita food production in the region are shown in world perspective in Table 1. The 67 percent increase in total food production in the Middle East over the past two decades may seem spectacular, but it has barely kept pace with an equally spectacular population expansion, resulting in less growth in per capita production than in the developed countries. While population growth may largely cancel the benefits of increased food production, and is the root of other development problems, the focus of this paper remains on production.

Grain production in the Middle East region over the past two decades has grown at an annual rate of 2.5 percent, lagging behind the world (2.7 percent) and the average of developing countries (3.0 percent). The region's slower growth in grain production compared to developing countries, as shown in Table 2 (2), is due to its smaller expansion of grain production area and a slower growth in yields. Particularly in the past decade, the region's improvement in grain yields has lagged far behind that of all developing countries, 1.2 and 2.5 percent, respectively.

The situation for meat production in the region, as shown by Table 3, is more favourable, the rate of growth having kept pace with that of other developing countries, at 3.9 percent, and surpassing that of the developed countries, which averaged 2.6 percent. This reflects the strong economic incentives for meat production in the Middle East. Meat prices have increased rapidly due to growing demand. Table 3 shows that Tunisia, Syria, Saudi Arabia, and Turkey had growth rates in meat production well in excess of other countries in the region.

Figure 1 shows that the developed countries exported food greater in net value than food imports over the last decade. In contrast, in the developing countries, the opposite was true. This implies the existence of a comparative advantage for food production in the developed countries relative to the developing countries. The deficit balance of food trade in the developing countries is even more pronounced for the Middle East, where the value of food imports has far exceeded that for food exports.

Figure 2 allows comparison of five countries in the region with respect to the trends in the nominal values of their food imports and exports. Because the values shown in Figure 1 and 2 are based on nominal prices, the effects of price inflation and quantity increases are lumped together as value increases. Nevertheless, valid comparisons can be drawn.

Syria and Tunisia have similar trends in gradually rising expenditures for food imports and low levels of food export. In both countries high domestic demand has taken large shares of domestic food production. Saudi Arabia, with its tremendous oil revenue, has shown an astronomical rise in food import expenditures. Food exports from this country are insignificant. Since 1973, Egypt has also greatly increased food imports while showing only slight increases in earnings from food exports. Perhaps a large part of these increasing trends are due to price inflation and not quantity increases.

1/ We wish to thank Thomas Nordblom who made a major contribution to this section and to Ahmed Mazid who helped assemble the tables and graphs.

Turkey is a large net exporter of food and stands in marked contrast to the other countries in the region. With the exception of 1974 and 1975, Turkey has had food export revenues far above those spent on imports.

The trends in imports and exports of animals and animal products for five selected countries are shown in Table 4. With the exception of Turkey, a net exporter of these products, most countries in the region have shown tendencies to import more and export less. The case of Syria provides a remarkable example. In the period 1968-1970, 44 percent of the value of Syria's food exports were animals and animal products. By the 1976-78 period this share had fallen to only 6.5 percent.

The differences in food production, consumption, and trade between the major classes within countries, between regions and between countries, illustrate the concept of comparative advantage. There are natural, physical infrastructure, and institutional reasons why comparative advantages exist. The natural aspects of comparative advantage include climate, soil, crop varieties, weeds, pests, and diseases. In addition to these natural aspects, there are the man-made infrastructures such as roads, ports, and grain storage and milling facilities. The presence or absence of these facilities may profoundly affect production costs and costs of food delivery and processing.

The ways in which the natural and man-made resources are exploited are heavily influenced by the existing institutions, i.e., the political and traditional framework of land tenure, agricultural credit, taxation and subsidization, market structure, and trade barriers. It is clear that these institutional aspects affect the costs of farm operations and, therefore, affect farmers' choices of crops and production practices. Given the natural resources available in a country, human institutions are developed to construct and manage them.

A partial picture of the natural and infrastructural contexts of agricultural production in the region is shown by the abundance of cultivated land and its division into irrigated and rainfed areas. Table 5 (3) shows that fully 80 percent of the cultivated land area in the Arab-speaking countries supports rainfed agriculture, although this varies from as much as 92 percent in Morocco and 90 percent in Syria to as little as 2 percent in Egypt. However, irrigated agriculture produces over 60 percent of the food in these countries and one can ill afford to neglect this; any future development plans must fully consider ways to help the region increase agricultural productivity on both rainfed and irrigated areas.

ICARDA's main thrust up to now has been to develop new technology that will give greater advantage to agricultural production in the region. The clearest examples of these are (i) the development of new plant varieties capable of high and stable yields, (ii) the discovery of efficient means to control diseases, pests, and weeds, and (iii) the determination of agronomic practices that are most efficient under local conditions.

"Local conditions" is the key phrase that encompasses all costs and constraints from the farmer's viewpoint: conditions that will change from one location to another. Farmers will adopt new methods, practices, and materials if, from their perspective, it is in their advantage to do so.

PRODUCTION POTENTIAL

There are many research efforts in the region that show dramatically the technical possibilities for potential productivity increases. To give just a few examples, however, one needs only to consider some of ICARDA's findings. This is a young centre, just entering its fifth year, and perhaps the most important achievement to date has been to demonstrate technical feasibility of achieving significantly higher yields under rainfed farming systems.

ICARDA's research activities are divided into four programmes, each of which can point to examples where large yield increases have been achieved. The Food Legumes Improvement Programme has developed chickpea cultivars that have shown resistance to ascochyta blight. This allows chickpeas to be planted two to three months earlier in Mediterranean climatic environments and thus make better use of limited available moisture. In the 1980/81 season, trials on farmers' fields showed dramatic differences (doubling of yields) between new cultivars planted in November/December and old cultivars planted in March.

In the Cereal Improvement Programme, the barley project is currently screening over 6,500 lines and has several hundred barley lines in preliminary and advanced yield trials. In the 1980/81 season, fifteen lines grown at ICARDA experimental stations in Syria and Lebanon in preliminary yield trials yielded six tons/ha or more. This should be compared to average yields on farmers' fields in a similar rainfall zone in Aleppo province of only 1.3 tons/ha. Not all of this increase is attributable to a variety effect, but it illustrates the gap that exists.

The Farming Systems Programme has research plots at five different locations along a rainfall transect in Aleppo province, and agronomic work on barley has also shown that a large potential to increase yields exists. Table 6 (4) suggests that increases are possible in all the rainfall zones but are highest in the drier zones 2, 3 and 4. It should be noted that the yield achieved in zone 4 is over 250 percent of that found on farmers' fields. This potential is even more encouraging because these drier zones contain some of the poorest families in rural areas of Syria.

The Pasture and Forage Improvement Programme is exploring the possibility for replacing the fallow crop in the prevalent cereal/fallow rotation with a forage crop. Preliminary results show that forages such as *Pisum*, *Vicia* and *Lathyrus* have yield potentials exceeding four tons, particularly when phosphorus fertilizer is applied. Because of the economic value of forage, such a change in rotation would more than compensate for a detrimental effect on the subsequent cereal crop. It is interesting to note that four tons of conserved forage is enough for six months of winter maintenance feed for 20 sheep.

Of course, these successes only indicate *technical* feasibility, some of which may not be economically feasible. This is a point that will be addressed in detail later, but indications are promising for these technical achievements to be economically attractive as well. Economic analyses of the response of barley to phosphorus application have been conducted by the Farming Systems Programme. For example, Table 7 shows that the costs of an application of P_2O_5 at 60 kg/ha were compensated for by more than 250 percent.

In spite of findings of this nature, agricultural production in the region has not grown as quickly as it could nor as it should. The next section explores some of the reasons for lagging productivity increases.

CONSTRAINTS TO AGRICULTURAL DEVELOPMENT

While the previous section drew solely on ICARDA's efforts, there are numerous examples from national research programmes and international organizations operating in the region that could have been used as well. In any case, the point that emerges should be clear: there are other constraints to increasing agricultural productivity in the region in addition to the technical ones. We need to look at the economic, social, and political institutions and the physical infrastructure to find the stumbling blocks. The major problem appears to be our inability to reproduce the research achievements, such as those mentioned in the last section, on farmers' fields.

Again, it is not necessary to restate the long list of constraints to the diffusion of new technology. These lists are readily available in the literature on development (5,6). Instead, only five issues are discussed, ones especially important to the Middle East.

Risk and uncertainty. The first of these refers to production variability in the rainfed areas of the region caused by extensive climatic variation. Consider, for example, barley production in dry villages in Aleppo province. Barley producers in the village were visited by ICARDA scientists on a regular basis for three growing seasons -- 1977/78 to 1979/80. By chance, the three years were very different from each other. The first year, 1977/78 was an average rainfall year (240mm); the second, 1978/79, was very dry (150mm); and the third 1979/80, well above average (270mm). Barley yields varied widely over these three years, as can be seen in Figure 3. The difference from year to year and also the differences among farmers in a given year should be noted. The inter-farmer difference is particularly striking in the best growing season, 1979/80. Only those barley plots that were harvested are shown in the figure. In the driest year, 27 of the 36 (75 percent) plots that were studied were grazed by sheep flocks and not harvested at all. In the average year, about 10 percent of the plots were grazed, while no plots were grazed in the wet year.

Farmers' responses to production instability are well documented (7). Most importantly, they reduce the amounts of costly inputs used in the production process. Furthermore, if they perceive that new techniques increase output instability more than current practices, they will adopt them less quickly or perhaps not at all. Research by ICARDA scientists in Jordan and Tunisia as well as in Syria (8, 9) shows that farmers consider production uncertainty to be one of their major problems. Even under irrigated conditions, e.g., faba bean production, yield instability would lead farmers to use fewer inputs than are economically profitable (10).

Farmers respond to risky production alternatives in several ways. One is to seek stable off-farm income, and this is very widely practiced in the Middle Eastern region. The classic response to uncertainty by producers averse to taking risks is to diversify activities by growing several crops. In zone three in Aleppo province, for example, wheat is the major source of income in a good year, but is less important in an average year when income from lentil by-products plays a larger role.

A more important form of diversification comes from adding animal production to the farming enterprise. This is virtually a universal practice in this region, and our lack of understanding of the interface between cropping and livestock systems is the second constraint that will be addressed.

Livestock-cropping interface. The conventional wisdom is that animals play a stabilizing role in the risky agricultural systems that are characteristic of the Middle East. They are a source of relatively liquid capital, they complement the inter- and intra-annual variations in cropping income, and they make it possible to extract some productivity out of uncultivated village common lands. Some form of this crop-livestock system is found in all the rainfed areas of the Middle Eastern region. Even in irrigated systems animals play an

DRA-I

important role, as is demonstrated by the amount of precious irrigated land allocated to the production of berseem clover in Egypt (11), where roughly half of the farmland is devoted to this crop in the winter months.

An example of a barley-sheep system in the dry zone in Syria nicely illustrates the interdependence of these two components. Currently research conducted by the Farming Systems Programme at ICARDA indicates that a farmer makes a series of decisions during the course of the barley-growing season. Each decision is made considering all currently available information, but acknowledging that future events are uncertain. Thus, each decision is made in a way so as to keep as many options as possible open, i.e., delay decisions until more information is available.

For instance, in November, the farmer must decide on, _inter alia_, land allocation, land preparation, planting date, variety, and phosphorus and nitrogen fertilizer use. He is likely to use little or no nitrogen fertilizer at planting, instead waiting until February to decide if there is a sufficient amount of accumulated rainfall to merit a nitrogen application and if so, how much. Some decisions are irreversible but some are not, and become part of a risk-reducing strategy. He may choose a variety that will have a good grain yield in a good season but one that will also have a reasonably good production of dry matter in a dry year. It should be recalled that, instead of harvesting, 75 percent of the farmers in a previous example mentioned earlier let their animals graze their barley. This grazing decision was due, in part, to a low potential grain yield that year, but also to the high grazing value of the crop.

Animals play other roles in Middle Eastern agriculture as well. They are a source of liquid capital, and in some cultures animal ownership may have social importance. Large numbers of animals in the region (300 million in 1980), huge areas of unimproved grazing land (natural grazing land is estimated to be twice the number of hectares of cropped land), and growing regional consumption of meat and animal products attest to the importance of animal production in its own right. This important sector has not received its fair share of research funds to date, and thus ICARDA intends to increase its efforts in animal production in the future.

Moisture use and management. In addition to irregular rainfall, much of the region receives precious little rain, even in a favourable year. We do not understand sufficiently well how best to use the little water that is available. This lack of understanding of this crucial topic is a major constraint to attainment of the region's production potential.

ICARDA research has shown significant increases in water-use efficiency by applying phosphorus and nitrogen fertilizers to barley production or by advancing the date of planting chickpeas (12). This is not surprising. On the other hand, as can be seen in Figure 4 (13), little or no moisture is stored on fallow plots according to farmers' current practices, which goes against conventional wisdom. Thus, perhaps a forage crop could be effectively introduced into this barley/fallow rotation, or perhaps the fallow could be managed more efficiently. There is considerable scope for improving the use of the moisture that is available, and new techniques must be developed.

Irrigated agriculture, which was the foundation stone of early Middle Eastern civilization and is still very important in the ICARDA region, is also plagued by problems. New lands that can be brought into agricultural production are becoming more scarce, so increases in total production will need to come from increased productivity per hectare. Increasing the cropping intensity is one way to achieve this if irrigation water is available. Yet there are large differences in how effectively this irrigated land is used. Compare, for example, the cropping intensity difference between Egypt and the Sudan. In Egypt, on average, each hectare of irrigated land has 2.85 crops per year, while irrigated land in Sudan has less than one crop per year (14).

To be sure, there are problems associated with these irrigated systems and they are falling far short of their potential. In many countries in the region land quality has deteriorated because of rising water tables, waterlogging of the soil surface, salt and sodium accumulation, etc. However, certainly one of the main problems is management and control of water delivery systems. In research being conducted by ICARDA in collaboration with the Agricultural Research Corporation in Sudan, 95 percent of the farmers in a survey of faba bean producers reported problems with the water delivery system, and yields were reduced as a result. As is the case with rainfed agriculture, it is a question of how to use water more efficiently. The region would benefit substantially from more research in this area.

<u>Equilibrium and adjustment</u>. No part of the developing world is more subject to change than the ICARDA region. Changes, both rapid and radical, are taking place all around us. Very few geographical locations in the Middle East come to mind where traditional agriculture is not affected by this. New machinery, different prices of both outputs and inputs, infrasturcture developments, etc. all affect agricultural production. It is helpful to think of agriculture as tending toward an equilibrium with numerous changes that disrupt the balance. Thus, continuous adjustments are required by the producer. Obviously, the more changes there are, the more complex the adjustment process is.

Consider two examples of these radical changes:

1. In the Syrian steppe, motorized transport has enabled Bedouin families to transport water to the sheep rather than vice versa, and consequently, the practice of sheep production in the steppe has been dramatically affected. Stocking rates have increased to the point that the steppe is rapidly deteriorating in the process (15).

2. In Turkey, mechanized land preparation that conserved soil moisture and allowed farmers to plant earlier enabled wheat production in the country to double in the space of a few years. Subsequently, energy prices were drastically increased and this has now put new pressure on high energy-using inputs. Thus, Turkish farmers have had to learn new techniques and also adjust to relative price changes within a short period of time.

These changes and the adjustments they require have created an even stronger need for an effective network of agricultural extension services than in the past. What is extension other than teaching farmers new methods, i.e., helping them adjust and move to a new equilibrium? Extension services are, in general, inadequate in the Middle East, yet this is an important phase of any development project if high adoption rates of new technology are to be achieved.

<u>Distribution effects of development</u>. An issue that goes hand in hand with the previous section on change is the question of who gains and who loses in the process. The benefits are often not shared equally. A final constraint to improving the lives of rural families in the region is the failure to develop projects that help improve the lot of poor families and reduce income inequalities. This is perhaps the point that brings us closest to the interest of our colleagues in human nutrition and food science.

Many studies of the Green Revolution (see also Somel article) have shown a net gain to regions or countries where the new rice and wheat varieties have been adopted. Ryan (16) argues that, while new wheat replaced pulses in India, per capita consumption of protein was no worse than before while per capita consumption of calories increased. These, however, are average figures and ignore the distribution effects. Brady (17) shows that there has been significant social gain for the new rice varieties in East Asia. This is illustrated in Table 8. However, these gains go to the consumer, while the producers lose as a result of producing more. Production gains that keep prices down allow the results of the new technology to go to consumers, most of whom live in the cities. One result of this is a degradation of the human condition and nutrition in rural areas.

Most technologies are "biased". Mechanized harvesting, for example, generally favours farmers with better landholdings, not the smaller holder with shallow, stony soil. Mechanization in general in the Middle East has replaced male labour, while the tasks done by females, e.g., weeding the fields and winnowing the grain, are still done by hand. Development projects, seeking high benefit/cost ratios, are drawn to favoured areas with higher production potential. As pointed out in Table 6, the relative potential for improvement may now be higher in disadvantaged areas, such as the drier marginal lands. Production priorities do not always coincide with objectives that consider human needs and meet human nutritional requirements.

This list of five constraints for improving the situation for agriculture and rural families in our region is by no means conclusive, but it is hoped that interesting and important issues that are special to the Middle East have been raised. Some suggestions for action on these points follow below.

SUMMARY AND CONCLUSION

Although the Middle East has made recent gains in increasing agricultural production, these are overshadowed by several other changes in the region. Some of these changes are prevalent in all developing countries across the world, but others are especially relevant to the Middle East. Two crucial changes that have caused an increase in the demand for food are the extraordinarily high rates of population growth and rapid increases in income in several countries in the region. This latter factor has manifested itself in an explosive demand for meat and other animal products.

Thus, food consumption for most of the people in the region has not improved in spite of considerable production gains. Fortunately, research at ICARDA and other organizations has shown the existence of large potentials for further increases in agricultural productivity, even in the lower rainfall areas. However, a number of constraints must be alleviated before this potential can be achieved.

Five such contraints, discussed in this paper, are particularly important to this region. They are:

1. Risky and uncertain production.
2. Lack of understanding of the complex interrelated cropping-livestock systems prevalent in the region.
3. Poor use of scarce moisture.
4. Radically changing economic environments that create agricultural problems in decision-making, and poorly developed or non-existent agricultural extension systems.

5. The inability to improve the income-distribution effects of introducing new technologies.

All of these constraints call for more research effort on our part. In considering possible solutions for each of these constraints, we can see that the task is not easy, but neither is it impossible.

1. Production is risky because the climate is variable. Solutions require agricultural techniques that are less sensitive to the vagaries of the weather as well as production diversification and other strategies to stabilize incomes.

2. Current livestock research suffers from the same problems that exist in current crop research, i.e., too much of it is done in isolation from other production activities. The strength of the rainfed agriculture in this region lies in the way the various components complement each other, but more research is needed on these interrelationships.

3. Moisture is a scarce resource in the region and using it efficiently requires a better understanding of soil/plant moisture dynamics; also, more work is required on moisture storage and conservation.

4. Due to the dynamic nature of Middle Eastern economies it is likely that agriculture producers will be faced with even greater adjustment problems in the future. Therefore, efforts are needed to seek ways to assist the farmer's decision-making process as he adjusts to new situations and conditions. For example, the effort to develop a methodology of on-farm testing that involves the farmers in the research process promises to be most useful.

5. Finally, we must improve the distributional impact of improved technologies. It is possible that efforts to find new technologies that are widely adaptable are destined to benefit those persons who are already relatively well-off. Thus, in order to help the poor farm families, it may take much more location-specific efforts. The need to improve agricultural productivity in shallow sloping soil is just one such example.

The impression we wish to impart is that we have much work to do. All of the suggestions made above require funds and scientific effort, perhaps with more and closer collaboration among the many disciplines that are represented. However, the outlook is positive and optimistic, as we have made great strides recently in more clearly identifying the problems. Now, the challenge is to find the solutions.

DRY AREA AGRICULTURE AND NUTRITION

1. T.W. Schultz, Transforming Traditional Agriculture (Yale University Press, New Haven, Connecticut, 1964).

2. U.S. Department of Agriculture, World Indices of Agricultural and Food Production (USDA Economic Research Service Statistical Bulletin No. 669, Washington, D.C., July 1981). Cited by T.N. Barr, "The World Food Situation and Global Grain Prospects," Science 214:1091 (1981).

3. A. Arrar, "The Role of Rainfed Agriculture in the Near East Region," in Proceedings of the FAO Regional Seminar on Rain-fed Agriculture in the Near East and North Africa, Amman, Jordan, 5-10 May 1979 (FAO, Rome, 1980).

4. D. Nygaard and A. Allan, "A Farming Systems Approach to Agricultural Research," paper presented at the Research Conference on Crop Production in Lebanon, December 1981.

5. H. Zandstra, K. Swanberg, C. Zulberti, and B. Nestel, Caqueza: Living Rural Development (International Development Research Centre, Ottawa, Canada, 1979).

6. T.W. Schultz, ed., Distortions to Agricultural Incentives (Indiana University Press, Bloomington, Indiana, 1978).

7. H. R. Anderson, J.L. Dillon, and J.B. Hardaker, Agricultural Decision Analysis (The Iowa State University Press, Ames, Iowa, 1977).

8. T. Roe and D. Nygaard, "Wheat Allocative Error and Risk: Northern Syria," Bulletin V, Economic Development Center, University of Minnesota, Minneapolis, Minnesota, 1980).

9. S. Arabiat, D. Nygaard, and K. Somel, "Issues for Improving Wheat Production in Jordan. Results of a Survey," Research Report, ICARDA, 1982.

10. G. Hawtin and C. Webb, eds., Faba Bean Improvement (Martinus Nijhoff, The Hague, 1982).

11. N.T. Habashy and J.B. Fitch, "Egypt's Agricultural Cropping Pattern," Micro-Economic Study of the Egyptian Farm System Project Research Paper No. 4, Ministry of Agriculture and Arab Republic of Egypt, Cairo, 1981.

12. ICARDA, In-House Review Documents, Aleppo, Syria, 1981.

13. P.J.M. Cooper, "Moisture Storage Under Summer Fallow in Syria as Affected by Winter Rainfall and Management," in press.

14. FAO, Near East Statistical Directory, Cairo, Egypt, 1975.

15. F. Bahady, "Recent Changes in Bedouin Systems of Livestock Production in the Syrian Steppe," in J.G. Galaty, D. Aronson, P.C. Salzman, and A. Chouinard, eds., The Future of Pastoral People (International Development Research Centre, Ottawa, Canada, 1981).

16. J.G. Ryan, "Human Nutritional Needs and Crop Breeding Objectives in the Semi-Arid Tropics," IJAE 32:3 (1977).

17. N.C. Brady, "Food and Research Needs of the World," in J.T. Manassah and E.J. Briskey, eds., Advances in Food Producing Systems for Arid and Semi-Arid Lands (Academic Press, New York, 1981).

TABLE 1. Changes in Total and Per Capita Food Production and in Population*

	1961-1963 to 1978-1980		Annual Rate of Increase (%)	
	% Total Increase	Annual Rate	1961-1963 to 1968-1970	1968-1970 to 1978-1980
FOOD PRODUCTION				
World	54	2.6	2.7	2.4
Developed countries	48	2.3	2.7	2.0
Developing countries	62	2.8	2.7	3.0
Middle East	67	3.0	2.9	3.1
POPULATION				
World	38	1.9	1.7	2.0
Developed countries	16	0.9	0.9	0.9
Developing countries	53	2.5	2.5	2.4
Middle East	58	2.7	2.7	2.7
PER CAPITA FOOD PRODUCTION				
World	12	0.6	0.7	0.6
Developed countries	27	1.4	1.7	1.2
Developing countries	9	0.5	0.2	0.7
Middle East	6	0.3	0.2	0.4

*Source: FAO Production Yearbooks, FAO, Rome, 1963, 1971, 1975, 1980.

TABLE 2. Growth in Grain Production* (Compound Annual Growth Rate, %)

	Production			Area			Yields		
	1961/62 to 1979/80	1961/62 to 1971/72	1971/72 to 1979/80	1961/62 to 1979/80	1961/62 to 1971/72	1971/72 to 1979/80	1961/62 to 1979/80	1961/62 to 1971/72	1971/72 to 1979/80
World	2.7	3.3	2.4	0.5	0.4	0.7	2.2	2.9	1.7
Developed countries	2.5	3.3	1.8	0.2	-0.2	0.8	2.3	3.5	1.0
Developing countries	3.0	3.3	3.2	0.8	0.9	0.6	2.3	2.3	2.5
Middle East	2.5	2.8	2.7	0.5	0.2	0.9	2.0	2.7	1.2

Source: Reference 2

TABLE 3. Growth in Total Meat Production (Thousand Metric Tons)

	Average 1969-71 *	Average 1978-80 *	% Total Increase	% Annual Compound to Growth Rate
World	105,865	138,630	30.9	3.0
Developed countries	70,806	89,281	26.1	2.6
Developing countries	35,059	49,349	40.8	3.9
Middle East	2,375	3,338	40.5	3.9
- Tunisia	55	88	60.0	5.4
- Syria	70	127	81.4	6.8
- Saudi Arabia	51	100	96.1	7.8
- Turkey	422	605	43.4	4.1
- Yemen A.R.	53	67	26.4	2.6
- Morocco	201	231	14.9	1.6
- Egypt	386	429	11.1	1.2

*Source: FAO Production Yearbook, 1980 (FAO, Rome)

TABLE 4. Export and Import Value of Live Animals, Meat, and Meat Preparations, Dairy Products and Eggs in Selected Countries*

	Average 1968-70			Average 1972-74			Average 1976-78		
	Import	Export	Difference	Import	Export	Difference	Import	Export	Difference
Value in US $ (000)									
Saudi Arabia	NA	NA	NA	97,654	706	-96,948	427,913	954	-426,959
Syria	10,773	25,286	+14,513	34,118	10,459	-23,659	62,644	3,334	-59,310
Tunisia	8,426	4,325	-4,101	21,834	1,772	-20,062	39,113	3,457	-35,656
Turkey	3,485	15,353	+11,868	6,506	42,772	+36,266	3,146	42,324	+39,178
Egypt	7,645	829	-6,816	23,034	2,253	-20,781	166,638	8,349	-158,289
Percentage of Food Trade									
Saudi Arabia	NA	NA		26.7	8.7		31.9	6.9	
Syria	15.7	44.0		18.3	23.5		19.9	6.5	
Tunisia	15.6	18.2		19.0	4.9		17.8	6.3	
Turkey	8.3	7.8		4.6	10.4		7.2	5.9	
Egypt	5.3	0.5		5.3	1.3		14.3	3.2	

*Source: FAO Trade Yearbooks (FAO, Rome, 1971, 1974, 1979)

TABLE 5. Present Land Use in the Countries of The Near East and North Africa*

Country	Cultivated Area Including Fallow Land			
	Total	Rainfed	Irrigated	% of Rainfed to Total
Algeria	7,000	6,750	250	96.4
Bahrain	2		2	0.0
Egypt	2,650	10	2,640	0.03
Iraq	5,920	3,000	2,920	50.7
Jordan	529	490	39	92.6
Kuwait	1		1	0.0
Lebanon	276	196	80	71.0
Libya	2,520	2,395	125	95.0
Morocco	7,040	6,590	450	93.6
Mauritania	263	260	3	98.9
Oman	36	4	32	11.1
PDRY	252	162	90	64.3
Qatar	2		2	0.0
Saudi Arabia	897	720	177	80.3
Somalia	960	800	160	83.3
Sudan	7,800	6,240	1,560	80.0
Syria	5,470	4,960	510	90.7
Tunisia	3,500	3,360	140	96.0
UAE	20	16	4	80.0
YAR	1,200	1,100	100	91.7
Subtotal	40,338	37,053	9,825	80.0
Afghanistan	4,900	1,816	3,084	37.1
Cyprus	433	389	44	89.8
Iran	16,000	5,550	10,450	34.7
Pakistan	19,200	5,700	13,500	29.7
Subtotal	40,533	13,455	27,078	33.2
GRAND TOTAL	86,871	50,508	36,363	58.1

*Source: Reference 3

TABLE 6. Barley Yields in Kilograms, Syria, 1980-1981

Rainfall Zone*	Yields on Farmers' Fields	Yields on Trials ICARDA	Potential Increase %
1	3,150	4,100	30
2	1,211	3,610	198
3	1,106	2,400	117
4	674	1,710	254

*Note:

Zone 1 - average rainfall between 350 mm and 600 mm

Zone 2 - average rainfall between 250 mm and 350 and not less than 250 mm in two-thirds of the years

Zone 3 - average rainfall over 250 mm and not less than this in half the years surveyed

Zone 4 - average rainfall between 200 mm and 250 mm and not less than 200 mm during half the years surveyed

Source: Reference 4

TABLE 7. Partial Budget for Phosphorus Fertilizer Application to Barley in Zone 3, Per Hectare (Rainfall 292 mm in 1980-1981 Cropping Season)

	No Phosphorus	60 Kg Phosphorus
Income (Syrian Lira)		
Grain yield (metric ton)	1.470	2.400
Grain revenue	882.	1,440.
Straw yield (metric ton)	2.340	5.340
Straw revenue	468.	1,068.
Total revenue	1,350.	2,508.
Expenses (Syrian Lira)		
Fertilizer		
Phosphorus	-	130
Labor for application	-	10
Credit	-	13
Harvesting		
Labor, equipment, transport, bag, etc.		173
Total change in expense	0	326
Net benefit	1,350	2,182
Benefit-cost ratio		2.55

Notes: Cost of phosphorus: 2.17 SL per kg
Price of barley grain: 0.60 SL per kg
Price of barley straw: 0.20 SL per kg
Labor for broadcasting: 10.00 SL per 120 kg of Triple

Both trials received 60 kg of N, at a seed rate of 90 kg with Beecher barley

Source: Reference 4

TABLE 8. Estimates on Annual Benefits of Rice Research

Period	Producers' Gain	Consumer Gain in Millions of Dollars	Social Gain
1961-1971	-345	702	357
1972-1975	-290	590	300

Source: Reference 17

Figure 1. FOOD* IMPORT AND EXPORT VALUE INDICES, 1964 to 1979

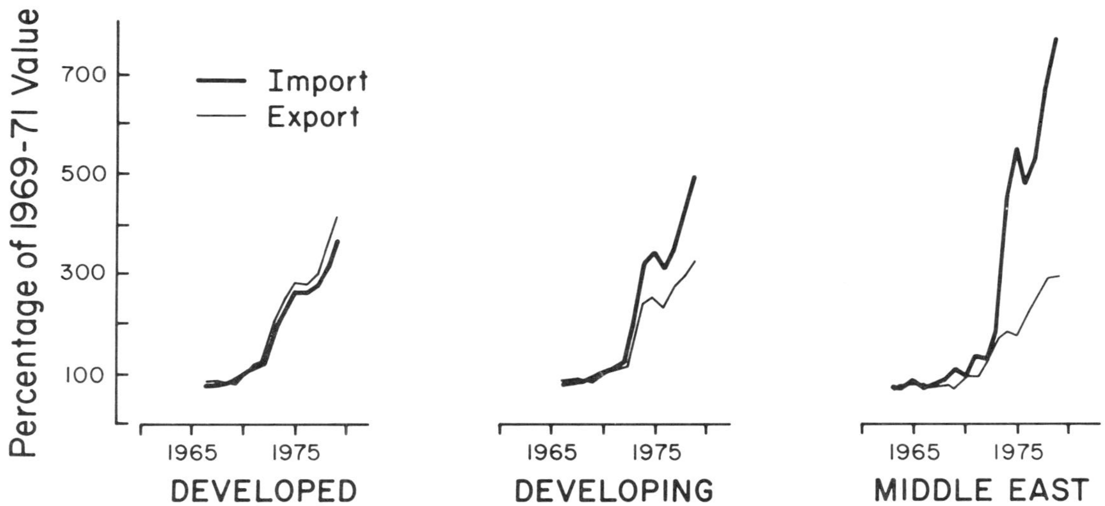

*Excluding fish

Source: FAO Trade Yearbooks, 1971, 1974, 1979. FAO, Rome.

Figure 2. FOOD AND ANIMAL IMPORT AND EXPORT VALUES IN SELECTED MIDDLE EAST COUNTRIES

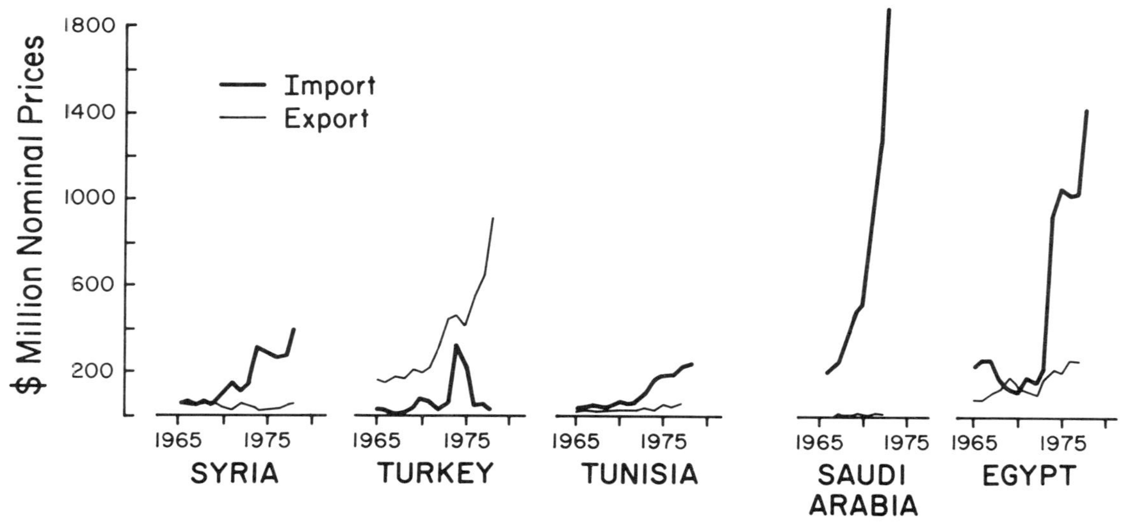

Source: FAO *Trade Yearbooks*, 1971, 1974, 1979. FAO, Rome

Figure 3. BARLEY YIELD DISTRIBUTIONS AT HAWAZ VILLAGE, SYRIA

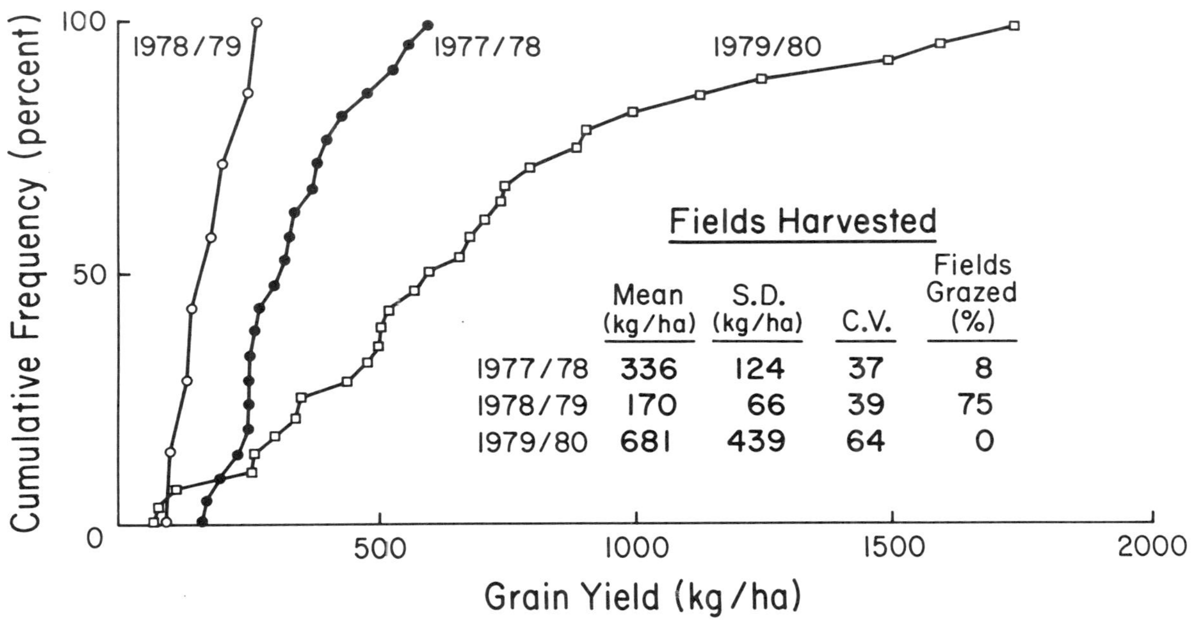

S.D. = Standard Deviation
C.V. = Coefficient of Variation

DRA-J

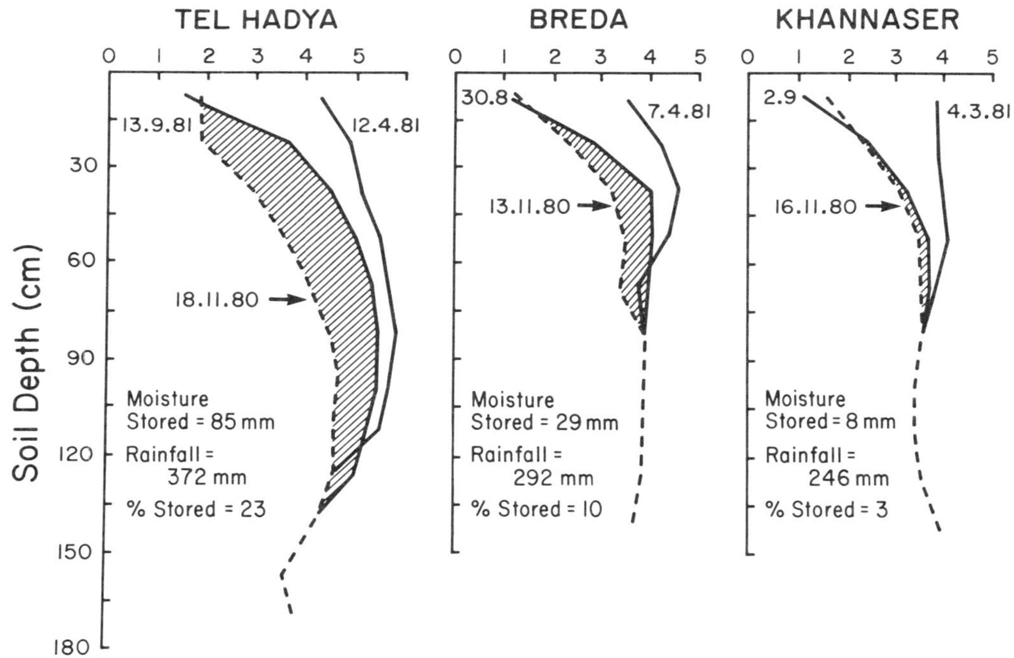

Figure 4. MOISTURE LOSS UNDER FALLOW DURING SUMMER MONTHS, 1981

Source: Cooper, Peter, J.M. Moisture Storage under Summer Fallow in Syria as Affected by Winter Rainfall and Management. Forthcoming.

FOOD AND NUTRITION IN THE MIDDLE EAST AND NORTH AFRICA

SAMIR MILADI AND PETER L. PELLETT

INTRODUCTION

The Middle East and the North African Region, as defined in this paper, consist of the Arabic-speaking countries in addition to Afghanistan, Cyprus, Iran, and Pakistan. In order to discuss the food and nutrition situation in the Middle East, it is necessary to consider a diverse population of 300 million from more than 24 countries. These range from some of the richest countries in the world to some of the poorest. Dietary patterns and nutritional problems not only vary from country to country and among socio-economic classes within a country, but also among members of a family. It is thus obvious that, while considerable generalizations are necessary, they may also be inaccurate.

The countries of the Region have some common historical, cultural, and environmental characteristics that reflect some similarities in their nutritional problems. However, variations do exist from one country to another, particularly in terms of resources, degree of development, availability of trained manpower, agricultural potential, and the population distribution. These variations are reflected in the food and nutrition situation in the individual countries of the Region and affect the priorities and active programs in each of these countries. A series of reports and reviews (1-18) have assessed the food and nutrition situation in the Region and further information has been extracted from major recent publications of FAO (19-21) and WHO (22).

The Region has certain special characteristics. Only six percent of the total land area is under cultivation, the rest being mostly arid or semi-arid. The rainfed and dryland agriculture represents 60 percent of the total agricultural land, and erratic rainfall frequently contributes to the instability of food production. Certain areas of the Region are also affected, from time to time, by severe droughts such as in Mauritania and Somalia. Therefore, rainfall affects food production, food availability and farm income and, to a certain degree, the national development plans of these countries. In the irrigated area, which constitutes a small part of the total land under crops, inefficient water control and inadequate water management, combined with poor drainage, have led to a progressive loss of cultivated land through increasing salinity and water-logging.

Livestock production, which contributes 30 to 40 percent of the agricultural GNP in a number of countries (Somalia, Sudan), has not improved significantly, since a high proportion of livestock continues to be raised under nomadic conditions. Overgrazing has led to a reduction in productivity of pastures. In addition, with the expansion in cereal cultivation, livestock has been pushed into still poorer pasturelands, and the off-take rates have been low. The productivity per head of stock for mutton/goat meat, for which the Region has a preference, has varied form 10 to 16 kg per annum.

Some countries of the Region have fragmented holdings that limit the possibility of introducing new technology (seed/fertilizer) for increasing food production.

Also there is a loss of a substantial proportion of food during the growth, harvest, and post-harvest periods. The marketing of the main crops, such as wheat, olive oil, cotton, maize, and sugar is mainly controlled by governments. The prices offered to the farmers are often much lower than those on the international market, so incentive to produce is low. In several countries of the Region, agriculture has not received its due priority in development plans, and accordingly, investments in this sector are still inadequate.

For the Region as a whole, 56 percent of the total population is involved in agriculture. In certain countries, such as Somalia and the Sudan, where the economy depends on agriculture, the number may be as high as 80 percent. In others, such as the Gulf countries -- with the exception of Oman -- the percentage of the population engaged in agriculture is very small. Generally, during the last two decades, the percentage of the rural population and the labor force in agriculture has been decreasing. Also, the rural exodus and emigration among countries of the Region continue to rise, leading in some cases to the abandonment of agriculture and the neglect of ongoing agricultural projects. It should also be noted that because of the male migration to the oil-rich countries, more women are engaged in agricultural production than before.

In several countries of the Region, the long-expected results of irrigation and reclamation projects are unfortunately not yet evident, even though ample potential for agricultural development exists. It is anticipated that each country will review its own agricultural development strategy. In such strategies, project implementation should be pursued on a continuing basis to ensure that the desired results are obtained.

THE REGION

To facilitate future discussion of the food and nutrition situation in the Region, the countries therein may be divided into three groups according to population, food and nutrition problems, and economic situation:

Group I: Oil-producing countries,
Group II: Oil-producing and agricultural countries,
Group III: Agricultural countries.

The relationship between wealth and infant mortality rates for the countries in these three groups is shown in Table 1.

Group I: Oil-producing countries. In the oil-producing countries the basic incomes are derived from oil, which represents the main export. These countries are Bahrain, Kuwait, Libya, Oman, Qatar, Saudi Arabia, and the United Arab Emirates. Some of the common characteristics are:

-- Cultivated land is very small compared to total area.

-- The majority of the countries are located in areas with scanty, unreliable rainfall, a very limited water supply, and hot weather throughout the year. Therefore, agricultural production is impeded by the scarcity of arable land and shortage of water and does not provide enough food to meet demand.

-- The countries are generally net importers of cereals, sugar, vegetable oil, meat, dairy products, and poultry.

-- Infant mortality is very high. It varies from 150 per 1000 live births in Saudi Arabia to 39 in Kuwait. Elsewhere in the Region, it is about 100 per 1000 live births.

-- Protein-energy malnutrition among preschool children is also widespread. This is apparently not because of the lack of food, but rather poor environmental sanitation and mothers' ignorance of nutrition principles.

-- Anemia is prevalent among preschool children, schoolchildren, and mothers.

-- Other nutritional deficiency diseases, such as hypovitaminosis A and rickets are becoming less common.

-- Obesity and coronary heart diseases are increasing among the adult population.

-- There is a notable lack of manpower (trained food specialists and nutritionists) and adequate institutions in the field of food and nutrition.

Group II: Oil-producing and agricultural countries. Algeria, Iran, and Iraq are important producers of oil and they also have a high agricultural potential. Some of their common characteristics are:

-- Generally large in size and population.

-- Annual population growth is very high, averaging 3.2 percent (among the largest in the Region).

-- The proportion of the population living in rural areas is very high and ranges from 55 percent in Iran to 37 percent in Iraq. Those engaged in agriculture represent more than 40 percent of the total labor force.

-- Cultivated land covers a large area and there is potential for expansion, especially in Iraq and Algeria.

-- Except in Iraq, most of the agricultural land is rainfed.

-- Agricultural production represents an average of 15 percent of the GNP. The share of agriculture in total investment is about 11 percent in Iran (no figures are available for Iraq, where large investments have recently been made in agriculture).

-- Annual average (1960-1975) growth rate is 18.7 percent in Iran and 15.8 percent in Iraq.

-- The countries import from 40 to 50 percent of their food, especially cereals, vegetable oil, sugar, meat, and dairy products.

-- Infant mortality is very high: 142 per 1000 in Algeria, 112 per 1000 in Iran, and 104 per 1000 in Iraq.

-- Protein-energy malnutrition is widespread, especially in rural areas where people have low incomes in addition to poor environmental sanitation. Illiteracy still exists and health delivery systems are inadequate.

-- Anemia is prevalent among vulnerable groups, including rural populations.

-- Trained manpower in nutrition exists, even if not very effectively used, especially in Iran and Iraq, which have national food and nutrition institutes.

Group III: Agricultural countries. This group should be divided into three sub-groups:

Sub-group A. This comprises Egypt, Syria, and Tunisia, which are basically agricultural countries, but are self-sufficient in oil and, to a limited extent, even oil exporters. Some of the common characteristics of this sub-group are:

-- They have not been adversely affected by increases in the price of oil; in fact, Egypt and Tunisia have benefited from increased export earnings from oil.

-- Egypt and Syria are exporters of a cash crop (cotton) and importers of foodstuffs.

-- The major crops produced in these countries (cereals, sugar cane, olive oil, cotton, rice) are usually sold to the governments at a fixed price.

-- In all three countries more than half of the population lives in rural areas and those engaged in agriculture comprise nearly half the total labor force.

-- Cultivated land in Egypt is only five percent of the total land area and is mainly irrigated, while in Syria and Tunisia most of the agricultural land is rainfed. This explains the fluctuation in agricultural production of these latter two countries from year to year.

-- The share of agriculture in total GNP ranges from 30 percent for Egypt to 22 percent for Syria, and 19 percent for Tunisia.

-- The population growth rate is relatively low in Tunisia (2.6) and Egypt (2.8), but extremely high in Syria (3.5).

-- Both Egypt and Tunisia import a large percentage of their food supplies, especially Egypt. Syria imports less.

-- Infant mortality is considered to be high in all three countries, ranging from 90 per 1000 live births in Egypt to 114 per 100 in Syria and 125 per 1000 in Tunisia.

-- Protein-energy malnutrition and iron-deficiency anemia are common. In Egypt, anemia caused by parasites constitutes one of the major public health problems in the rural areas.

-- Trained manpower in food and nutrition activities and specialized institutions are available in these countries. However, they need better support and necessary orientation to meet their objectives.

-- These countries receive a substantial amount of food-aid assistance, especially through the World Food Programme (WFP). Evaluation of the impact of this assistance would be worthwhile.

Sub-group B. Cyprus, Jordan, Lebanon, Morocco, and Pakistan are basically agricultural, but have no oil resources. There are variations among these countries in terms of population, degree of development, socio-economic structures, diversification of the economy, education level, and distribution of population and incomes. Some of the common charactersitics are:

-- Agriculture plays an important role in their national economies; however, land fragmentation is one of the main problems facing this sub-group. For example, in Pakistan, 88 percent of the holdings are less than 10 hectares, while holdings in Cyprus and Jordan are 85 and 65 percent, respectively, are under 10 hectares.

-- The rural population is relatively large, ranging from 40 percent in Lebanon to 72 percent in Pakistan.

-- The annual rate of population growth ranges from 3.3 percent in Jordan and Pakistan to 2.9 percent in Lebanon.

-- The countries vary in quantity of food imported. However, they all export food, and this constitutes an important share of their foreign exchange earnings.

-- Infant mortality rate is generally moderate.

-- All these countries receive food aid, espeically from the WFP.

Sub-group C. This sub-group consists of needy countries: Afghanistan, Mauritania, People's Democratic Republic of Yemen (PDRY), Somalia, Sudan, and the Yemen Arab Republic. These countries share the following characteristics:

-- The basis of the economy in all is derived from agriculture.

-- The rural population is very high, varying from 70 percent for PDRY to 90 percent in the Yemen Arab Republic and Afghanistan.

-- The average GNP is generally very low.

-- The infant mortality rate is excessive, ranging from 141 per 1000 live births in the Sudan, to 187 per 1000 in Mauritania.

-- Anemia, vitamin A deficiency, and goiter are prevalent.

-- Foreign exchange is derived mainly from agriculture.

-- These countries are receiving substantial food aid.

-- Trained manpower in the fields of food and nutrition is very limited, except in the Sudan and Somalia.

DRY AREA AGRICULTURE AND NUTRITION

FOOD SITUATION IN THE REGION

Food Production

In spite of the constraints facing food production in the Region, during the last decade (the 1970s), the percentage of annual increase in food production was 3.5 percent. This was the highest regional percentage of increase in the world (Table 2). However, the general situation is far from satisfactory for both the Near East Region and Africa when population growth is also taken into consideration.

The potential problems of some countries are shown in Table 3 in terms of annual rate of growth in food production in relation to population growth. For some countries, notably those towards the bottom right of the Table, food production is greater than population growth. Others are in a much more serious situation, where their population growth exceeds, sometimes by a large degree, the increase in food production. This is shown in more detail in Table 4 where the rates of population growth and food production are compared for individual countries in the 1960s and mid-1970s. Low and negative values are indicative of unsatisfactory conditions. In some countries, the causes were clearly the effects of war, liberation stuggles or internal conflicts, and it could reasonably be hoped that when these crises were over, food production would increase sharply. In others there were valid economic reasons based on the comparative advantages of exporting agricultural or even non-food products and importing the balance of food required. However, in certain countries, the high rates of population growth, ranging between three and four percent per year, far outweigh the growth in food production. There is no clear indication as to how and when this problem will be resolved (20,21).

Some selected indicators pertaining to food production in the Near East Region, compared to Africa and world and regional data, are shown in Table 5. For many of these indicators, Near East values are greater than those for world data and often exceed the mean value for developing nations as a whole. This is particularly noticeable for fertilizer production and fertilizer consumption, a factor not unrelated to the oil wealth of the Region. The various types of crops for which production increases have been obtained are shown in Table 6; the average annual increases of nearly five percent for wheat over the previous decade are notable (21).

Food Exports and Imports

In several countries of the Region where the economy depends on agriculture, food exports play an important role in foreign exchange earnings, e.g., fruits and vegetables for Cyprus, Lebanon, and Jordan; olive oil for Tunisia; livestock and bananas from Somalia; groundnuts and sesame from Sudan; and durum wheat (in years of good harvest) from Syria. There is also a great deal of exporting among the countries, especially to the oil-producing countries. The indices of value of imports during the last decade are shown in Table 7. The percentage of annual increase for food exports is 13.7 percent in comparison with 15.6 percent in developing countries. The figures, however, refer to value, which does not always give a good indication of quantity, since price and inflation play a major role.

One of the main problems in the Region is the rapidly increasing food demand that cannot be met through local production, thus increasing dependence on food imports. The indices of value of imports during the 1970s increased approximately sevenfold for food and ninefold for feed. This represents an annual increase of 31 percent for food, which is considered to be the highest in the world (22 percent in the developing countries and 17 percent in the developed). The net imports of cereals into the Region increased from 4.4 million tons during 1961-65 to 12.6 million during 1974-76. Imported wheat --the staple food of the Region -- accounted for the bulk of these, amounting to 11 million metric tons during 1974-76. While the Region was an exporter of rice during 1961-65, it became an importer during 1974-76. The same was true for coarse grains, primarily because of the increased demand for feed and pulses. Among animal products, net imports of milk increased from 690 thousand tons during 1961-65 to about 2 million during 1974-76, and egg imports rose from 4 thousand tons to 44 thousand (21).

Among other foods, the increase in net imports of sugar and vegetable oil has been the most marked. Net imports of sugar increased from 1.9 million tons during 1961-65 to 2.5 million during 1974-76, and vegetable oil imports increased more than fourfold from 156 thousand to 946 thousand tons. The total value of imports reached almost 12 billion dollars in 1979.

This substantial growth in food imports in the 1970s was not only a reflection of the high rate of population growth, but also of the rise in national per capita income, which led to greater expenditures for consumer goods, especially food. This was true not only in the oil-exporting countries, but also in some non-oil producing countries, such as Egypt, Syria, and Tunisia. Thus, with the expanding populations, the demand for the traditional staple foods -- cereals, pulses and vegetable oil -- increased rapidly and, in the countries with rising per capita incomes, a new demand developed for foods previously considered luxuries, such as sugar, meat, milk, and other dairy products. Rapid population growth, urbanization, and rising incomes have all led to a dependence on food imports.

Food Availability and Food Consumption

Food availability in the Region is calculated in the traditional way from production plus imports, minus food exports. Consideration is also given to the feed produced for livestock, fodder, or manufacture (for food and non-food use), and to losses during storage and transportation. Data on food availability for the Region are presented by FAO in food balance sheets (19). However, the amount of food actually consumed may be considerably lower than the quantity shown in food balance sheets, depending on the degree of losses of edible food and nutrients in the household, i.e. during storage, in preparation and cooking, as plate waste, or as quantities fed to domestic animals and pets, or thrown away. Food balance sheets do not give any indication of the differences that may exist in the diets consumed by different population groups, e.g. different socio-economic groups, in different ecological zones and geographical areas within a country; neither do they provide information on seasonal variation in the total food supply.

Nutritional and food balance data for the Middle East Region are shown in Tables 8 to 11. Table 8 shows the daily per capita availability of protein and food energy from various food groups. The data in Table 9 show the estimated average daily availability of selected nutrients for the same countries. Also shown in Table 9 are some adult requirements for food energy, protein, and the same minerals and vitamins. Table 10 represents per capita dietary energy supplies in relation to nutritional requirements for the countries of the Middle East Region. The nutrient availability figures are averages for the whole population and thus are not directly comparable to the requirement figures shown in the right-hand column.

(The information in Table 11 is calculated on the basis of the data in Tables 8 and 9, and shows some indices of quality of the diet. Also shown in the Table are the major cereals consumed in the various countries, with the proportions these constitute of the total calories coming from cereals. If comparison is made to developed countries, it can be seen that most countries of the Middle East Region consume most of their calories from cereals and also have a much smaller proportion of their protein from animal sources. The value for Pcal% (protein calories as a percentage of total calories), however, is far more constant, but two of the poorest countries, Mauritania and Somalia, show high values, reflecting their much greater consumption of milk than is common for the other countries of the Region. Also in Table 9 the importance of cereals is readily apparent; most countries consume wheat as their main staple cereal. The major exceptions to this are Mauritania, People's Democratic Republic of Yemen, Somalia, the Sudan, and Yemen Arab Republic where sorghum and millet are important in addition to wheat.

Food energy availability for most of the countries of the Region shows some increase, as do the developing country and world data. However, certain countries -- Iraq, Jordan, Mauritania, and Somalia -- show a rather static picture with little increase over the period. In contrast, Libya has shown a dramatic increase in per capita food energy availability, currently approaching that in the developed countries. Food balance sheet data are not available for the Gulf States because of their size and very high level of imports, but similar dramatic intakes would be anticipated. Cyprus also shows food energy intake near the levels in developed countries, and there were steady but less dramatic increases in food energy availability in both Syria and Tunisia. In some countries where increased food energy intake has been recorded, the proportion from cereals has also increased, e.g. Tunisia. On the other hand, for a country such as Libya, the cereal calories have remained rather constant despite the enormous increase in total calories. A similar situation has occurred in Saudi Arabia where cereal calorie intakes have declined despite a modest increase in total calores.

In general, protein availability parallels the availability of food energy with dramatic increases ocurring in the same countries. For animal protein, values remain rather static in most countries with the exception of Cyprus, Libya, and Saudi Arabia. There are relatively high proportions of animal proteins in both Mauritania and Somalia, whose dietaries in other respects are more typical of poorer countries. In both of these countries, milk consumption is considerably higher than usual for developing countries.

Despite the limitations of food balance sheet data, it is possible to draw reasonably valid conclusions concerning protein, fat, and food energy availability. Yet, minerals and vitamins, since their content can vary widely according to soil and climatic conditions even within a single country, nutrient availability from food balance sheets is less reliable. Certainly deficiency syndromes exist, and inadequate intakes of vitamin A, zinc, iron, and iodine have been demonstrated in various areas. The most common deficiency, however, is that of total food rather than of specific nutrients, and most diets are probably adequate in their protein energy value (1-5, 8).

THE NUTRITION SITUATION IN THE MIDDLE EAST REGION

The nutrition situation in the Region varies greatly among countries and within population groups in the same country and also among family members (11). Certain indicators are used for determining and comparing the nutritional status of various populations. Examples are infant morbidity and mortality, anthropometry, biochemical and clinical signs, and prevalence of nutritional diseases of public health importance.

Infant mortality. Infant mortality varies from country to country in the Region. It is 17 per 1000 in Cyprus and up to 187 per 1000 in Mauritania. Even within a country, mortality among infants of rural populations is partially caused by the lack of social services, clean water supply, environmental sanitation, education, low socioeconomic status of the family, etc. There is thus no correlation in the Middle East Region as a whole between average GNP and infant mortality. This is evident from consideration of certain oil-producing countries, where the infant mortality rate remains very high (Saudi Arabia -150, UAE - 138, and Libya - 130 per 1000), compared to Lebanon and Jordan (65 and 97 per 1000, respectively). Almost 60 percent of infant deaths in some countries in the Region result from undernutrition combined with infection. Mortality at ages 1 to 4 years is much lower in all populations than infant mortality, but the infectious diseases of childhood, such as measles and pertussis, as well as pneumonia, begin to appear in the second half of the first year or in the second year of life.

Low birth-weight of infants. The poor nutritional status of the mother can contribute to low birth-weight infants (2500 g or less). The incidence of low birth-weight has a close correlation with socioeconomic status. Ninety percent of the countries averaging less than 2800 calories per capita per day for the Middle East Region present a high incidence of low birth-weight infants. Calculations from WHO data estimate that some 2.5 million children born in 1982 weighed less than 2500 g. Low birth-weight infants, having experienced retardation in fetal growth, show a tendency toward hypoglycemia, hypothermia, frequent and severe infections, loss of subcutaneous fat, high mortality rates, and sub-optimal postnatal development (24,25).

Protein-energy malnutrition. Using the prevalence data from Bengoa and Donoso (26) and current population estimates (21), the world incidence of protein-energy malnutrition among preschool children has been estimated to be 104 million cases, among which some 10 million live in the Middle East. These numbers probably represent a minimum. In the first place, many children are reported to have died from an infectious disease, when indeed, malnutrition was the underlying or associated cause. In the second place, malnutrition is subject to seasonal variation. Table 12 gives some anthropometric indicators of nutritional status of children aged 1 to 5 in some Middle East countries (10, 27-30). Wasting (acute undernutrition) is a significant public health problem in Oman (27) and is of serious dimension in Pakistan (28). Stunting is a serious problem in all the countries except Kuwait (29), and of considerable importance in Egypt, Oman, and Pakistan (10,27,28).

Iron deficiency anemia. Iron deficiency is by far the commonest nutritional disorder and the most frequent cause of anemia. Prevalence studies in the Near East Region leave no doubt that nutritional anemias are serious and widespread. Some recent surveys are summarized in Table 13. It has been estimated that 20 to 25 percent of children, 20 to 40 percent of adult females, and up to 10 percent of adult males suffer from varying degrees of anemia in the Middle East (31). In the vulnerable groups -- infants, pregnant and lactating women -- the proportions with anemia reach 70 to 90 percent. Anemia appears to be a public health problem in Oman where 60 percent of mothers surveyed had hemoglobin levels below 12 g per dl (27). Anemia was also highly prevalent in the pre-school child in Oman, ranging from 40 to 56 percent, depending on the standard used and age distribution of the population (23). It was also high in Bahrain for mothers (30). The Egypt survey showed that anemia was considered an important problem in preschool age children (10).

Vitamin A deficiency. Vitamin A deficiency is believed to be a public health problem in several countries in the Region despite consumption of wheat as a staple (31,32). In Pakistan and Jordan, serum retinol levels were shown to be low or deficient in up to 76 percent of preschool children (31). Xerophthalmia was declared a notifiable disease in Jordan, and several notifications were received.

Goiter and iodine deficiency. The prevalance of goiter in the Region has been reviewed (31,33). High prevalence was cited for Afghanistan, Egypt, Ethiopia, Iran, Iraq, Jordan, Lebanon, Pakistan, and the Sudan. Lack of citation most probably indicates the absence of a survey rather than the absence of goiter. A survey in Pakistan showed the incidence of goiter among schoolchildren to be as high as 68 percent (34). Population incidence followed the expected patterns, with goiter being more prevalent among older children and adults, and affecting women more often than men.

Rickets and vitamin D deficiency. Rickets, which is still significant in the Middle East, is unlike most nutritional disorders in that it is more determined by cultural factors than by social or economic ones. As has become clearer in recent years, vitamin D functions more as a hormone than as a vitamin. The importance of vitamin D in human nutrition lies in its role of regulating calcium and phosphate metabolism. In spite of constant sunshine, rickets has been reported from several countries of the Region, including Egypt, Iran, Libya, Tunisia, and Iraq (31).

Disease of affluent societies. Heart disease is one of the three major causes of death in all age groups beyond adolescence in both developed and less developed countries. Recent data for Kuwait show heart disease to be the major cause of death. In the US, between 1968 and 1975, there was a decline in CHD mortality of about 20 percent, while in Kuwait, mortality from ischemic heart disease increased from 5.7 percent of all deaths in 1970 to 10.5 percent of all deaths in 1977 (35). Fat calorie intake as a percentage of total calories has increased as countries of the Region have become richer. For example, in Saudi Arabia the Fcal percent has increased from 12.5 percent in the early 1960s to 22 percent in 1977 (19). Obesity and lack of physical activity are also correlated with CHD.

CONCLUSION

The nutritional status of a population is an integral part of its historical, ecological, environmental, and cultural background. Factors that affect positively or negatively the relationship between food consumption and the nutritional status of a population are multiple and vary from country to country, and any change in one or more of these factors may introduce a new dimension to the situation at a particular time. These factors are the political structures of the country, the nature of development strategies; the economic policy, the social service delivery system, for example, education, health, social welfare and security; the basic infrastructures (roads, housing, water, sanitation); population distribution and related policy; the participation of the community; the distribution of investments (among social/economic classes and between rural and urban sectors); agricultural policy (reform, credit, marketing and seed/fertilizer/energy availability); application and adoption of technology, migration, and refugees; and last but not least, foreign aid and foreign technical assistance.

All the above factors have been found to have a large effect on several countries in the Region. The changes that have occurred during the last decade illustrate this relationship. As an example, in Group I countries, several of these factors have produced high investments in infrastructures (Kuwait, Saudi Arabia, United Arab Emirates), and have resulted in population migration by nomads and fishermen from the rural to urban areas (Bahrain, Oman, and the United Arab Emirates). Social services have been expanded, especially in education and health, with more emphasis in the latter on cure and less on prevention. However, the political structures remain (except recently in Kuwait and Libya), in which people particpate in planning and decisions through their national assembly. In Group I, the food consumption patterns have changed and, accordingly, nutritional status, with the apparent paradox of obesity now occurring among adults while undernutrition still exists among preschool children.

In Group II (Algeria, Iran, Iraq), the development strategies adopted by Algeria, in which investments favored industries with a limited share for agriculture, had a negative impact on food production and consequently on the rural population. In Iran, the development strategy, which leaned more towards intensive capital with less social justice and low investments in rural areas, has resulted in a revolution. Iraq favored agricultural development for the benefit of the rural poor in its development strategy.

In Group III, sub-group A (Egypt, Syria, and Tunisia) whose national development plans raised the average GNP, food demand increased, and consumption patterns changed for certain population groups. The problem of disparity in income still remains, as in Tunisia where 20 percent of the population uses 50 percent of the consumer goods. In sub-group B (Cyprus, Jordan, Lebanon, Pakistan), the development strategy during the last decade was based on maintaining agriculture as a priority with more diversification of the economy into tourism, such as in Cyprus, Lebanon, and Jordan, and providing technical expertise to the neighboring oil-producing countries. In Cyprus, with an average GNP of only $3000 per capita, and very limited natural resources, the infant mortality rate is only 17 per 1000, the lowest in the Region. Problems of undernutrition have disappeared in this country where people and community participate in planning programs, making decisions, and implementing projects.

In sub-group C (Mauritania, PDRY, Somalia, Sudan, YAR), representing needy countries, development -- especially in the Sudan -- should perhaps be directed more towards infrastructure, especially roads. Small surveys showed that changes in the price of one food item increased tenfold at a distance of 200 km. This demonstrates the gap between the producers who get the minimum and the consumer who pays the maximum. The discovery of new resources such as oil in one of these countries would, however, completely change the food consumption and nutritional status of the population.

1. P.L. Pellett, "Food and Nutrition Situation in the Near East Region," MIT International Food and Nutrition Program Discussion Paper No. 20, Center for International Studies, MIT, Cambridge, Massachusetts, 1983.

2. D.S. McLaren and P.L. Pellett, "Nutrition in the Middle East," World Rev. Nutr. Dietet. 12: 43 (1970).

3. V.N. Patwardhan and W.J. Darby, The State of Nutrition in the Arab Middle East (Vanderbilt University Press, Nashville, Tennessee, 1972).

4. P.L. Pellett, "The Nutritional Quality of the Available Food in the Middle East," Indian J. Nutr. Dietet. 7: 366 (1970).

5. P.L. Pellett, "Nutritional Problems of the Arab World," Ecol. Food Nutr. 5: 205 (1976).

6. N.S. Scrimshaw, E.B. Skolnikoff, W.H. Mosley, J.E. Rohde, S.P. Caper, D.S. DeHaan, and J.M. Tinker, World Hunger, Health and Refugee Problems: Summary of a Special Study Mission to Asia and the Middle East (U.S. Government Printing Office, Washington, D.C., 1976).

7. N.S. Scrimshaw and M. Gabr, eds., Practical Approaches to Combat Malnutrition with Special References to Mothers and Children (IUNS Conference, Cairo, Egypt, May, 1977, Ministry of Health, Cairo, 1977).

8. M. Autret and S. Miladi, Food and Nutrition Situation (with Particular Reference to Children) in the Gulf Countries (FAO, Rome and UNICEF, Abu Dhabi, 1980).

9. O. Koksal, Nutrition in Turkey - National Nutrition, Health and Food Consumption Survey of Turkey (Hacettepe University, Ankara, Turkey, 1977).

10. Nutrition Institute, Arab Republic of Egypt, USDHEW, Egypt AID, USAID, Nutrition Status Survey, Egypt (USAID, Washington, D.C., 1978).

11. A. Bornstein, "Food and Society in the Yemen Arab Republic," FAO, Rome (1974).

12. Food and Agriculture Organization, The Sudan: Applied Nutrition Project Findings and Recommendations (FAO, Rome, 1973).

13. M. Siraj-ul-Haq, "Nutrition Planning - Problems and Prospects," Nutrition Cell Planning and Development Division Workshop, Islamabad, Pakistan, 1976.

14. M. Siraj-ul-Haq, M. Ullah, and N. Shah, "Bibliography on Food and Nutrition," Nutrition Cell Planning and Development Division, Islamabad, Pakistan (1978).

15. Europa Publications, The Middle East and North Africa, 1980-81, 27th Edition (Europa Publications, London, U.K., 1980).

16. M. Riad El-Ghonemy, Agrarian Reform and Rural Development in the Near East (FAO, Rome, 1979).

17. A. Hussain, "Women in Arab Society," Middle East J. 7: 440 (1953).

18. A.R. Omran, Population in the Arab World: Problems and Prospects (Carolina Population Center, Chapel Hill, North Carolina, 1981).

19. Food and Agriculture Organization, Food Balance Sheets, 1975-1977, Average and Per Caput Food Supplies (FAO, Rome, 1980).

20. Food and Agriculture Organization, The Fourth World Food Survey, FAO Food and Nutrition Series No. 10 (FAO, Rome, 1977).

21. Food and Agriculture Organization, The State of Food and Agriculture, 1979, FAO Agricultural Series No. 10 (FAO, Rome, 1980).

22. World Health Organization, Sixth Report on the World Health Situation, Part I, Global Analysis, and Part II, Review by Country and Area (WHO, Geneva, 1980).

23. Food and Agriculture Organization and World Health Organization, Handbook on Human Nutritional Requirements, FAO Nutrition Studies No. 28 and WHO Monogr. Ser. No. 61 (FAO, Rome, 1974).

24. World Health Organization Division of Family Health, "Low Birth-Weight Infants," World Health Statistics Quarterly 31: 74 (1978).

25. World Health Organization Division of Family Health, "The Incidence of Low Birth-Weight - A Cricital Review of Available Information," World Health Statistics Quarterly 33(3): 197 (1980).

26. J.M. Bengoa and G. Donoso, "Prevalence of Protein-Calorie Malnutrition," PAG Bull. 4(1): 24 (1974).

27. E.K. Amine, Oman: Nutrition Status Survey (UNICEF Gulf Area Office, April, 1980).

28. M.A. Anderson, "Comparison of Anthropometric Measures of Nutritional Status in Preschool Children in Five Developing Countries," Amer. J. Clin. Nutr. 32: 2339 (1979).

29. S.A. Mostafa and H.Y. Nuwayhed, "Growth Pattern of Kuwaiti Children from Birth to 60 Months (1979) and Nutrition Status Assessment of Pre-School Children (1980), Preventive Health Section, Ministry of Public Health, Kuwait.

30. E.K. Amine, Bahrain: Nutrition Status Survey (UNICEF Gulf Area Office, April, 1980).

31. L.S. Rao, "Panorama of Malnutrition in the Eastern Mediteranean Region," Report to Second Regional Seminar on Food and Nutrition, FAO, Cairo and WHO, Alexandria (1973).

32. World Health Organization, Vitamin A Deficiency and Xerophthalmia: Report of a Joint WHO/USAID Meeting. WHO Tech. Rep. Ser. No. 590 (WHO, Geneva, 1976).

33. F.C. Kelly and W.W. Snedden, Prevalence and Geographical Distribution of Endemic Goiter. WHO Monogr. Ser. No. 44 (WHO, Geneva, 1960).

34. M. Siraj-ul-Haq, A.H. Maan, and H. Ulla, Goiter in Pakistan (Nutrition Cell Planning Division, Government of Pakistan, Islamabad, 1978).

35. Department of Public Health and Planning, Ministry of Pubic Health, Kuwait. Vital and Health Statistics Division, Annual Report, Kuwait, 1978.

TABLE 1. Relationship Between Income, Literacy and Infant Mortality in the Middle East

Group/Country	Population Millions 1979	Average Annual Increase 1970-1979	GNP at Market Prices Billion $	GNP per capita $	Literacy Rate 1975	Infant Mortality Rate per 1000
Group I Oil-Producing						
Kuwait	1.27	6.1	18.04	14,890	60	39
United Arab Emirates	0.91	3.4	11.44	14,230	--	138
Qatar	0.21	3.2	2.84	12,740	--	138
Saudi Arabia	8.06	3.0	63.06	7,690	15	150
Libya	3.13	4.1	18.66	6,910	45	130
Bahrain	0.34	2.9	1.51	4,100	--	78
Oman	0.87	3.1	2.16	2,570	--	142
Group II Oil/Agriculture						
Iraq	12.40	3.2	22.69	1,860	26	104
Algeria	18.79	3.2	22.18	1,260	35	142
Group III Agriculture						
A) Tunisia	6.37	3.3	5.70	950	38	125
Syria	8.37	3.3	7.53	930	53	114
Egypt	41.80	2.7	11.48	280	40	90
B) Cyprus	0.62	1.0	0.91	1,520	76	17
Jordan	2.90	3.3	3.15	1,050	59	97
Pakistan	77.90	3.0	17.78	230	21	142
Yemen P.D.R.	1.80	3.2	0.70	390	27	155
Sudan	17.76	2.5	5.57	320	20	141
Mauritania	1.49	2.6	0.41	270	17	187
Somalia	3.89	2.6	0.48	130	50	177

Sources: J. Econ. Coop. Islamic Countries Vol. I, No. 4, and Vol. II, No. 1, 1979-1980, and U.N. Statistical Yearbook, United Nations, New York, 1978.

TABLE 2. Food Production in the Near East Region as Compared to Africa and to World Data

	Near East	Africa	Developing Nations	Developed Nations	World
Food Production Index* 1979	131	115	128	121	124
Annual Percent Increase 1970-1979	3.5	1.6	3.0	2.2	2.5

*1969-1971 Average = 100.
Source: FAO, The State of Food and Agriculture (21)

DRA-K

TABLE 3. Annual Rate of Change of Food (Crops and Livestock) Production in Relation to Population Growth for Selected Countries of the Near East 1970-1979*

Food Production (%)	Population Increase (%) <1.5	1.6--2.0	2.1--2.5	2.6--3.0	3.1--3.5	>3.5
Minus						
0.1--2.0				Morocco Mauritania	Algeria	
Plus						
0.0--0.9	Cyprus		Lebanon Egypt	Somalia	Iraq	Jordan
1.0--1.5		Yemen A.R.				
1.6--2.5						
2.6--3.6			Yemen PDR		Pakistan	
>3.6			Tunisia	Sudan Turkey Iran	Syria Saudi-Arabia	Libya

*Source: FAO, The State of Food and Agriculture, 1979 (21).

Most Seriously Affected (MSA) countries are underlined.

TABLE 4. Rates of Growth of Population and Food, Agricultural and Cereal Production 1961-65/70 and 1970-76 for Individual Countries of the Near East and North Africa*

Country	Period	Population Increase	Production			Production per capita		
			Food	Agri-cultural	Cereals	Food	Agri-cultural	Cereals
Afghanistan	1	2.3	1.3	1.3	0.6	-1.0	-0.9	-1.6
	2	2.6	4.5	4.7	5.7	1.9	2.0	3.0
Algeria	1	3.4	2.6	2.7	5.2	-0.8	-0.6	1.8
	2	3.2	2.5	2.5	4.5	-0.7	-0.7	1.3
Cyprus	1	1.1	7.3	7.1	-2.0	6.1	5.9	-3.1
	2	1.2	-4.5	-4.4	2.0	-5.7	-5.6	0.8
Egypt	1	2.5	3.5	3.3	3.3	1.0	0.7	0.8
	2	2.4	2.1	1.4	1.4	-0.2	-1.0	-1.0
Iraq	1	3.2	3.8	3.9	5.0	0.5	0.7	1.7
	2	3.4	-0.2	-0.5	-3.6	-3.5	-3.8	-6.9
Jordan	1	3.0	-10.4	-9.8	-12.3	-13.4	-12.8	-15.3
	2	3.4	0.4	0.5	-4.8	-3.0	-2.8	-8.2
Libya	1	3.7	0.8	1.1	-2.1	-2.8	-2.5	-5.8
	2	3.1	10.2	9.5	27.8	7.1	6.3	24.7
Mauritania	1	2.0	1.8	1.8	0.1	-0.3	-0.3	-1.9
	2	2.0	-3.9	-3.9	-6.2	-5.8	-5.8	-8.2
Pakistan	1	2.8	6.2	6.0	9.1	3.4	3.1	6.3
	2	3.2	2.9	2.0	3.1	-0.2	-1.1	-0.1
Saudi Arabia	1	2.7	2.5	2.5	1.8	-0.2	-0.2	-0.9
	2	3.0	4.6	4.6	6.5	1.6	1.6	3.5
Somalia	1	2.2	2.8	2.8	0.2	0.5	-0.5	-2.0
	2	2.6	-0.6	-0.6	0.3	-3.2	-3.1	-2.3
Sudan	1	2.9	3.9	4.3	4.4	0.9	1.3	1.5
	2	3.1	5.4	4.1	5.4	2.2	1.0	2.2
Syria	1	3.2	-0.6	-0.4	-4.8	-3.7	-3.7	8.0
	2	3.1	11.4	9.0	20.7	8.3	5.8	17.6
Tunisia	1	2.1	1.3	1.4	-1.0	-0.7	-0.6	-3.0
	2	2.3	6.5	6.4	7.9	4.1	4.0	5.5
Yemen A.R.	1	2.8	-2.5	-2.5	-1.9	-5.3	-5.3	-4.7
	2	2.9	9.2	9.5	13.0	6.3	6.6	10.1
Yemen P.D.R.	1	2.7	2.5	2.0	2.9	-0.2	-0.6	0.2
	2	3.0	3.8	3.3	1.8	0.8	0.4	-1.1

*Source: FAO, The Fourth World Food Survey, 1977 (20)
Note: 1 refers to period 1961-1965/70, and 2 refers to 1970-1976.

TABLE 5. Some Selected Indicators Pertaining to Agricultural Production in the Near East Region as Compared to Africa and World Data

	Near East	Africa	Developing Nations	Developed Nations	World
Cereal area	1.2	0.9	1.2	1.2	1.1
Cereal yield	2.2	0.2	1.7	1.5	1.6
Cereal production	3.4	1.1	2.9	2.6	2.7
Fertilizer production*	17.2	3.6	13.0	4.4	5.5
Fertilizer production** % of world total	1.6	0.7	17.5	82.5	100.0
Fertilizer consumption	11.5	7.6	10.2	4.3	5.6
Tractors in agriculture	14.7	3.9	9.2	2.5	3.2

*N, P_2O_5, K_2O (including ground rock phosphate for direct application)
**World total production ca. 113 million metric tons
Source: Reference (21) All data except where indicated are percentage of annual increases, 1970-1979

TABLE 6. Volume of Production and Rate of Increase of Major Food Crops in Near East Region

Food	Production*	% Increase**
Total Cereals	54,000	3.4
Wheat	31,000	4.9
Rice	4,600	0.2
Barley	8,000	2.7
Maize	5,500	3.4
Total Root Crops	5,800	5.5
Potatoes	5,400	6.0
Cassava	110	0.2
Total Pulses	1,800	1.8
Citrus fruit	3,500	4.7
Bananas	300	2.9
Apples	1,700	7.3
Vegetable oils	1,600	3.4
Soybeans	210	36.5
Ground nuts	920	10.9
Sunflower seed	530	3.0
Sugar	2,600	4.5
Total meat	3,200	3.9
Milk	14,000	2.9
Eggs	610	7.9
Marine fish	550	3.6
Crustaceans	40	6.0

*Production 1978: metric tons x 10^3 rounded figures
**Average increase per year, 1969-1978
Source: Reference (21).

TABLE 7. Indices of Value of Imports and Exports of Agricultural Products for Near East and African Regions as Compared to Developing and Developed Countries

	Agricultural Products		Food		Feed		Raw Materials		Beverages		Fishery Products	
	I	%	I	%	I	%	I	%	I	%	I	%
Near East (Developing)												
Exports	214	10.4	303	13.7	63	5.2	164	8.3	210	9.6	249	13.6
Imports	653	29.3	692	30.8	935	32.8	427	21.8	488	20.4	845	32.9
Africa (Developing)												
Exports	264	13.5	262	12.3	130	6.4	179	8.7	318	17.5	290	15.3
Imports	456	22.2	489	23.0	677	25.3	357	19.2	264	16.9	345	19.2
Developing Countries												
Exports	293	15.3	298	15.6	462	23.0	209	9.8	344	17.4	432	20.6
Imports	418	20.7	436	21.5	656	28.1	352	17.4	311	16.3	326	16.8
Developed Countries												
Exports	346	17.5	354	18.0	392	18.3	264	13.2	423	19.8	359	16.8
Imports	308	16.0	318	16.6	354	18.1	220	10.3	378	18.7	365	17.3

*I = Index 1969-1971 Average = 100
**% = Annual percentage change 1969-1978
Source: Refernce (21)

TABLE 8. Protein (g) and Food Energy (Kcal) as Supplied by Various Food Groups - Per Capita per Day for Some Countries of the Near East and North Africa, 1975-1977 Data

Country	Total		Cereals		Roots/ Tubers		Sugar/ Honey		Pulses		Nuts and Oilseeds		Vege- tables		Fruit		Meat and Offals		Eggs		Fish/ Seafood		Milk		Oils/ Fats	
	C	P	C	P	C	P	C	P	C	P	C	P	C	P	C	P	C	P	C	P	C	P	C	P	C	P
Saudi Arabia	2108	58.9	1140	30.1	11	0.2	152	-	24	1.6	38	1.6	40	1.9	262	2.7	116	10.1	12	0.9	10	1.4	125	7.3	162	-
Libya	2948	74.9	1193	33.8	41	0.9	457	-	55	3.8	99	3.2	91	4.3	214	2.6	133	12.3	5	0.4	17	2.1	197	9.5	54	0.1
Iraq	2323	61.5	1441	39.5	10	0.1	349	-	53	3.4	10	0.3	62	3.6	67	1.0	79	5.7	11	0.9	5	0.8	69	5.4	155	-
Cyprus	2964	90.0	1235	35.8	74	1.7	200	-	78	5.2	113	3.2	44	2.4	163	2.2	388	21.6	26	2.1	12	1.7	205	12.5	317	0.1
Algeria	2357	63.1	1485	44.7	53	1.1	214	-	47	3.1	6	0.2	20	0.9	90	1.1	42	3.4	5	0.4	5	0.8	128	6.8	246	-
Jordan	2060	56.0	1253	35.5	27	0.6	252	-	51	3.1	23	0.7	29	1.6	46	0.6	76	5.3	20	1.6	6	0.8	84	5.5	192	0.1
Tunisia	2658	72.5	1465	44.1	31	0.7	248	-	72	4.7	39	1.0	73	3.9	76	1.1	94	7.8	10	0.9	10	1.5	96	6.0	421	0.1
Syria	2618	73.3	1356	38.8	28	0.7	245	-	132	7.7	90	3.0	109	6.0	134	2.0	87	5.8	17	1.3	3	0.4	89	7.0	314	0.1
Yemen A.R.	2260	67.9	1529	43.9	24	0.6	179	-	118	7.6	8	0.2	19	1.2	115	1.0	85	5.9	8	0.6	9	1.3	75	5.1	87	0.1
Yemen P.D.R.	1919	58.0	1160	31.5	1	-	143	-	14	0.4	20	1.3	56	3.7	178	1.8	56	3.7	3	0.3	80	13.0	63	4.2	171	0.1
Sudan	2226	67.0	1245	39.6	45	0.6	185	-	38	2.6	67	2.7	22	1.2	63	0.8	120	10.5	3	0.3	3	0.4	134	7.5	272	-
Egypt	2779	76.1	1851	49.9	37	0.7	236	0.2	102	7.7	22	0.9	84	3.8	91	1.2	61	5.2	6	0.5	8	1.2	41	4.2	229	0.1
Mauritania	1895	68.0	1023	26.0	11	0.2	141	-	99	6.5	17	0.9	1	0.1	38	0.4	113	10.5	4	0.4	42	6.6	321	16.3	80	0.1
Pakistan	2255	62.0	1439	39.2	12	0.2	263	0.5	73	4.1	6	0.5	18	1.0	41	0.5	37	3.4	3	0.2	3	0.4	160	11.5	194	0.1
Somalia	2137	73.9	939	25.1	28	0.2	177	-	9	0.6	65	2.3	9	0.5	51	0.6	275	24.2	2	0.1	2	0.3	432	19.3	141	0.1
All Developing Countries	2260	57.3	1369	31.8	162	1.9	156	-	95	6.0	50	2.7	33	1.9	48	0.6	102	5.8	9	0.7	16	2.5	49	2.9	134	-
All Developed Countries	3395	99.1	1036	29.4	159	3.7	441	-	29	1.9	45	2.2	62	3.3	87	1.1	478	26.8	53	4.2	50	7.1	295	17.5	468	0.2
World	2571	69.8	1278	31.2	161	2.3	234	-	77	4.8	48	2.5	41	2.3	59	0.7	205	11.5	21	1.7	25	2.8	116	6.9	225	0.1

C = Food Energy Kcal/capita/day
P = Protein g/capita/day, as provided by the various food groups
Source: Food Balance Sheets, 1975-1977 Average (FAO, Rome, 1980) Reference (19).
Note: Food Balance Sheet data are not available for the Gulf countries.

TABLE 9. Estimated Average Daily Availability of Selected Nutrients and Adult Requirements for Some Countries of the Near East and North Africa, 1977

Country	Food Energy Kcal	Protein Total g	Protein Animal g	Fat g	Calcium mg	Iron mg	Retinol Equiv. ug	Thiamine	Riboflavin mg	Niacin mg	Ascorbic Acid mg
Saudi Arabia	2233	63.0	24.9	54.8	560	14.3	834	1.11	1.07	15.1	78
Libya	2985	75.0	25.2	86.9	655	17.3	970	1.48	1.35	17.2	121
Iraq	2155	57.4	13.0	31.6	375	14.8	1137	1.36	0.82	12.3	74
Cyprus	3054	92.8	40.4	105.3	797	21.5	1038	1.97	1.55	19.8	117
Algeria	2372	63.8	11.6	45.1	410	12.5	341	1.30	0.81	11.2	53
Jordan	2107	56.0	13.8	41.4	349	10.8	280	1.15	0.72	9.8	42
Tunisia	2674	73.0	17.5	73.6	437	16.5	1058	1.53	1.05	13.6	128
Syria	2685	77.6	15.4	59.8	575	20.4	944	1.94	1.14	15.3	150
Yemen A.R.	2311	69.4	14.2	38.1	405	19.6	444	1.63	1.04	16.3	35
Yemen P.D.R.	1975	60.7	22.7	38.5	466	15.6	374	1.08	0.81	14.2	32
Sudan	2274	68.3	19.0	63.2	496	19.0	551	1.53	1.13	16.8	44
Egypt	2787	76.5	11.2	50.1	427	19.9	745	1.89	0.95	16.4	112
Mauritania	1963	69.9	34.7	47.3	768	15.0	484	1.03	1.30	12.1	11
Pakistan	2281	62.9	15.8	41.6	544	17.7	648	2.14	1.02	19.5	44
Somalia	2228	75.9	44.2	75.7	905	16.1	856	1.41	1.85	17.6	32
All Developing Countries	2260	57.3	12.0	38.4	348	16.1	609	1.32	0.79	13.7	77
All Developed Countries	3395	99.1	55.7	125.3	843	18.5	1055	1.79	1.79	20.9	130
World	2571	68.8	23.9	62.2	483	16.8	730	1.45	1.06	15.7	92
Requirements											
Adult male (65 kg) (moderately active)	3000	37	-	-	400-500	5-9	750	1.2	1.8	19.8	30
Adult female (55 kg) (moderately active)	2200	29	-	-	400-500	14-28	750	0.9	1.3	14.5	30
Pregnancy (latter half)	+350	38	-	-	1000-1200	-	750	+0.1	+0.2	+2.3	50
Lactation (1st 6 months)	+550	46	-	-	1000-1200	-	1200	+0.2	+0.4	+3.7	50

Source: References (19) and (23)

TABLE 10. Per Capita Dietary Energy Supplies in Relation to Nutritional Requirements for Countries of the Near East Region and North Africa

	Averages 1966-68	1969-71	1972-74	1975-77	Requirement
		% of Requirements			Kcal/capita/day
AFRICA	92	94	93	95	2334
Algeria	77	79	89	98	2400
Mauritania	85	83	75	82	2310
Morocco	96	102	103	106	2420
Somalia	95	96	96	92	2310
Tunisia	85	90	107	111	2390
NEAR EAST	98	99	102	108	2455
Afghanistan	98	81	82	81	2440
Cyprus	112	120	126	123	2480
Egypt	104	104	103	108	2510
Iran	95	97	110	132	2410
Iraq	87	91	95	96	2410
Jordan	87	93	89	84	2460
Lebanon	100	100	101	101	2480
Libya	93	105	124	126	2360
Saudi Arabia	89	89	93	102	2420
Sudan	84	92	89	95	2350
Syria	95	98	101	105	2480
Yemen A.R.	86	81	87	90	2420
Yemen P.D.R.	93	89	85	79	2410
ASIA	88	94	93	93	2216
Pakistan	89	95	95	98	2310

Source: Reference (21)

TABLE 11. Some Indices of Quality of the Diet as Derived from Food Balance Sheet Data for Countries of the Middle East and North Africa

Country	Pcal %*	% Animal Protein to Total Protein	Fcal %**	Cereal Cal %	Sugar Cal %	Thiamine/ 1000 Kcal	Riboflavin/ 1000 Kcal
Saudi Arabia	11.3	39.5	22.1	54.1	7.2	0.50	0.48
Libya	10.0	33.6	26.2	40.5	15.5	0.49	0.45
Iraq	10.7	22.6	13.2	62.0	15.0	0.63	0.38
Cyprus	12.2	43.5	31.0	41.7	6.7	0.64	0.51
Algeria	10.8	18.2	17.1	63.0	9.1	0.55	0.34
Jordan	10.6	24.6	17.7	60.8	12.2	0.55	0.34
Tunisia	10.9	24.0	24.8	55.1	9.5	0.57	0.39
Syria	11.6	19.8	20.0	51.8	9.4	0.72	0.42
Yemen A.R.	12.0	20.5	14.8	67.6	7.9	0.70	0.45
Yemen P.D.R.	12.3	37.4	17.5	60.4	7.5	0.55	0.41
Sudan	12.0	27.8	25.0	55.9	8.3	0.67	0.50
Egypt	11.0	14.6	16.2	66.6	8.5	0.68	0.34
Mauritania	14.2	49.6	21.7	54.0	7.4	0.52	0.66
Pakistan	11.0	25.1	16.4	63.8	11.7	0.94	0.45
Somalia	13.6	58.2	30.6	43.9	8.3	0.63	0.83
All Developing Countries	10.1	20.9	15.3	60.6	6.9	0.58	0.35
All Developed Countries	11.7	56.2	33.2	30.5	13.0	0.53	0.52
World	10.7	34.7	21.8	49.7	9.1	0.56	0.41

*Protein calories as percentage of total calories
**Fat calories as percentage of total calories
Source: Reference 19 calculated from data presented in Tables 8 and 9

TABLE 12. Anthropometric Indicators of Nutritional Status of Children Aged 1 to 5 for Some Near East Region Countries

		Percentages of Children											
		Weight for Age				Height for Age				Weight for Height			Number of
Country	Reference	<60	60-75	75-90	>90	<85	85-90	90-95	>95	<80	80-85	>85	Children
Kuwait	(29)	0	2	33	65	1	3	22	58	1	3	96	1611
Bahrain	(30)	2	16	50	32	2	12	28	58	4	12	84	300
Oman	(27)	6	20	37	37	9	15	25	51	22	17	61	428
Egypt	(10)	1	8	39	53	5	17	40	39	1	2	98	8016
Pakistan	(28)	34		66		30		70		8	46	46	1202

Note: For Pakistan, weight-for-age data are only reported as above or below 75%, height-for-age above and below 90%, and the cut-off point for weight-for-height is 90%, not 85% as in the other countries.

TABLE 13. Percentage Distribution of Hemoglobin and Prevalence of Anemia in Some Recent Surveys

Country and Group	Number Examined	Percentages <9	9-10	10-11	11-12	>12	Anemic*
Bahrain (Ref. 30)							
preschool <60 m	295	2	9	23	33	33	11(10):34(11)
mothers	212	<1	5	10	34	50	49(12)
Oman (Ref. 27)							
preschool <60 m	428	18	21	27	14	20	39(10):56(11)
mothers	303	10	10	17	22	41	59(12)
Kuwait (Ref. 29)							
preschool <7 m	288	7	13	56	16	8	20(10
7-24 m	332	19	23	33	18	8	42(10)
25-60 m	552	7	12	22	29	30	41(11)
Turkey (Ref. 9)		<7.9	8-10	10-11	>11		
preschool <60 m	2976	16	33	24	27		49(10):73(11)
females (pregnant)	322	16	35	23	26		74(11)
(lactating)	420	9	33	24	35		66(11)
Egypt (Ref. 10)			9.5	<9.5-11.0	11-12		
preschool survey <60 m	1609		12	26	62**		28(10 and 11)
preschool special <60 m	359		2	15	83**		17(11)
mothers	1478		4	8	15	73	27(12)

*Shows percentage defined as anemic using criterion shown in brackets (g hemoglobin/100 ml)
For Egypt a dual standard was used: 10 g/100 ml when below 2 years and 11 g/100 ml when above.
**Includes those >12 g/100 ml

DISCUSSION

SESSION III - FOOD PRODUCTION AND NUTRITION IN THE MIDDLE EAST

JOHN D. GERHART

Nour mentioned a number of factors that constrain agricultural production in the ICARDA region. I think there is an item that he omitted -- one that affects rural economies and households, consumption and production in the Middle East, and I think it would be remiss not to deal with it a little more systematically. This is the question of labour migration.

Beginning with the oil price boom in 1973, the countries of the Gulf became extremely wealthy and a very large and complex labour migration, which already had existed for some time, became even more important. This is particularly significant for those populous countries that are agricultural producers but not oil-producers, or not major oil-producers, such as Syria, Egypt, Jordan and the Sudan. Even for the smaller countries, for example, Yemen, labour migration to the Gulf states is very important. The size of remittances in the Yemeni economy is greater than gross domestic product and I think this is the only country in the world that can say that.

The numbers involved are enormous, although nobody knows the exact figures. Egypt's estimate is that from one to three million Egyptians are working outside the country. Jordan has a very large proportion of the prime male labour force working abroad and, in fact, Jordan has to import migrant labourers to replace them. Seventy-thousand Egyptians are now working in agriculture on the East Bank of the Jordan river and Pakistanis are living in tents and planting tobacco in rainfed areas of the country. This unprecedented migration is not limited to the Arab countries by any means; it is very important to Pakistan and India, and it is becoming increasingly important to East Asia and Southeast Asia. It certainly compares with the earlier migration of workers to Europe that affected Turkey and Algeria very heavily. It compares with the largest worker migration in the world, which is from Mexico and Central America to the United States. It may be as large as that, although we do not exactly know the size of the labour migration in either case.

In any event, this migration has an impact in a number of ways, and I would like to mention some of them. In production, it has a very startling impact on rural wage rates. The real wage rate for agricultural labour in Egypt has been rising at nine per cent a year since 1975. That is the real wage, not the normal wage rate, and this is quite unprecedented in any rural situation. There are critical labour bottlenecks, there is high turnover of employment among factory workers, and there is a tendency towards mechanization, both in factories and in agricultural production, in order to deal with these labour bottlenecks.

It also has implications for decision-making in agricultural production at the farm level. There are many cases as in Jordan and Egypt where the male head of the household is absent and the farm is being managed by his wife, son, wife's father, his father, or some other combination of people. There is a much more divided decision-making process than there was previously. Also, it has caused substantial changes in the gender of the labour force who do particular tasks as demonstrated by factory workers in Egypt. Even in agriculture, women are driving tractors and doing things that were virtually unheard of ten years ago. No one really knows what is happening because no one has studied household labour practices in much detail. Now that these households are in considerable flux, the relationships are even more complex.

There is also an increase in incomes that results in a much higher effective demand. This can be seen in the increasing demand for meat in many countries as a result of high incomes and high income elasticity for meat. It has resulted in enormous inflation rates in some circumstances because an increase in purchasing power is chasing the same amount of goods or even fewer goods, and as a result prices rise. If you visit Aqaba in Jordan or Suez or Alexandria in Egypt and look at the ports, you can see what is happening to imports, and this is not just food imports but imports of durable goods as well.

This has had a very complex and probably damaging effect on consumption. Myntti mentioned this in a previous session and I hope she will comment further about it. There has been a large increase in convenience foods and in packaged products. You can buy milk from Denmark, Italy, and France. There has been a much greater commercialization of food consumption in some countries. In countries like Egypt and possibly Syria, this may not be so serious because there is a substantial amount of domestic production and a higher demand for local products. However, in smaller countries like Jordan and Yemen, agricultural production has dropped considerably in many respects and people are substituting imported products for local ones. The resultant changes in dietary intake are likely to affect the overall nutritional value of the diet in both positive and negative ways that we cannot yet evaluate.

There are other issues that are not yet apparent but may well be developing. My own background has been in Sub-Saharan Africa and in countries in that part of the world where labour migration is much older. Workers in South Africa have been going to the mines in Zimbabwe and northern Zambia for 50 to 60 years. In these cases, there are early signs of certain social pathologies that result from divided families because of the migration of part of the family. There is an increase in divorce, abandoned families, certain juvenile delinquencies, and problematic child behaviour owing to the absence of the father. These problems, which are very profound in Africa, appear to be very small in the Middle East, but large-scale migration is a recent phenomenon. Here it is less than 10 years old, but if you look at western Zambia or Botswana where migration has been taking place for 50 years you find that 40 to 60 per cent of households have no male in the home and in half of these, the women have never been married. These were societies that once had even stronger family structures than the Middle East has today. Therefore, it is possible that such social pathologies may result from this large-scale migration in the future. It seems to me that this is an added factor that complicates the interrelationships between human nutrition, food production, and farm management.

One more problem we should add to the picture -- one that has an impact on the receiving countries as well -- is the very serious question of health and nutrition among migrant workers themselves. There are also the questions of human rights, labour rights, and wage protection and exploitation. This is perhaps less important because the receiving countries are wealthy enough to afford to pay; they certainly do not have a balance of payments problem. Second, the migrant labourers are generally at the peak of their physical capacity; that is why they are there. They are able-bodied, young male workers and so the damaging effects are probably not as permanent or serious in the receiving countries as they may be in the sending countries. However, I am more concerned with the impact on the labour-exporting countries and particularly on the effects on agricultural production.

Labour migration is the only factor that I thought was not included in the two papers I am discussing. Now, I would like to change the subject slightly and ask how ICARDA views nutrition within its mandate. What are the things ICARDA would do differently if it had had the kind of knowledge of nutrition in the Middle East that the experts have now given us? Since the rest of the workshop is concerned with this specific question, I thought it might be worthwhile if I listed seven areas where I think ICARDA should be conscious of nutrition and can have a major impact on the nutritional status of populations within the region.

There are areas where nutrition is directly related to ICARDA's present activities and to some activities it may become more involved in. To help guide the subsequent discussion, I will try to list these. What could ICARDA do, or for that matter, what could any national programme do, in this regard? If nutrition receives a higher priority from these research institutions what does this imply for staffing?

Of course, the first goal is to achieve higher food production through higher yields, greater acreage, higher cropping intensity, and so forth. This will lead to greater home consumption and higher incomes through producing a surplus for sale. Alternatively, higher yields per hectare could lead to reduced cropping area for cereals or diversification into animal products, tree crops, and vegetables. These are all things that would improve the quality of the diet by reducing the amount of labour and the size of areas used to grow basic foodstuffs. Labour is in many cases the real constraint in rural farming systems, and technologies that require reduced time or that spread time requirements more evenly throughout the year can result in freeing labour for other paid employment, leisure, better child care, better food preparation, or many other things that relate to the quality of nutrition. Higher food production also usually results in lower consumer prices. So on the production side, although we are properly critical of research where the only goal is to increase yields, higher production is one area in which we could expect to get results that would have beneficial effects on nutrition.

The second area where ICARDA may or may not be active is to lower food losses. This refers to reducing losses in the fields and during harvesting, storage, processing and perhaps even during cooking or food preparation when nutrients are lost. We hear that these losses are very high, yet we do not know how much time ICARDA and/or other research institutions devote to reducing these food losses.

A third area is better food quality. This is not an area I know very much about. This could include improved nutritional quality of the grains themselves, which Scrimshaw pointed out can have a macro effect. It can also refer to better digestibility, and more ready assimilation.

A fourth area is higher food acceptability, either through changes in taste, colour, consistency, or whatever it is that makes varieties desirable to consuming populations. We all know cases of people refusing to eat certain foods imported under food aid schemes. Yellow corn in Africa is one example of a food that is very unpopular with local populations. These first four research areas are well understood and part of ICARDA's mandate; the three that follow are areas that may require more breadth of effort.

The fifth area is greater production reliability. Nour mentioned water management in his paper and this falls into my fifth area. Other items include the maintenance of natural resources, less erosion, less waterlogging, less salinity, more salt-tolerant varieties, and more cold-tolerant varieties. The heavy pressure on good land in many countries, most recently in Egypt, has severely damaged potential productive capacity. Although there have been improvements in food production over the last 20 years, the cost has often been heavy exploitation of the resource base. In Sudan, you have to drive almost 100 miles from Khartoum to find natural vegetation, because nearer to the city it has been devastated by firewood collection, overgrazing, and overexploitation.

Also under this heading of greater production reliability would be to strive for less seasonal variability and less annual variability among crops. In other words, what can you do to maintain the production system and fertility while reducing variability in the system? If you want to take an historical look, you can go back to the search for Troy. When the archeologists were seeking the actual site of Troy, they looked on the sea coast where it was reputed to be. Then they realized that when Troy existed, 1000 BC, the sea coast was in a different place, so they took satellite maps and went farther inland and found Troy 30 miles from the present sea coast. Soil from the mountains of Turkey had eroded down and extended the deltas of the rivers into the ocean to add to the landmass. Similarly, in the case of Babylon, a contributing factor to the fall of the Babylonian civilizations was soil salinization. This could well happen to Egypt and is a major problem in Iraq and Syria today. So resource maintenance is a very important component for agricultural research because it now affects, and will increasingly affect, nutrition in the future.

A sixth area is easier adaptation to farm circumstances; we normally call this farming systems analysis. How do you develop crops, interventions, technologies that fit the real, as opposed to the ideal, circumstances of farm families? This area includes labour-saving factors, energy saving factors, sequencing or spreading labour requirements across the year, and recognizing that livestock play a very important role. Nour mentioned livestock in his remarks; livestock is the money-spinner, where the cash comes from in the cereal-livestock systems, and it is also the savings mechanism for many pastoral societies. If you do not consider livestock in the system, you cannot explain very important things like half the acreage going to berseem clover in Egypt, or the stripping of corn or maize stalks in Egypt in order to provide fodder for the animals. Agricultural experts deplored this maize-stripping for years until they actually did an analysis and found that the value of fodder was greater than the loss of grain yields. Why is this? It is basically because meat prices are not controlled while grain prices are. Therefore, meat is profitable, and people will do anything to keep their animals healthy and productive.

The last area of importance is the question of food policies. We certainly would not want to rely on IFPRI alone to deliver the goods in this field. It seems to me that every good agricultural centre, just like every good agricultural producer, ought to be lobbying for improved farm policies. We have seen in Farming Systems Research how you can affect research priorities, but you could also affect macro policies and support policies for agriculture. If you do economic trials and demonstrate that nitrogen, phosphate, early planting, machine drilling, or some other piece of infrastructure or activity is profitable, then there has to be a support system that can deliver that. You have to be able to buy fertilizer and the value of the increased production has to be enough to pay for the fertilizer. Research stations carrying out experiments that do not reflect or pin-point objectives are not doing a sufficient job. The international centres have, in the last ten years, made much progress in this direction and are clearly leaders in virtually the whole field of agricultural policy.

The final comment I would like to make concerns Turkey. I attended the ICARDA/CIMMYT cereal meeting recently and there was a discussion about the wheat production programme in Turkey where total wheat production has recently increased from 9 to 17 million tons. We were told that this production was valued at about two billion dollars a year. Look at what that is worth to the economy of the country where the money goes to their own farmers rather than to foreign farmers. For a large country, this is an extremely important factor. What happened in Turkey was that there was a conjunction of a successful agronomic package with favourable price incentives. Somel says this was because the policy makers did not know what the wheat was worth; had they known that, they could have tried to turn the tap down. Nevertheless, it was profitable and it achieved an important increase.

There may be other areas I have not mentioned, but there is a positive answer to what ICARDA can do to improve the nutritional status of populations in the region, and I have cited some of the areas in which ICARDA could have an impact.

I would now like to invite open discussion of the papers presented in this session:

Amir: Figure 1 of Nour's paper shows a drop in the import and export curves for the developed, developing, and Middle Eastern countries between 1973 and 1975. I can understand the explanation of that drop in the Middle Eastern countries. Is this reflected in other countries? If so, do we have figures that show the deterioration of the nutritional status of the world during that period, or was the world able to manage with local resources without any such deterioration? My personal feeling is that because of maldistribution, the more food we import, the more we waste.

Nour: Thank you for asking a question for which neither I nor Nygaard have a reliable answer. There is certainly an anomaly there that is worth examining. You are interested in the nutritional effects of that particular situation. I do not believe that ICARDA, being only five years old, has data or capacity to analyze the nutritional aspects of such shortfalls and will put the matter to the floor.

Parpia: I have two questions for Nour. First, we have been discussing interdisciplinarity in order to increase resources so that more food will be available and poverty will be reduced. A question arises from one of the important points of Nour's paper. In Egypt, the imports of food have gone up, but he did not refer to other commodities. I recall a study carried out under Nour's own leadership in FAO that recommended that the production of food whould not be encouraged as much in Egypt because it was felt that greater income could be generated through cotton. Therefore, by exporting cotton, more food could be imported than could be locally produced. So the question of food is related, on the one hand, to production of other commodities and on the other to the contribution food and non-food agricultural production make towards the transformation from an agriculturally dependent society to a balanced agro-industrial society. In regard to Saudi Arabia, the imports of food have gone up considerably because of affluence. Table 4 in the Nour-Nygaard paper gives figures only in monetary terms, yet it is fairly likely that substantial amounts of money are being spent on junk food and processed food.

The second question arises out of the Nour-Nygaard and Miladi-Pellett papers. Many times governments have to make a decision as to what they should import and what they should process. If, like Egypt, they begin to import large amounts of processed food, then an indigenous industry that was already in the early stages of development would be completely crushed by cheap, imported products. At the same time, this results in a considerable deficit in trade balance. How can we use food and agricultural commodities to stimulate economic development and transform society?

DRA-I

Nour: Your first question is about Egypt. I left Egypt three or four years ago so I hope Gerhart, who lives there now, will comment as well. I think the issue you have put your finger on is found not only in Egypt but in many other countries in the developing world. This is the question of food security. The problem that confronts these governments is the balance between what is known as food security (which is almost the same as political security) and economic feasibility of crop production. My feeling in this matter is that in Egypt, the balance has been tipped by the government in favour of cotton production at the expense of food crops and animals. There is a grey area where potential conflict exists between food policy and national policies on import and exports. I would welcome other comments on whether there is a good balance in Egypt on these agricultural policies.

I agree with your suggestion about imports of food by Saudi Arabia. It is absolutely correct that the Saudis are also embarking seriously on a national food security policy, where they are using scarce ground and underground water to produce wheat. This is a policy that appears to be neither rational nor enlightened. Nevertheless, it is a question of Saudi Arabia's considering itself a major country in the region. It is a question perhaps of national pride and security that makes it want to grow wheat from very scarce water resources at extremely high costs. A kilogram of wheat produced in Saudi Arabia costs over one dollar. That is, of course, a very high price to pay for food security.

Your second question could better be answered by more competent persons because it impinges on post-harvest work and resulting food losses. Maybe Nygaard would like to make an interjection here as well as Gerhart.

Gerhart: If we could just focus for a minute on this question of food security versus comparative advantage. This is of course a source of some pain to all economists.

Nygaard: I would like to use an example from Tunisia that I think nicely illustrates the importance of agricultural policies and the possible pitfalls of such policies. It also impinges on the issue of self-sufficiency. In Tunisia, in the late 1960s, there was a growing interest in increasing bread wheat production, and this was encouraged by CIMMYT and others. Tunisia produces a high-quality durum wheat that is used to make macaroni products in Italy or other European countries. That money can be used to import more bread wheat because bread wheat is cheaper than durum. For reasons of food security or self-sufficiency, Tunisia, acting on expert advice from others, tried to increase bread production at the expense of producing less durum wheat. In fact, there was no economic reason for doing so unless they were worried that trade lines would be cut with the outside world. Therefore, they adopted a policy of self-sufficiency, in the very strongest sense of the word, and went a long way with a breeding programme in bread wheat before they gave their durum wheat programme any attention. When they realized this error and finally developed their durum wheat programme, the adoption rates for new durum varieties were substantially higher than the adoption had been for new bread wheat varieties introduced before.

Miladi: In response to Parpia's first question, the case of cotton in the Sudan is interesting. The price of cotton on the international market has been decreasing in the past five years, while the price of food commodities has increased tremendously. The government developed a cotton policy in order to get foreign exchange. Similarly, in Egypt the farmer is obliged by the government to grow cotton, and the price offered to farmers is always much less than that on the international market. The farmer is not in favour of growing cotton, but the government needs to get foreign exchange. Due to the recent price changes, these governments are suffering severe balance of payment problems.

The other question Parpia raised is concerned with imports of 'junk' food versus the protection of locally processed foods. It is true that the lack of a food policy in the different countries of the Near East disturbs the food system. In Egypt a law was passed that all food could be imported tax free and without foreign currency restrictions. As a result, you now see chocolate cakes and potato chips even in a country that produces and exports potatoes. You find imported Uncle Ben's rice available while Egypt is a rice-exporter. All kinds of foods such as these are found on the market, and unfortunately, they are readily purchased by the Egyptian public. Now the government is trying to change this law, but the basic foods are not available to replace the junk foods. It is a question of Egypt's lacking a food policy that could make more basic foods available instead of foods that are not needed. Parpia was quite right in saying that industrial development in Egypt suffered from this kind of import policy. Recently, many issues have been raised in the Egyptian press about the question of a food import tax and how the traders are taking advantage of the system and are bringing in poor-quality foods -- foods not fit for human consumption, such as animal or cat foods being used for humans -- at the expense of locally processed food.

Pinstrup-Andersen: You are raising the question of self-sufficiency versus comparative advantage in agricultural production. One has to be very careful not to take too naive a point of view at a time when food is, in fact, being used as a political tool by one of the biggest food exporters in the world. I think that a country that depends on the import of basic staples for its population is in a very uncomfortable situation, even though the cost of domestic production may greatly exceed the current import prices. The comparative advantage argument has somehow to be modified by political realities.

Let me mention a few examples. We saw strong reactions in the beginning of the 1970s when fertilizer prices went up dramatically, and there was great panic insofar as actual availability was concerned. We saw a large increase in investment, or at least investment plans, for fertilizer production in importing countries. Fertilizer had suddenly become a strategic commodity and countries could not afford to depend on imports. This is obviously more important in the case of staple foods. We also see similar reactions in the case of energy dependence. Brazil is greatly expanding its production of alchohol from sugar cane, primarily to reduce the dependence on imports. So, I do not think we should be surprised when traditional food importers at least try to reduce their dependency on food imports. Additionally, I think we have seen important problems arise out of the dependency on imports of commodities that cannot easily be produced in the importing country. I am referring here to wheat, not only wheat imported through the PL 480 and similar USAID programmes, but also through commercial channels. This was discussed in the previous session.

To add one other thing, I am wondering to what extent we are overstating the problem of importing convenience foods and 'junk' foods. I think it is an important issue at the household level, but I wonder whether, in fact, countries that are short on food and long on foreign exchange are not primarily importing staple foods. And if they are not, if they are putting emphasis on milk from Denmark, which by the way is a very good commodity, if they are emphasizing convenience foods and high-priced calorie foods, then what is wrong with the system? Is it because the additional incomes are not really distributed well in society so that there is a great accumulation of wealth and therefore a greater increase in the demand for processed foods by some segment of society, or are governments making decisions on food imports that go against the demands of the population? I am concerned as to whether we are overstating the problem, or whether governments are making some strange import decisions.

Gerhart: That would be worth future study. Are these imports really 'junk' foods or basic staples?

Salameh: Up to this point in the workshop, we have dealt with potential in agriculture and food production. We have collected great columns of information and data about population growth and nutrition problems in the Middle East and other areas in the world, but we have not considered governmental bodies and structures that are concerned with agricultural and nutritional affairs, particularly organizations that plan and evaluate activities in nutrition. In the Middle East, to what extent can these structures cope with the potential and the problems to insure significant food and nutrition policies?

Miladi: This is a valid question. Unfortunately, food in the Middle East has no identity and there is nobody to deal with food. Ministries of Agriculture only deal with production. Food is only a commodity of agriculture and they are not concerned with what happens with the production or who will consume it. The Ministries of Supply are concerned with imports. The Ministries of Economy are concerned with prices and inflation, while the Ministries of Health treat diseases caused by poor nutrition. Food and nutrition are rarely the major concerns of anybody and are not receiving enough priority.

If you go to a country and ask about the food and nutrition situation, there is no information. If you ask about trends in consumption, again there is no information. If you ask about the impact of certain policies, the question will not be answered, nor would questions about the impact of food price subsidies on nutrition. The main problem is that there is no identity within government structures to deal with the food situation, and the personnel do not exist either. There are only two or three institutions in the world that deal with food and nutrition policy from the socioeconomic and political aspects. Food does not have an identity, in spite of the amount of money that the consumer spends on it every day.

Allan: In many cases, new enterprises demand large amounts of energy, and in Egypt one can see many new enterprises involving livestock, poultry, beef cattle, milk production, etc. All of these enterprises are poor converters of energy if you take the overall picture into account. Gerhart said in an earlier session that the Egyptian energy policy is in an extremely poor state, with huge subsidies that cause structural distortions throughout the economy. It is also importing a huge amount of energy. We have heard about Saudi Arabia and how it is importing large amounts of food, some of which may be 'junk' food. Here is a country exporting its oil to another country that processes it into food to the benefit of its industries and population and returns it to Saudi Arabia. In order to combat this, Saudi Arabia is developing large agribusiness enterprises whose ecological and economic apects are dubious and whose energy aspects are absolutely appalling.

This leads to the next point. We have been discussing food, but food depends largely on energy. A number of workshop participants have been hinting at this in their statements, but I would like to bring it a little more out into the open and encourage more discussion on this point. I think that we should be considering the energy aspect of food production in this area. The economists are good about providing inputs, outputs, profitabilities, value-cost ratios, and all sorts of graphs and equations, but from some of the books I have been reading recently, I gather economics and its devotees have no real mechanism for coping with situations of resource depletion. This is certainly the situation with regard to energy stocks. They are a finite resource, representing the world's capital, and if we use them up, that is it, they are gone! Economists should be trying to come to grips with this situation. An aspect policy makers could look at and give more emphasis to is the question of energy balances of various food production technologies.

Nahal: I would like to make a few comments on a subject I think is very important in the region concerning the relationship between the rapid growth of population and the conservation of natural agricultural/industrial resources. I will take Syria as an example because I know it very well.

Syria is currently undergoing very rapid population growth, increasing by between 3.5 and 4 percent annually. At this rate, the total population will reach 18 million by the year 2000. The implications of this growth for agriculture and natural resources are clear and alarming. Indeed, just to approach the country's goal of self-sufficiency in food, Syria will have to more than double its present output of basic food and fiber commodities within 20 years, using a land base that will not expand enough, even including the projected new land in the Euphrates project. Such rapid population growth will put severe strains on the country's agricultural resources, particularly on soil, water, forest and land management. This presssure, indeed, could lead to agricultural resource degradation and deterioration and also to accelerated desertification if sound and integrated management, conservation, and development of agricultural resources are not followed.

This example could be applied to the other countries in the region, particularly Lebanon, Iraq, and Jordan. Indeed, this accelerated desertification and a deterioration of the natural and agricultural resources is currently taking place in both rainfed and irrigated agricultural zones. For this reason, I think that any project of developing agriculture and food production in this region should take into consideration the very important problems of water and soil conservation. In the Euphrates Basin in Syria the irrigated lands are deteriorating because of waterlogging and salinization that have led to a loss of 5,000 hectares per year. If we do not take this into consideraton, after 20 years 100,000 hectares will be out of production. The same danger exists in rainfed agriculture on hillsides. Some studies have shown that in Syria, 50 to 80 tons of top soil per hectare per year are lost in these sloping areas. We are improving soil fertility by using fertilizers to improve yields, but we are not protecting the soil from degradation.

I would like to summarize what I think ICARDA can do in the future in this field. First, it can develop research projects to control desertification in rainfed agriculture and prevent wind and water erosion. Second, it can develop sound management principles of irrigated agriculture in order to protect the environment. Third, it could develop a research programme on land use capacity to identify erosion, topography and flood-control problems. This is a part of sound water and soil management. Fourth, it could develop a programme for recycling organic materials in order to increase the fertility of the soil.

El-Achkar: I would like to point out some social and economic factors behind the low productivity that explain the slow expansion of food production in the agrarian regions of Syria.

The first factor is related to marketing problems. Farmers sometimes fail to expand their production of certain kinds of fruits and vegetables because the demand for them is limited, although the climate and other conditions are favourable for doing so. If there were some food industries using these fruits and vegetables as ingredients, farmers could produce larger quantities of them. Tomatoes and onions are examples of this.

The second factor is related to migration from rural to urban areas. The migratory movement disturbs the distribution of the labour force and creates problems in the villages as well as in the cities. In particular, some agrarian regions in Syria have become short of labour because of this migration. This hinders the process of carrying out economic development programmes in these rural areas. The only way to solve this problem is to improve the living conditions of farmers and to increase the provision of social services in the villages.

The third factor, as noted by Nahal, is demographic. Large family size and high dependency ratios in Syria seem to decrease the potential for savings and investments in rural areas that are essential for improving living conditions and raising productivity. Introducing new agricultural technology needs capital that is not available to farmers with many children. Expanding fruit trees, for example, requires farmers to sacrifice land revenue for several years. Poor people cannot afford to do this.

The last factor is related to property and land tenure. If farmers operate on small holdings they will not be in a position to take advantage of this division of labour in farming. Small holdings do not enable farmers to raise productivity from economies of scale as larger holdings do. Small holdings do not stimulate the introduction of new and expensive machinery in agricultural work. Combining the money of neighbouring farmers into one productive cooperative may be helpful in this case to increase productivity. Therefore, it is important, in carrying out investigations at the regional level, to consider these and other social and economic problems if we are to improve food production in the area.

Halila: In the last session, Nygaard threw the ball to the plant breeder and the agronomist. In this session we have heard statements from Miladi suggesting what plant breeders and agronomists should do. I do not pretend to speak on behalf of the scientists at the international centres, but let me give the point of view of an agronomist in a national programme.

The problem is not that simple. When we start development programmes at the national level, say improvements of cereal or legume production, there are priorities that we have to consider. When people have empty stomachs, they are not going to look for the nutritional quality of the product. Therefore, the first priority is to increase yield, and after we have achieved high and stable yields we can then look at the nutritional properties of the agricultural product. We have to reach self-sufficiency first, and give people enough to eat before attending to nutritional quality.

However, I do agree with most of the discussants who have made comments so far in the workshop. A multidisciplinary approach is necessary -- a global approach to the problems should be used to increase agricultural production and improve nutrition. In this context, I would like to say that I am delighted to be attending this conference because it is the first of its kind in the region. We have the nutritonist, the agronomist, and the agricultural economist grouped around one table, the first step in achieving the multi- and interdisciplinary approach.

I would like to give an example that occurred last year in Tunisia to demonstrate this approach. To enhance nutrition education, the government put some publicity spots on the radio encouraging people to eat (especially women who were breast-feeding their babies) such and such a food. One of the publicity items asked the population to eat lentils. Six months later a high demand for lentils was created and the Department of Cereals came to the

National Institute and asked what we had done or could do with this crop because large quantities of lentils were having to be imported in order to satisfy the local demand. We found that the problem had been neglected for a long time. In examining the production figures we noticed that the area devoted to lentils had decreased by 80 percent from 1975 to 1981 -- from 5,000 hectares to 1,000 hectares. We asked agricultural economists to make a survey to find out why this happened. They found that the farmers were stopping lentil production because the prices were not good and because there was a problem in harvesting the crop. At harvest, pod-shattering was a big problem. Therefore, the farmers were switching to other crops. This example, from my point of view, clearly illustrates the multidisciplinary approach: the nutritionists who put the spot on the radio and encouraged people to eat lentils, the agronomist who had to increase production through breeding for high and more stable yields, the economist who identified the production problems and price constraints, and the mechanical engineer who will have to devise the appropriate machines to harvest lentils without pod-shattering once the high-yielding varieties are achieved.

My second comment is on the paper presented by Miladi. I agree with him that agriculture has been neglected in Tunisia in terms of investment, and the government is trying to bridge this gap. As a point of information, 17 percent of the total amount of the money that will be invested in the current development plan in Tunisia will be devoted to agriculture. This has never happened before.

Miladi: We are not really looking to plant breeders to increase protein quantity. In North Africa we have couscous and chickpeas if nothing else. In Egypt we have the faba beans, bread, rice, lentils and oils. Here in Syria we have the hommos bi-taheeni. We have a lot of traditional foods with high nutritional value, and we have to retain these foods. There is no protein gap per se. One cannot find kwashiorkor (protein-deficient) children in our society. It has to be made clear to the plant breeder that he does not need to look at only lysine and methionine, but the whole diet.

Mansour: I would like to go back to this radio publicity spot and explain why we formulated this campaign because it was an accident. One day there was a woman waiting in the Institute of Nutrition to see us. She said that 10 years ago she used to eat lentils when she became pregnant because it was good for the baby. We agreed with her and it gave us the idea for this radio spot. However, we did not know that lentil production in Tunisia was decreasing. Why? Because we did not have any relationship with the Ministry of Agriculture. This was perhaps our fault, but one kind of problem a workshop of this sort should address is how to get different specialists from Ministries of Agriculture, or Health and Nutrition, etc. together. This is one of the problems that most of the countries in the region face.

Srivastava: I would like to highlight with several examples what is happening in North Africa and the Middle East with respect to consumer uses of the crops that are already being cultivated. Previously, barley was used by the population for food, but slowly, in most of the countries, human consumption of barley has decreased. In Syria, I have been told that previously there were a number of nutritious local products in the diet, such as freekia or cracked wheat. In North Africa a major use of wheat was for couscous and bulgar. Today, can we go to a market and find a kilo of these products readily available for the housewife to purchase? I have been told that the nutritional value of freekia is exceptionally high, but nowadays it has become expensive to make freekia and no technology has been developed to prepare it quickly and cheaply. Therefore, it is not now available. Western technology has arrived. The bread in Syria is made from flour that has an extraction level of 83-85%; the most nutritious part of the grain is thrown away because the flour mills here were developed elsewhere to produce yeast bread, not the local flat bread. Saudi Arabia traditionally grew a sizeable amount of durum wheat. Recently, the Saudis have built very sophisticated flour mills and the policy now is to grow only bread wheat because the millers say that is the only kind they can mill. We are gradually losing some of the most nutritious of our traditional foods. We certainly should work for yield increases and stability in barley, durum and bread wheat production, but can we not think about developing local technology for local products?

For example, we are looking at what we can do to make better local bread, bulgar, or couscous. But it seems that even if we knew how to make better bulgar, we lack the small-scale industry that could be set up in the village next to our research station. Who can produce bulgar with durum wheat so that the local products that were so good nutritionally in the past can be revived? In the absence of this technology, I am afraid we will have to import canned foods. If we want to restore barley to the diet and use durum wheat, let us return to historical uses of these products in the Middle East. We at ICARDA are willing to carry on research, but we also need to develop the technology for small-scale industries within the region. I do not see this developing yet. Parpia has done an excellent job at CITRI in India, where they are successfully developing small-scale industries to make food products Indians like. There is a need in the Middle East and North Africa for such industries.

Scrimshaw: The remark on traditional technology deserves support but I want to comment on the intervention of Halila. One of the purposes of this interface workshop was to indicate some agricultural realities to nutritionists so that they would not make nutrition education recommendations that are not feasible, and at the same time make sure that agriculturalists would not work towards nutritional goals that are trivial or unimportant. The intervention suggests a difference between nutritional considerations in agricultural policy and nutritional considerations in plant-breeding goals. I think most nutritionists would agree with him that a goal of increasing cereal production, with protein quality and quantity at the bottom of the list, is a perfectly good set of priorities. An emphasis on legume production and a small increase in legume intake can have a far greater impact on protein status than would any increase in protein level that could be achieved in a cereal-breeding programme. Essentially, we would recommend exactly what he said, except that there should be coordination between the nutritional advice for increased legume consumption and local agricultural practices.

I would also like to comment on Gerhart's emphasis on the migration of workers in the Middle East to the Gulf states. Miladi discussed the very high birth rates and population increase. In emphasizing this pull part of it, there should also be emphasis on the push part of it. Some of the reasons for the migration are because these rates of population increase obviously have serious implications for agricultural demand, policy, and ultimately the nutritional status of people in the region.

Khattab: Both Nour and Gerhart mentioned the importance of animals in the farming systems in the region. I would like to emphasize this point and add to it. It is very important to consider animal husbandry and animal production in these farming systems, especially since a large section of the population is engaged in forage or pasture production for animal feeding. ICARDA should concern itself more with this aspect, and I am glad to note that it has a programme on forage legumes. This programme should be developed further to include other types of pasture plants and to evaluate them, not only from the point of view of increasing dry matter, but also for the utilization of these grasses by farm animals. These forage crops should be evaluated by digestibility analysis and other methods to determine the true nutritive value of these grasses for animals. This is particularly important because in this region much of our animal protein is imported from abroad. There is good potential here if we emphasize animal production in future research at ICARDA and other similar institutions. Perhaps we can reverse the current practice of importing meat, milk, and other products from abroad. I think this would go a long way to serve the majority of the people who are engaged in animal husbandry and forage production.

Pellett: The term "junk food" has been used several times. It is a very emotive term that is applied to items like carbonated soft drinks that supply only calories, as well as to fast-food meals that may include hamburger and salad, or fish and chips. Obviously, spending money for "useless" calories is wasteful, but fast-foods can make a considerable addition to the good nutrition of people and often give good value for money spent.

I should like to add to Srivastava's comments concerning traditional foods. In the very early stages of planning for this workshop, we discussed having a session on local food industries. It was not possible because of the difficulty in obtaining this type of information. In general, food habits in the Middle East are excellent because of the balance of the many types of food used and the way they are mixed together. A sound rule of nutrition is that the more food components are combined into a meal or a dietary, the better the nutritional balance; this is the hall mark of Middle Eastern diets. If many of the traditional foods are allowed to be replaced by use of imported products, there will be a nutritional loss for the region.

Myntti: On the subject of consumption, allow me to give you an example from a village in North Yemen where I lived for two years, working in my field of anthropology. The economy of the community was dominated, not by agriculture, but by the migration of its men and the inflow of remittances. As elsewhere in Yemen, agriculture in this village was limited to sorghum production on rainfed lands, and was a risky undertaking. Nour has already pointed to the constant problem of risk in the rainfed zones of the Middle East. With the labour shortages caused by migration and general inflation, inputs for agricultural production were very expensive. Given the risk and the inflated costs of growing sorghum, I saw that farming households were making decisions -- indeed rational, economic ones -- on whether to cultivate their lands or not. The decisions were made considerably easier in that it cost the farmers less to buy imported wheat than to grow their own sorghum. Moreover, deciding not to cultivate had a secondary effect on animal production since the main source of fodder -- sorghum stalks -- was no longer available. The villagers therefore sold their animals and were deprived of dairy products. The main point is that international and national economic trends have clear effects, not only on production in remote "subsistence"-level agricultural areas, but also on consumption and nutrition at the household level.

What is more, cultural attitudes influence how people behave in any given economic context. To consider the women and children left behind in the Yemeni village, thanks to remittances from their migrant male kin, they can, in theory at least buy meats, fresh fruits, vegetables, and a range of imported foods. But this is not what happens. First, the physical mobility of Yemeni women is restricted. It is not considered proper for a village woman to walk into the market town where fresh produce is available and unless she has an efficient messenger service via her children or neighbours, she, as the acting household head, might not be able to reach the nutritionally valuable goods available in the market. Instead she buys staples available from a nearby village shop:

sweets, soft drinks, macaroni, rice. Second, a woman alone with her children might not think it appropriate to eat high-status foods like meat and fresh fruits in the absence of the household men.

During my years in rural North Yemen I witnessed significant changes in the diet. People were eating fewer local dairy products, sorghum breads, porridges and beans, and more sugar, white breads, macaroni, rice, and potatoes. These changes have taken place in less than five years. Do nutritionists have a methodology for measuring the nutritional consequences of such rapid dietary change?

Miladi: If changing dietary patterns have an effect on nutrition from a public health viewpoint, then nutritionists can play a role. If, however, people are shifting from sorghum to wheat and there is no sign of deficiency in their diets, one should not feel a human being has to eat certain things. Nutritionists intervene only when public health is endangered. Changing dietary patterns that cause obesity or coronary heart disease in the oil-producing countries, and the change from breast-feeding to bottle-feeding with its consequences of increased preschool child mortality -- are situations where nutritionists should intervene.

Pellett: To answer Myntti's questions, the methodology is fully available, but often the will to do the surveys and the money are limiting. There are a number of organizations doing what is now called nutritional surveillance and projects are being set up in various parts of the world. For example, there is a group at Cornell that has a large AID grant to implement these projects. They do not have much activity in the Middle East as yet, although I believe they were working in Yemen. The idea behind nutritional surveillance is that at the government level there should be the ability to follow inter alia changing dietary patterns within the community and to monitor whether these changes are beneficial or not. If diets appear to be going in the wrong direction in that adverse effects are appearing, the team can then suggest changes before nutritional disease occurs. The methods are there, but the application is limited.

Karrar: In Sudan we are formulating homemade weaning foods, and we have tried most of the legumes consumed in the region. We found that chickpea is of high biological value, and I see from Nour's presentation that ICARDA is paying a lot of attention to this crop. I am wondering if ICARDA has any intention of doing a biological evaluation of legumes? If not, on what grounds do you increase the production of these legumes? Is it only because of the demand? Why do not we also improve the nutritional value of these legumes? If there is no unit in ICARDA to do these evaluations, I suggest you have a small laboratory evaluate the nutrients in these legumes.

I did some work on anemias in the U.A.E. and would like to make a comment on Miladi's remarks about anemia in the Middle East. In this study we found that, even though the people in U.A.E. have one of the highest incomes in the world, anemia among preschool and school-age children is very high and most of the children are infested with parasites. Scrimshaw has written extensively about relationships between infection and/or infestation and malnutrition. If we want to improve the nutritional status of a population, it is not only the diet but other factors like infection and sanitation that are important.

Our colleague from Tunisia said that the agronomist may not be able to do much about nutritional objectives in a breeding programme. We have found that the staple diet in most areas is rice and the iron in rice is found to be poorly utilized. Therefore, breeders have a great role to play if the staple diet is of low biological value. They could introduce cultivars with more nutritionally available iron. If we can orient breeders and also agricultural economists toward nutritional issues the role they play might be even more useful.

Williams: I have three small points to make. The first is that we have a very active forage evaluation programme at ICARDA. There is a comprehensive laboratory for determining the nutritional quality of the crops -- forages, legumes, and cereals. Evan Thomson and the forage programme scientists are in the process of doing livestock evaluation studies as well, so laboratory analysis is being done.

Second, there has been much discussion about priorities of increasing yield or the nutritive value of crops. There is no real reason why the two cannot be done at the same time. All international centres that I know of have laboratories, and it is simply a matter of doing some additional chemical analysis of protein quantity or amino acid balance, which can go hand in hand with efforts to increase yields. There is no reason why there should be any diversion in priorities as far as improving nutritional value is concerned.

Third, to support Scrimshaw's comments, I certainly agree that we should do much more work on local, specialized foods -- foods that you do not hear much about; kisht in Egypt is an example. Can we produce these foods economically? Quite likely we can. We are certainly going to investigate this possibility at ICARDA. One of the things we need to know is why these foods have suddenly stopped being made. If there is a reason why people have stopped using local foods, perhaps they do not want us to start making them again. We must ask these questions first.

Pinstrup-Andersen: Following-up our discussion in the previous session, I believe we agreed that if we were going to have anything useful to say about priorities in agricultural research from a nutrition point of view, we must know what poor and malnourished people consume and how they react to changes in the prices of these commodities. We must also know what poor, malnourished farmers produce and how they would react to new technology. My question is to the two speakers in this session who presented excellent data on national averages. Do we, in fact, in this region know anything about what poor people are eating? Do we know how they would react to changes in prices of given commodities? The only comment that I heard to that effect in this session was the comment on the Tunisian food survey, but I am aware of similar surveys in the Sudan, Egypt, and Kuwait. There may well be surveys of this nature in all of the countries in the region, and if so, we should try to pull the data out of the surveys.

Gerhart: I think that is partly the answer to Williams' question about local foods as well. We need to look at what is happening to household labour. The special local foods require a long time for preparation, the men are no longer there, and the women have many new economic functions that they did not have previously. Thus, their time to prepare these foods is significantly altered, and we know very little about household budgeting under these circumstances.

Nygaard: I would like to make two comments. The first is to add to what Nahal said. In the pre-conference mailing, participants received an article by Lester Brown in which he recounted many of the things Nahal said about the loss of soil and deterioration of natural resources, etc. The loss of agricultural land to development and to urban expansion is obviously a problem in Syria. If you drive from Aleppo to Afrin you cross some of the best agricultural land in Syria, and it is being turned into a suburb this very minute. I believe there is a real need for some rural zoning to preserve that land.

I would like to respond to Halila's comments in which he addressed a very interesting problem of declining lentil production. The Ford Foundation has made some money available to the Farming Systems Program at ICARDA and about $10,000 of that money was designated for just such a research project.

<u>Nour:</u> My task has been made easier by Nygaard's last remarks. Neither do I wish to make a summation of this two-and-a-half-hour session; I simply could not do it. But I would like to say how thoroughly enjoyable the discussion has been and how useful it is to ICARDA. We have learned a great deal from the contributions and participation of the various people, including the distinguished array of priorities that Gerhart gave to us as the discussant of this session. We have taken copious notes.

I do want to address a point raised by Pinstrup-Andersen concerning food security and issues related to the political and social aspects of that function. I entirely agree that we should not oversimplify that situation, but there are certain countries that are, in fact, overdoing it. I agree that we ought to have a reasonable balance. We have to keep a very careful watch on how we criticize the food security policy of countries like Egypt, Sudan, Syria, Jordan, Iraq, Pakistan, and others. But when it comes to a country like Saudi Arabia, I think there is a certain amount of extremism exercised there that ought to be recognized. If grain were stored, it would be a much cheaper and a much more permanent way to sustain our food security. We would save scarce natural resources, particularly water, and also energy in the production of food at such high costs.

I am particularly impressed with the statement made by Myntti on her experiences in Yemen. Yemen is a country in which ICARDA would like to develop a project. We would like to draw on your experience on this issue because when we set our policy for outreach work, it is contributions of this nature that we ought to consider in advance.

I would also like to say that the contributions of Khattab and Nahal on recommendations for ICARDA are much appreciated, and we will certainly bear these in mind as we develop our long-term objectives. The remarks on local industry are much needed and, of course, this is not news to ICARDA. Scrimshaw brought this up here to get a reaction, and we are delighted to see unanimous support for the need to study local foods.

SECTION IV

GENETIC IMPROVEMENT AND NUTRITION

NUTRITIONAL GOALS FOR PLANT BREEDERS WITH PARTICULAR REFERENCE TO FOOD LEGUME RESEARCH AT ICARDA

RICARDO BRESSANI

INTRODUCTION

The number of basic foods that are now providing the main nutrients for mankind is relatively small. These include some eight cereal grains and about 14 food legumes. Furthermore, the protein quality and nutritive value of these foods leave much to be desired, particularly for specific population groups. Cereal grains are low in protein and in the essential amino acids lysine, tryptophan and threonine, while food legumes are low in total sulfur amino acids.

The quantity produced may not be sufficient, but even that available is often subjected to losses that may be qualitatively, technologically and nutritionally very important. It is therefore urgent and important to upgrade in whatever way possible all the components of productivity.

As shown in Figure 1 these factors are included in a multivariable equation, made up of three main factors: a production factor, a postharvest technology factor, and a nutritional factor. Furthermore, these factors are made up of a series of components that are the expression of the genetic makeup of the food crop, be it a cereal grain or a food legume. Thus, if these components are chemical entities and have a genetic base, they probably show variability and one could, therefore, select for them.

The production factor (kilograms/hectare) is made up of a number of components, including plant characteristics, resistance to disease and insect attack, environmental conditions and agricultural practices. Their interactions are very well known by agronomists and plant geneticists, and will not be further discussed here. The postharvest technology factor in the equation also has many components. These include those that interact during handling and storage, those of importance in industrial or home processing, the effects on product production or development, cooking quality, and acceptability by the consumer. The final factor in the equation, that of nutritional quality, includes components such as protein and amino acid availability or digestibility, presence of antiphysiological factors and fiber, vitamin, mineral, and carbohydrate utilization. It is important to note that these three main factors in the productivity equation are not independent of each other, and the interactions that exist may affect one more than the other.

Therefore, in breeding and production programmes of any particular food crop, all factors must be considered together. It is, however, necessary to select the most important component in the postharvest technology and nutrition factor and to develop rapid screening procedures useful to the plant breeder and geneticist. This will be possible if communication between scientists exists and if basic knowledge is developed to understand the biochemical basis of the results observed. Some of the components within each factor, and in particular the postharvest technology and nutrition factors, are food-crop-specific and specific for end-use by the consumer; therefore, it would not be expected or desirable for plant breeders to include all of them in breeding programmes. Furthermore, it is important to obtain basic knowledge on the biochemical basis for the development of the component of interest within each factor as a means to control it in the particular food crop in which it is present. A classical example is high-lysine or opaque-2 corn. A gene increased the protein quality of the corn, but it also resulted in low yields and poor postharvest conservation and processing.

This paper will discuss those postharvest technology and nutrition factors that are of importance in food legumes, with particular reference, whenever possible, to the food legumes of interest to ICARDA, so as to be able to propose nutritional objectives for these food legumes.

Production: The First Priority

Food legumes are considered to be relatively good sources of protein, particularly when consumed together with cereal grains, whose protein is very well complemented by legume protein. The problem, however, is that because of a relatively low and unstable yield per unit of land area, availability of food legumes is also low and thus increases cost to the consumer. This is reflected in a low frequency of intake as can be seen from dietary surveys conducted in Guatemala, shown in Table 1 (1). The frequency of intake by most people is from three to four times per week, but is less for those who need it most (1). This, of course, has nutritional implications because, as shown in Table 2, the protein quality of the diet will shift to a lower value as the frequency of legume intake falls. In this particular example, rats were fed a basal corn diet combined with common beans. As bean intake was gradually decreased to zero, both weight gain and the amount of total nitrogen in the carcass of the animals also decreased (2,4).

Similar observations have been made in children who were fed cooked corn and beans at different time intervals. The nitrogen retention values obtained are shown in Figure 2, which clearly indicates a reduction in protein complementation as evidenced by lower nitrogen retention as the bean intake time interval increased from 3 to 12 hours (1,2). Obviously, the effect of lower frequency of intake on nutritive value will be more important for those population groups needing more and higher protein-quality diets, such as children and pregnant and lactating women.

As mentioned earlier, legume protein is an excellent supplementary source of protein when combined with cereal grains. This is evident from an analysis of the protein quality response curves shown in Figure 3 for different food legumes mixed with different cereal grains. In all cases there is an improvement in protein quality as the legume protein increases in the diet. A maximum is reached, to decrease again as less cereal or less legume protein is included in the diet. The peak value may be broad as for mixtures of rice with common beans, or it may be sharp as with corn and common bean mixtures.

The same situation occurs with faba bean and whole wheat mixtures, as is shown in Figure 4. Maximum protein quality in this food consumption system takes place when intake of faba beans and whole wheat is in a ratio of about three to seven by weight. If the actual consumption for a population is at point A, increasing bean intake will result in protein quality B. For this to be achieved, production and availability must increase and costs must decrease. On the other hand, consumption to give quality B may never be reached because of factors other than availability and cost. These could include undesirable physiological effects, low acceptability, or excessive cost of preparation. In any case, the low consumption frequency and the low intake level seem reasons enough to indicate that increased production may be a first priority in breeding programmes for all legumes.

Postharvest Technology Factors: A Second Priority

Postharvest technology factors of the productivity equation are used here in a broad sense, and include both components in food legumes inherited by the seed itself and those acquired after harvest. The various aspects considered relate to storage and handling, processing at the industrial level, and to factors of importance at the home level. These may be highly significant as far as the consumer is concerned. Agricultural programmes in many developing countries introduce improved seed selected on the basis of high yield per unit area, in the belief that producers will benefit from using them, because higher production implies higher income. However, the disregard of factors such as industrial or home processing and of acceptability by consumers has often resulted in disappointment and losses to the producers, who then return to cultivating the seed they have selected and are familiar with, even though yields are lower. For illustration, three factors will be discussed. These are: (i) storage and handling; (ii) milling characteristics, and (iii) the hard-to-cook condition that is very common in most food legumes.

Storage and Handling. A great deal more attention should be given to the processing of food legumes in order to increase their importance as sources of nutrients for the world population. Important problems in industrial or home processing of food legumes are to be found not only in their physical inherited characteristics, but also in those that often develop during storage and handling after harvest. If storage conditions are not adequate, at least three problems may arise: i) insect and mould infestation, ii) losses during milling or home preparation, and iii) increased cooking time. All these may cause high physical losses as well as reduction in nutritive value.

Studies carried out in India (3), which are shown in Table 3, indicate that infested chickpeas or pigeon peas lost about 18 percent of their protein quality. The loss may be due to contamination from uric acid, a protein metabolite of insects, as well as to increases in fat acidity and microbial infestation, and even to losses of grain fractions. Besides a qualitative loss there is also a quantitative loss, as is shown in Table 4, for chickpea subjected to milling to produce dhal. The infested grain yielded 65 percent dhal, while the control gave values of 82 percent, which is close to the theoretical figure. Resistance to insect attack has been reported for common beans (4). Faba beans are also attacked by insects, and a report indicated that infestation for local cultivars was 37.0 to 76.6 percent (5). It is possible to conclude, therefore, that natural resistance to insect infestation exists, so a closer cooperation between plant breeders and food technologists should be established. Results of such cooperation could be improved resistance, thus alleviating storage problems, reducing chemical treatment for insect control, maintaining nutritive value, and increased efficiency of processing.

Milling. Most food legumes are consumed with the seed coat. An exception is cowpeas in both India and Africa. However, increased production and use of food legumes will generally result only if such foods are processed into flours or other products. If this is the case, removal of the hull may be an important problem to be solved. Legume species vary in the amount of dhal they yield. This may be partly because of the amount of seedcoat in the seed (3). Some further relevant information is shown in Table 6, demonstrating high variation within and between species with respect to the percentage of seed coats in various food legumes (3). Storage conditions influence milling efficiency for removal of the seed coat. Although milling processing conditions can be adjusted to increase yield of the edible fraction, this may be facilitated by selecting for lower seed coat percentages in the grain or by changing the shape of the seed, because regular-shaped grain varieties can be milled more easily than irregular varieties. The development of loose-husked varieties should be given priority in order to improve milling outputs, increase quality, and reduce processing costs. Furthermore, as will be discussed later, it may also improve protein quality.

Cooking Quality. Storage and handling factors may also affect appearance and cookability of food legumes, and therefore these broader areas of concern that have economic and social significance should not be overlooked in food legume research. It is well known that food legumes take more time to cook than cereal grains, but it has been observed that even longer cooking is necessary when food legumes are stored under adverse climatic conditions, in comparison to recently harvested seed. In addition to the inherent characteristics of food legumes, the "hard-to-cook" condition seems to be influenced by time, temperature, and relative humidity during storage.

This effect is shown in Figure 5 which shows cooking characteristics of common beans stored for up to nine months at 35° C. Samples withdrawn at 0, 3, and 9 months were cooked at atmospheric pressure in water (1 part beans to 3 parts water) and their hardness was measured using an Instron Texturometer. A value of about 90 g-force was chosen as the acceptable degree of hardness by consumers. Cooking time for the same hardness increases with storage time. As indicated previously, moisture content in beans seems to increase the problem as is shown in Figure 6. These studies reported by Burr and Kon (6) demonstrated clearly that moisture content, temperature, and length of storage influence how much cooking time is required for presoaked beans to become tender. In addition to increasing cooking time, storage also affects protein quality. This is shown by the results in Figure 7, in which common beans were stored up to six months (7). The beans were soaked for 16 hours prior to cooking under 15 lbs pressure (121° C) for the time shown. Besides a decrease in quality because of longer cooking time, storage also decreases protein quality through heat damage, resulting in a lower available lysine (8). Because beans become hard with increased storage time, it is also possible that ten minutes of cooking were not enough to destroy antiphysiological substances.

Cooking time is also a problem affecting Faba beans and chick peas. With Faba beans, Youssef and El-Tabey (9) demonstrated the significance of various physical properties of the seed itself in relation to cooking quality, as shown in Table 7. They found the seed coat to be of importance as were the chemical constituents of the cotyledons, such as starch and protein.

As early as 1921, Glover (10) described the problem and suggested that in food legumes, two types of hardness are found: hardshell and sclerema. Hardshell was described as a physical condition in which the seed failed to absorb water. Sclerema, on the other hand, took place in the cotyledons and was induced by various factors that are still under investigation today. In this situation the cotyledons become very hard and often dark in colour.

A working diagram on the general process of bean-hardening is shown in Figure 8, which indicates that the hard-to-cook condition is inherent in the seed and may be affected by both pre-and post-harvest handling. Under poor storage conditions the problem seems to increase. Various theories have been proposed, including: polymerization of polyphenolic compounds in the seed coat where these substances are found (11), and changes in the microchemical structure of the cotyledons involving carbohydrates, pectic substances, phytic acid, and K, Ca, and Mg ions (12, 13).

Nutritional Quality: A Third Priority

The third factor in the multifactorial equation of productivity is the nutritional quality of the food product. For purposes of discussion this has been divided into positive and limiting components, as shown in Table 8.

Positive factors. Food legumes in general contain relatively high levels of protein; for *Phaseolus vulgaris* this ranges from 19 to 31 percent with an average of 24 percent (1). With respect to *Vicia faba*, average values are closer to 30 percent. In addition to their high protein content, food legumes are also excellent sources of lysine, with a reported range of 207 to 607 mg/g N. Lysine values for *Vicia faba* have been reported to be about 400 mg/g N, which is similar to the average value for Phaseolus of 464 mg/g N. Since food legumes are relatively high in lysine, the amino acid deficient in cereal grains, it follows that they are excellent complementary proteins to cereal grains. This is indicated by the results shown in Figure 9. In every case, the combination giving the highest protein quality is that in which the two component systems are around a weight ratio of seven parts cereal to three parts food legume. This ratio seldom changes, but higher levels of either lysine or methionine increase the quality at the best ratio. These results, known for some time, are brought about by the lysine contribution of the food legume protein to that of the cereal protein, which in turn supplies the sulfur amino acids lacking in legume food protein. Thus, on the cereal side of each figure, lysine is the most limiting amino acid, while on the legume side, sulfur amino acids become first limiting.

The mixture giving the highest quality can still be improved by the simultaneous addition of lysine and methionine, as shown in Table 9. *Vicia faba* responded to methionine supplementation and wheat to lysine addition as expected. Furthermore, both amino acids added together to the 7:3 mixture of wheat and faba beans resulted in increased protein quality. Such an increase can also be obtained by adding 10 percent milk to the 7:3 mixture, as is also shown in Table 9. These results suggest, therefore, that some nutritional benefit could be derived if beans had a slightly higher sulfur amino acid content. Selection for the most appropriate legume for complementing a cereal should be based on methionine content. The results also suggest that the nutritional goals for either food legumes or cereal grains must be based on food consumption patterns as they exist in regions or countries.

Limiting factors: Antiphysiological substances. The presence of antiphysiological substances in common beans has been known for some time. Much attention has been given in the past to the trypsin inhibitors, lectins, and the flatulence factors in comon beans, but only recently have the polyphenolic compounds also been considered (11). In Figure 10 (left) the changes are shown in trypsin inhibitors, hemagglutinins, and polyphenolic compounds relative to cooking time at atmospheric pressure. In this case, 500 g of black-coated beans were placed in 1,500 cc of boiling water and small samples were withdrawn at specific times, freeze-dried, and chemically analyzed. Both trypsin inhibitors and hemagglutinins disappear at about 90 minutes; however, polyphenolic compounds, although decreasing with time, are still found in the cooked material. Relatively high amounts are found in the cooking liquor, equivalent to about 20 per cent of the total. The significance of this in common beans is still not well known, but preliminary evidence suggests they decrease protein digestibility and quality (11) The beneficial effect of heat on the destruction of the trypsin inhibitors and lectins is shown in Figure 10 (right) by a significant increase in protein quality. Again, excess heat destroys the quality of bean protein.

With respect to the antiphysiological factors in Vicia faba, available evidence suggests that vicine is located in the cotyledons in amounts varying from 0.23 to 0.61 percent, with up to 0.07 percent in the seed coat (14), so far as known, this substance is not affected by processing in the same way as trypsin inhibitors and haemagglutinins. However, it is important to stress the variability reported, which suggests the possibility for breeders to select for lower vicine values in the cotyledons.

The role of condensed tannins in faba beans has received some attention (15, 16). As is the case with common beans, phenolic compounds are present in the testa of faba beans. This is shown in Table 10. The data demonstrate that white cultivars are very low in tannins compared to colored seeds. Tannins interfere with nutrient utilization, as has been demonstrated for faba beans in studies with experimental animals (15, 16). In the case of common beans, the intake of phenolic compounds decreases protein digestibility and increases faecal nitrogen output (11). Table 11 shows regression equations of tannin intake to faecal nitrogen output and of tannin intake to apparent protein digestibility in experiments using young adult human subjects (11). Therefore, the significance of developing varieties with a testa easier to remove is recommended, because the removal of the seed coat containing the polyphenolic compounds would increase the nutrient availability from the beans.

Sulfur amino acid deficiency and protein digestibility. The significance of other limiting nutritional factors in beans is shown in Table 12. This refers to the deficiency of sulfur amino acids in bean protein. The upper part of the figure shows that the importance of methionine in beans, when consumed with a cereal grain, depends on the proportion in which both protein sources are consumed. When corn predominates, methionine addition has no nutritional importance. However, the importance of methionine is evident when the amount of beans in the mixture increases, as is shown from the PER values in the lower part of the Table.

The significance of a higher sulfur amino acid level in food legumes becomes more important when they are consumed in diets based on starchy roots such as cassava, or fruits such as plantain. This is indicated in the figure in Table 12. Here, a basal cassava diet was fed with increasing levels of common beans with and without addition of methionine. The results show that body weight maintenance is possible with lower levels of bean intake when methionine was added compared to the weight change associated with consumption of unsupplemented common beans. This was at about 15 percent beans when no methionine was added and 10 percent when 0.2 percent methionine was added. These results suggest, therefore, that some increase in sulfur amino acid content would be desirable in food legumes, especially when they are components of food consumption systems based on starchy foods (17).

Finally, one of the most important nutritional problems is the low protein digestibility of beans. Some information from adult human studies is shown in Table 12. The values found range from 50 to 62 percent for apparent digestibility, depending on the color of the seed. This can be compared to values for animal protein sources determined at INCAP that show digestibilities of 76 percent for cheese and 86 percent for meat. The protein digestibility for faba bean is also low. Explanations for these low digestibilities and their significance remain unclear.

Other Nutritional Factors

Up to now emphasis has been placed on protein in food legumes because of its nutritional significance as a component in diets. However, other nutritional factors should also receive attention as nutritional goals for plant breeders. An example is shown in Table 14. Animal models were used to evaluate mixed diets, one based on a mixture of corn and beans in a weight ratio of 87:13 and a second on a weight ratio of 70:30 (18, 19). These diets were offered *ad libitum* to five-week old pigs in individual pens for a 12-week experimental period. The diets were supplemented with groups of nutrients as shown. The 70:30 mixture induced better weight gain and feed utilization than the 87:13 mixture. The addition of all nutrient groups caused an improvement in animal performance except when the diets were increased in calories. Furthermore, the effects on feed efficiency were higher for the 87:13 than for the 70:30 mixture. It is of interest that the effect of added mineral mixture was the greatest among individual dietary treatments.

These results were interpreted to mean that, in increasing yield of grain legumes or in selection programmes, attention should also be given to nutrients other than protein, which may also be limiting in food legume-cereal based diets. Diets completely suplemented with all nutrients were, however, never as good as the control diet. This was a result of limitations in feed intake by the young animals even though feed was available at all times. These results suggest the need to increase nutrient concentration in the components of such mixed diets.

CONCLUSIONS

Some recommendations are given in Table 15 on several nutritional goals for the upgrading of food legumes. First, yields must be increased or should remain stable, because current trends seem to indicate decreases in per capita consumption of food legumes. It is, however, important that the increases in yield should not be at the expense of consumer acceptability in marketing systems that include processing, and also they should not be at the expense of protein or lysine content. Furthermore, slightly higher levels of sulfur amino acids would be desirable. Research is needed on the problem of low protein digestibility that may be associated with polyphenolic compounds. Finally, attention must be given to other essential nutrients, cooking characteristics, storage stability, and breeding for higher acceptability to the consumer, as well as to characteristics favouring processing either at the home or industrial level.

REFERENCES

1. Bressani, R., M. Flores and L.G. Elias. Aceptabilidad y valor nutritional de las plantas leguminosas y grano en la dieta humana, p. 13-29, 1979. In: Seminario sobre el Potencial del Frijol y de otras legumino-sas de grano comestible en America Latina. Feb. 26 - Mar 1, 1973. CIAT, Cali, Colombia. Pub. Ser. CS-2, Agosto, 1975.

2. Bressani, R. and L.G. Elias. The world protein and nutritional situation, p. 3-23, 1979. In: Seed Protein Improvement in Cereals and Grain Legumes. Vol. 1. Proc. Symp. Sept 4-8, 1978. Int. Atomic Energy Agency, Vienna, 1979.

3. Parpia, H.A.B. Utilization problems in food legumes, p. 281. In: Nutritional Improvement of Food Legumes by Breeding. Proc. Symp. PAG/FAO, July 3-5, 1973.

4. Pabon R., L.A.; C.J. Aguirre, y J.A. Reyes Q. Resistencia de diez y siete variedades comerciales de frijol (*Phaseolus vulgaris* L.) en almacenamiento al ataque del gorgojo pintado de los granos (*Zabrotes sub-fasciatus* Boh). Acta Agronomica 26: 39-47, 1976.

5. Tahhan, O. and G. Hariri. Infestation of faba bean seeds by *Bruchus dentipes* Baudi (Coleoptera: Bruchidae), p. 58 FABIS Newsletter No. 3 April 1981. ICARDA.

6. Burr, H.K. and S. Kon. Factors influencing the cooking rate of stored dry beans, pp. 50-52. Report of 8th Dry Bean Research Conference. Bellaire, Michigan, Aug. 11-13, 1966. ARS-USDA, 74-41, 1966.

7. Molina, M.R., G. de la Fuente and R. Bressani. Interrelationships between storage, soaking time, cooking time, nutritive value and other characteristics of the black bean (*Phaseolus vulgaris*) J. Food Sci. 40:587-591, 1975.

8. Bressani, R., L.G. Elias and A.T. Valiente. Effect of cooking and of amino acid supplementation on the nutrition value of black beans (*Phaseolus vulgaris*). Brit. J. Nutr. 17:69, 1963.

9. Youssef, M.M. and A.M. El-Tabey. Cooking quality of faba beans (*Vicia faba*). FABIS Newsletter No. 3. April 1981. ICARDA

10. Glover, W.O. Sclerema and hard-shell, two types of hardness of the bean. Prc. Amer. Assoc. Offic. - Seed. Analyst 13-60, 1921.

11. Bressani, R. and L.G. Elias. The nutritional role of polyphenols in beans, p. 61-72, 1979. In: Polyphenols in Cereals and Legumes, J.H. Hulse, ed. Proc. Symp. 36th Annual Meeting of IFT St. Louis, MO, 10-13 June 1979. IDRC 145e.

12. Crean, D.E.C. and D.R. Haisman. The interaction between phytic acid and divalent cations during the cooking of dried peas. J. Sci. Food Agro. 14:824-833, 1963.

13. Sefa-Dedeh, S., and D.W. Stanley. The relationship of microstructure of cowpeas to water absorption and dehulling properties. Cereal Chem. 56:379-386, 1979.

14. Jamalian, J. Favism-inducing toxins in broad beans (*Vicia faba*). Determination of vicine content and investigation of other non-protein nitrogenous compounds in different broad bean cultivars. J. Sci. Food Agro. 29:136-140, 1978.

15. Martin-Tanguy, J., J. Guillaume and A. Kossa. Condensed tannins in horse bean seeds: Chemical structure and apparent effect on poultry. J. Sci. Food Agr. 28:757-765, 1977.

16. Marquardt, R.T., J.A. McKirdy and A.J. Ward. Comparative cell wall constituent levels of tannin-free and tannin-containing cultivars of faba beans (*Vicia faba* L.). Canad. J. Anim. Sci. 58:775-781, 1978.

17. Bressani, R. and L.G. Elias. Cantidad minima de proteina de frijol para mantenimiento de peso en ratas en crecimiento alimentadas con tuberculas y platano. INCAP, Guatemala City, Informe Anual 1980.

18. Bressani, R. and L.G. Elias. Development of new highly nutritious food products, p. 251-274. In: *Man, Food and Nutrition*, M. Rechcigl, Jr., ed., CRC Press, 1973, Cleveland, Ohio 44128.

19. Contreras, G., L.G. Elias and R. Bressani. Limitations of corn (*Zea mays*) and common beans (*Phaseolus vulgaris*) diets as protein and calorie sources. Qual. Plant. Plant Food Hum. Nutr. 30:145-153, 1980.

TABLE 1. Frequency of Common Bean Intake per Family in Rural Areas of Guatemala

Frequency Days/Weeks	Number of Families	Percentage Distribution
2	10	12.7
3	20	25.3
4	36	45.5
5	10	12.7
6	3	3.8

Source: Reference 1

TABLE 2. Effect of Frequency of Common Bean Intake on Weight Gain and Carcass Nitrogen in Rats

Frequency of Bean Intake Day/Exptl Period	Average Weight Gain (g)	Average Carcass Nitrogen (g)
28 of 28	103	4.02
20 of 28	75	3.23
12 of 28	74	3.17
0	46	2.47

Source: Reference 2

TABLE 3. Protein Quality of Chick Pea and Pigeon Pea Infested by Insects

Protein Source	PER
Chick pea dhal (control)	2.21
Chick pea dhal (infested)	1.83
Pigeon pea (control)	2.04
Pigeon pea (infested)	1.66

Source: Reference 3

TABLE 4. Effect of Insect Infestation on the Yield of Dhal from Bengal Gram

% Kernel	% Dhal Damage	Yield
Chick pea (control)	2	82
Chick pea (infested)	15	65

Source: Reference 3

TABLE 5. Yield of Dhal from Different Commercial Strains of Red Gram Grown in India

Strain	% Average Yield	
	Traditional Method	Improved Method
Lathur white	75	84
Hyderabad red-white mix	72	81
Bihar red-white mix	70	81
U.P. gray	68	80
Mysore red	64	79

Source: P.P. Kurien et al., CFTRI, unpublished data, 1970, cited in Reference 3.

TABLE 6. Percent Average Yield of Dhal from Legumes by Different Processes

Legume	Home-Scale Process	Conventional Commercial Methods	Improved CFTRI Process	Maximum Theoretical Yield
Chick pea (*Cicer arietinum*)	75	75	82	89
Pigeon pea (*Cajanus cajan*)	68	75	83	89
Black gram (*Phaseolus mungo*)	69	71	82	88
Green gram (*Phaseolus radiatus*)	64	65	82	89

Source: P.P. Kurien et al., CFTRI, unpublished data, 1970, cited in Reference 3.

TABLE 7. Correlation Coefficients between the Physical Properties and the Cooking Quality of Stewed Faba Beans

Properties	Portion of Seed*	Correlation Coefficient
Weight of 100 seeds	S	+ 0.68**
Lightness (color by C.I.E. method)	H	+ 0.78**
Specific gravity	S	+ 0.66**
Percent of hulls to seed	S	- 0.95**
Percent of fraction easy to mill	H	+ 0.85**
Percent of fraction hard to mill	H	- 0.93***
Viscosity (by Visce/amylograph)	C	+ 0.72**
Transition temperature (at beginning of response of amylogram)	C	- 0.91***
Hydration coeffiecient after stewing	S	+ 0.75**
Total solids in stewing liquor		+ 0.80***
Soluble solids in stewing liquor		+ 0.85***
Insoluble solids in stewing liquor		+ 0.74**
Lightness (color by C.I.E. method)	C	- 0.24

*S = whole seed; H = hulls; C = cotyledons
**Least significant values for r equals 0.66 at 0.05
***Least significant values for r equals 0.79 at 0.01

TABLE 8. Principal Nutritional Characteristics of Food Legumes

---

Positive factors

- high protein content
- high lysine content
- excellent supplementary protein to cereal grains

Limiting factors

- antiphysiological substances:
  - trypsin inhibitors
  - hemagglutinins
  - polyphenolic compounds
  - flatulence factors
  - those particular to each fod legume species:
    - vicine, convicine, dopa-glucosidase (faba beans)
- nutritional factors:
  - sulfur amino acid deficiency
  - low protein digestibility

TABLE 9. Protein Quality Improvement of the Wheat/Faba Bean Mixture (7:3) by Amino Acid and Protein Supplementation

Treatment	Weight Gain (g/14 Days)	Net Protein Ratio*
Faba beans	8	1.62
Faba beans + methionine**	53	3.19
Whole wheat	26	1.93
Whole wheat + lysine***	46	2.55
Wheat/faba bean mixture (7:3)	38	2.76
Wheat/faba bean mixture (7:3) + methionine**** + lysine***	56	3.05
Wheat/faba bean mixture (7:3) + 10% skim milk	57	3.10
Casein (control)	65	3.91

*Mean values for eight rats (four male and four female/group)
**0.3% DL-methionine
***0.2% L-lysine HCl
****0.2% DL-methionine

TABLE 10. Tannin Content in Common Beans and in Faba Beans

Material	Testa Color	Whole Seed	Cotyledon	Testa	Ref.
Phaseolus vulgaris	white	3.85	4.15	1.30	2
	black	7.95	5.25	42.50	2
	red	9.30	5.00	38.00	2
Vicia faba	Diana	-	0.10	4.40	16
	triple-white	-	0.1	0.10	16

TABLE 11. Regression Equations between Absolute Intakes of Tannic Acid and of Catechin and Fecal Nitrogen and Protein Digestibility in Young Adult Humans

F.N. = 38.03 + 0.008 (Abs. T.A. intake)	r = + 0.33
F.N. = 40.24 + 0.147 (Abs. Cat. intake)	r = + 0.37
P.D. % ap = 65.54 - 0.010 (T.A. mg %)	r = - 0.32
P.D. % ap = 62.71 - 0.20 (Cat. mg %)	r = - 0.35

F.N. = Faecal nitrogen
P.D. = Protein digestibility
T.A. = Tannic acid
Cat. = Catechin equivalent

TABLE 12. Protein Digestibility of Common Beans in Adult Human Subjects

Bean	No. of Subjects	Apparent Protein Digestibility (%)
Black beans	8	54.6 ± 4.1
Ground meat	5	86.0 ± 1.2
Black beans	12	49.6 ± 2.9
Red beans	12	55.7 ± 4.6
White beans	12	62.1 ± 2.9
Cheese	12	72.2 ± 1.4

TABLE 13. Average Weight Gain and Feed Conversion Efficiencies of Young Pigs Fed Corn Bean Diets under Different Dietary Treatments

Dietary Treatment	87/13		70/30	
	Wt. Gain Kg/Day	Feed Efficiency	Wt. Gain Kg/Day	Feed Efficiency
None	2.35 ± 1.6 (d)	20.3	10.88 ± 1.9 (c,d)	5.9
Lysine, methionine, tryptophan	14.25 ± 1.2 (c,d)	5.3	13.63 ± 1.9 (c,d)	5.4
Vitamins	8.50 ± 1.9 (c,d)	7.7	15.88 ± 1.8 (c,d)	5.0
Minerals	14.63 ± 6.9 (c,d)	5.7	17.88 ± 5.8 (c)	4.4
Fat	6.00 ± 2.3 (c,d)	9.1	8.63 ± 3.6 (c,d)	6.9
All nutrients	35.00 ± 4.7 (b)	3.4	37.00 ± 6.5 (b)	3.2
Control	54.88 ± 3.6 (a)	2.4	----------------------------	

Source: Reference 19

TABLE 14. Recommended Nutritional Goals for Food Legumes

1. Increased and stable yield of accepted varieties
2. Maintain protein and lysine content
3. Increase sulfur amino acid content
4. Reduce antiphysiological factors, including polyphenol compounds
5. Improve protein digestibility
6. Improve storage stability
7. Consider cooking characteristics, acceptability, and processing efficiency

FIGURE 1

AGRONOMIC AND NUTRITIONAL PRIORITIES FOR BASIC FOOD CROPS

Productivity = Production (kg/ha) x Post harvest technological quality x Nutritional quality

FIGURE 2

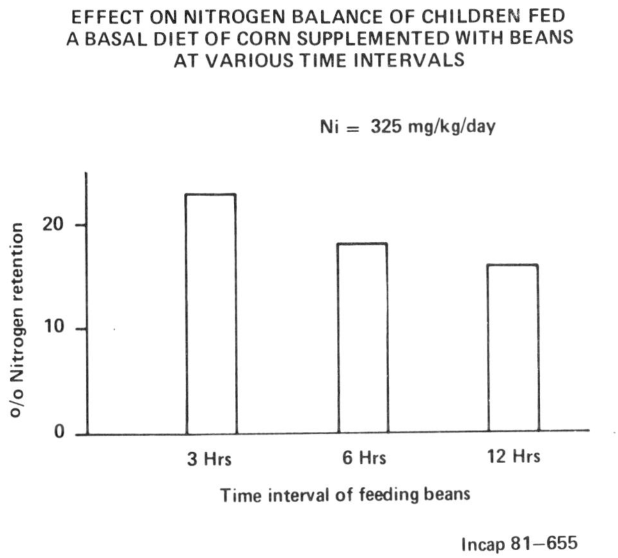
EFFECT ON NITROGEN BALANCE OF CHILDREN FED
A BASAL DIET OF CORN SUPPLEMENTED WITH BEANS
AT VARIOUS TIME INTERVALS
Ni = 325 mg/kg/day
o/o Nitrogen retention
20
10
0
3 Hrs
6 Hrs
12 Hrs
Time interval of feeding beans
Incap 81–655

FIGURE 3

PROTEIN QUALITY OF CEREAL GRAIN/FOOD LEGUME MIXTURES

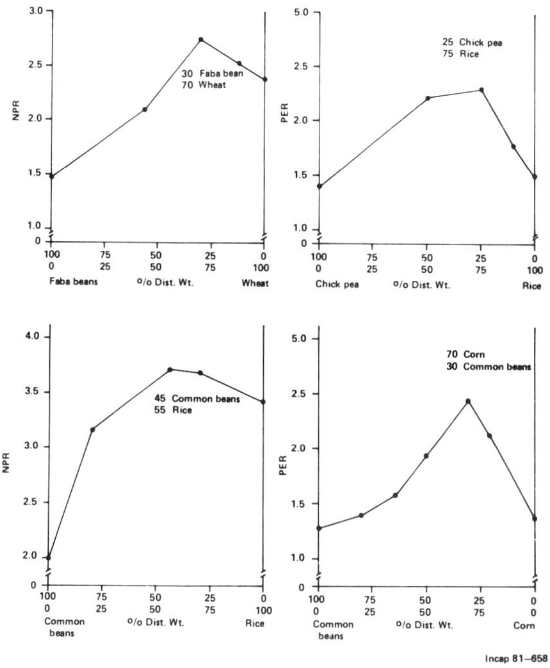

FIGURE 4

PROTEIN QUALITY OF MIXTURES OF FABA BEANS AND WHOLE WHEAT AND SIGNIFICANCE OF INCREASED PRODUCTION, ACCEPTABILITY AND NUTRITIVE VALUE

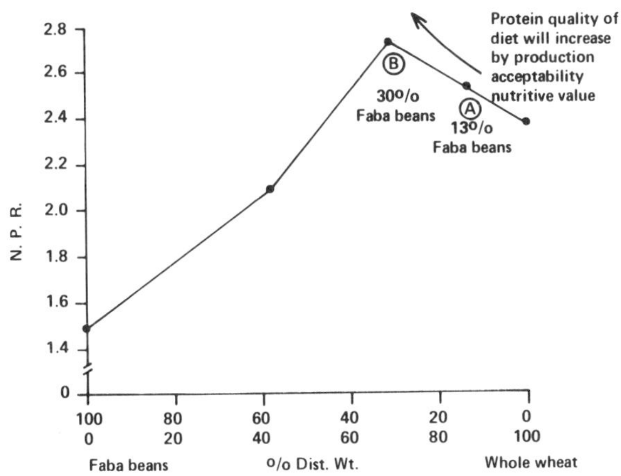

Incap 81–656

FIGURE 5

LIMITING NUTRITIONAL FACTORS OF COMMON BEANS

A. PHYSICAL FACTORS: HARD–TO–COOK

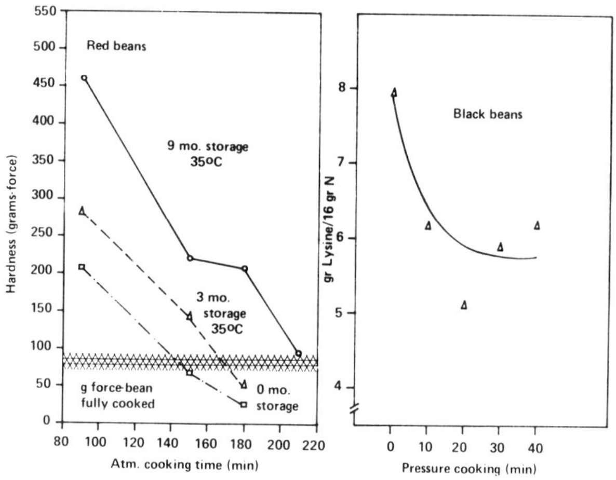

Bressani, 1981

Incap 82 - 139

FIGURE 6

EFFECT OF MOISTURE AND STORAGE TIME ON COOKING TIME OF COMMON BEANS

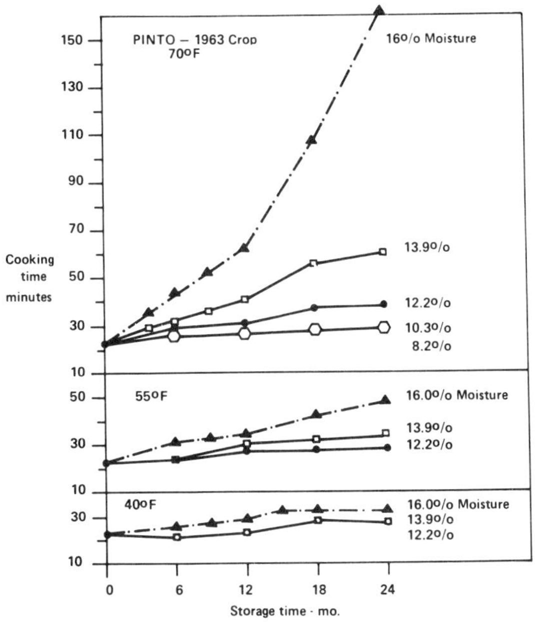

Burr & Kon, 1966.

Incap 81–664

FIGURE 7

EFFECT OF STORAGE ON THE PROTEIN QUALITY COMMON BEAN COOKED DURING 10, 20 AND 30 MINUTES

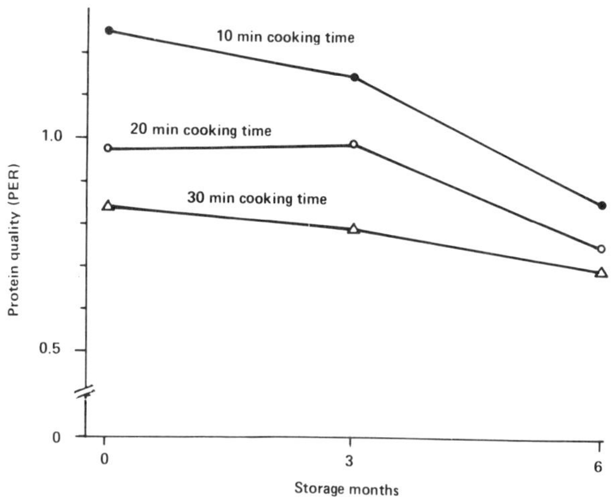

Incap 82–115

FIGURE 8

HYPOTHESIS ON THE GENERAL PROCESS OF BEAN HARDENING

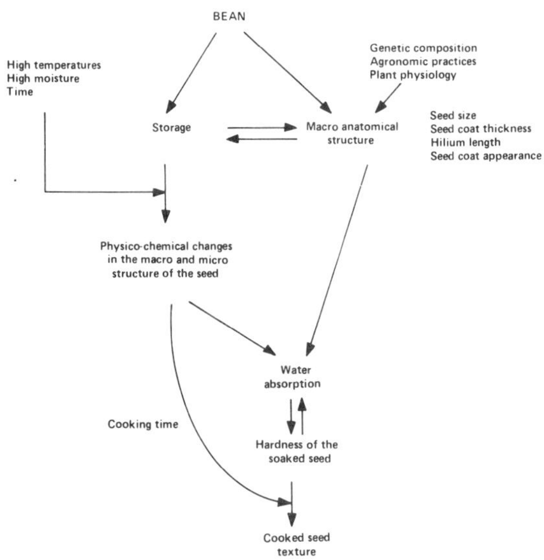

Incap 81–663

FIGURE 9

COMPLEMENTATION EFFECT BETWEEN FABA BEAN AND WHOLE WHEAT PROTEIN AND LIMITATIONS

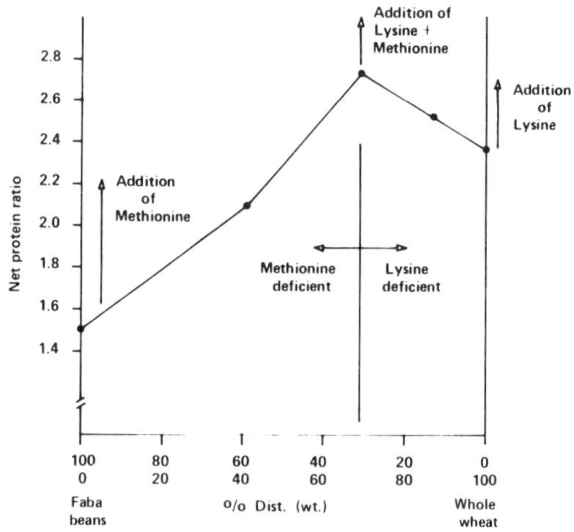

Bressani, 1981

Incap 81–657

FIGURE 10

LIMITING NUTRITIONAL FACTORS OF COMMON BEANS

B. ANTIPHYSIOLOGICAL SUBSTANCES – TRYPSIN INHIBITORS
– HEMAGGLUTININ COMPOUNDS
– POLYPHENOLIC SUBSTANCES

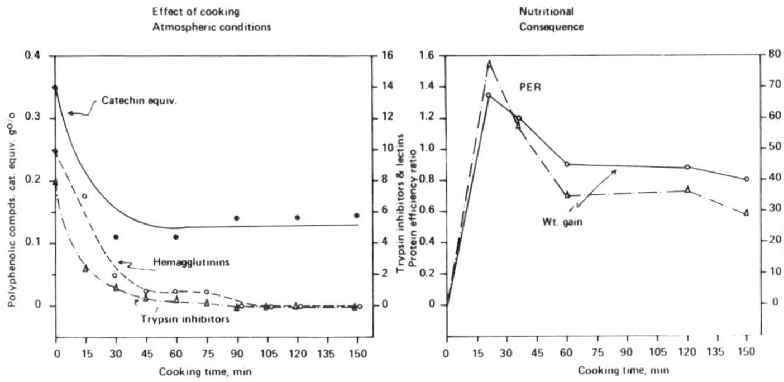

Bressani, 1981

Incap 81 660

FIGURE 11

LIMITING NUTRITIONAL FACTORS OF COMMON BEANS

C. SULFUR AMINO ACID DEFICIENCY. Ave. 125 mg/g N
SIGNIFICANCE: SOME FOR CEREAL/BEAN MIXTURES
HIGH FOR TUBER/BEAN MIXTURES

CEREAL/ BEAN FOOD CONSUMPTION SYSTEM

	PER
Corn (87) + Beans (13) = Basal	2.11
Basal + Lys + Try	2.64
Basal + Met	1.93
Basal + Lys + Try + Met	2.69
Corn (70) + Beans (30) = Basal	2.41
Basal + Lys	2.35
Basal + Met	2.60

CASSAVA/BEAN FOOD CONSUMPTION SYSTEM

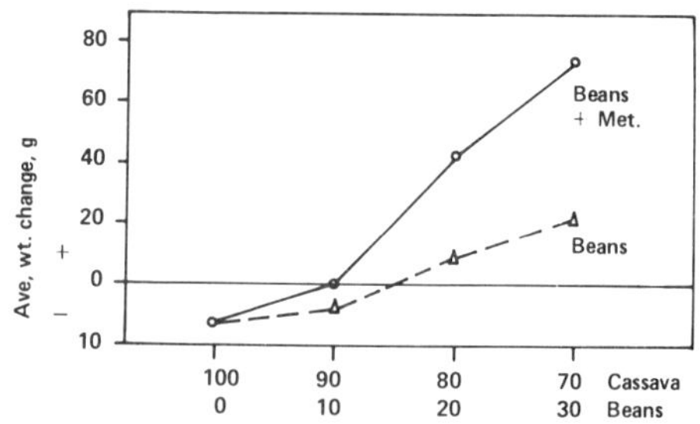

Bressani, 1981.

Incap 81–659

BREEDING FOR NUTRITIONAL QUALITY IN CEREALS

MOHAMED S. MEKNI and MOHAMED M. NACHIT

INTRODUCTION

Cereals have been the pillars on which many civilizations have developed since ancient times. They are still the world's largest crops and the main staple food for man and animals. Johnson *et al.*, (1) estimated that wheat alone sustains at least one billion humans, and Swaminathan *et al.*, (2) indicated that in India alone, cereals contribute 60.2 percent of the protein supply. Cereals were grown in 1977 on 739 million hectares (Table 1) and produced more than 14 billion quintals, corresponding to an average yield of 19.5 q/ha. Wheat remains the world's main cereal crop. Production for the 1979-1981 crop seasons is presented in Table 2.

There are important genetic, morphological, and physiological differences among cereal crops, but they constitute a fairly homogeneous groups and improvement in one has generally interested other researchers to apply the same techniques to additional cereals even though some crops have been neglected in many parts of the world. Because of their productivity, cereals are increasing in economic importance, and while rye and oats have shown a notable decline, barley has registered the highest increases in terms of area and production since 1968. Wheat and barley, in particular, give very high yields under favourable growing conditions and would be expected to continue to play a leading role.

The organoleptic technological properties of cereals are diversified and meet consumers' desires better than other crops. From a small volume they bring a raw substance rich in calories, easily planted, harvested, transported, stored, processed, and cooked using countless recipes. They also supply a large portion of the required protein to many communities. Grown mainly for their seed, cereals have a valuable straw that is either fed to animals, used for bedding, or processed by the paper industry. Finally, they can be grown alone or in association with other crops.

The growing of high-quality cereals is a complex process and many aspects must be considered.

1. The nutritional value is itself complex. Many factors, including the amount of crude protein and its essential amino acid composition, amount of oil, the vitamins, and carbohydrate constituents, are all of importance.

2. Cereals breeders have, for a long time, concentrated on yield and agronomic characteristics first -- characteristics that are often negatively associated with nutritional quality.

3. The success of plant breeding in terms of quality has been achieved mainly to suit the needs of the cereal industries. This is particularly true of the milling and baking industries for wheat and the malting industries for barley.

The discovery in the early 1960s of mutant genes that increased lysine (3) or tryptophan in the maize endosperm (4) raised hope for similar discoveries in other cereal crops. The nutritional quality of cereals is limited by their short supply of certain essential amino acids, mainly lysine, and when used for food or feed, cereals are often supplemented with other proteins from animal or other vegetable sources. Supplementing the diet with vitamins and minerals is often required as well. An increase in the nutritional quality of cereals is generally accompanied by decreases in the amounts of supplements required. In most cereal crops, nutritional quality is often considered synonymous with protein content, and breeding for higher quality seldom means more than breeding for a higher level of protein or for higher percentages of the essential amino acids in the protein.

Protein Variability

Mutants similar to those in Opaque-2 and Floury-2 maize that improve the nutritional quality and increase the proportion of limiting amino acids are desirable in other cereals, but differences have never been obtained of the order of magnitude found in the maize mutants (2). Interest in breeding for higher protein content is not new, but varietal differences in wheat protein are, with few exceptions, not known (5,6). Protein increases in the range of two to three per cent have been accomplished in selections from Atlas 66 x Hard Red Spring Wheat crosses (1). Hageberg and Karlsson (7), using one-thousand cultivar samples from the USDA world collection, also found that total content of lysine, histidine, and arginine increased with higher yield, even though they decreased with higher protein percentage. In the same samples, protein content varied from 8.8 to 16.9 percent, and this indicates a wide genetic variation for protein *per se*. Sixteen lines of barley were reported to have protein above 16 percent in the 1978-1979 preliminary observation nursery (ICARDA, In-House Review Research Highlights, 1980).

Quality of cereals and consequently their nutritional value is lower when fibre content is increased. This is especially true for oats and barley. It is possible to produce naked barley seeds because the hull inheritance is controlled by a single recessive gene. Naked barleys, as a group, are higher in protein content than types with hulls (8).

Nutritional Quality of Cereals

In many cereals, particularly wheat, quality depends upon the physical properties of the grain, mainly its size and plumpness, and on its protein content. However, like most plant proteins, the nutritional quality of cereal proteins is known to be limited by a small proportion of the essential amino acids and thus a large proportion of the nonessential amino acids as compared to animal proteins. In many cereal proteins, lysine is the essential amino acid most limiting. There are indications that high levels of protein bring about greater imbalances among protein fractions and that breeding for increased protein percentage often leads to smaller fractions of essential amino acids and poorer quality (9, 10). Munck (8) indicated that when protein levels in cereals increased, the non-essential amino acids increased faster than the essential amino acids, and therefore protein quality became poorer. However, he showed that more of the amino acid lysine and the other essential amino acids were available due to an increase in yield per hectare, which compensated for the decrease in protein quality. The two relationships were verified by Johnson *et al.*, (11) using the USDA world collection of 12,613 common wheats as well as by Hageberg and Karlsson (7).

Environmental Effects

The nutritional value of cereal proteins is therefore dependent upon their amino acid composition. The latter is in turn influenced by the genetic background, the environment, and agronomic practices that influence availability of nutrients, mainly nitrogen. Several researchers have demonstrated that the inheritance of protein content is strongly influenced by the environment (12-14). However, although increments of nitrogen fertilizer have brought about higher contents of protein in the grain (11), it has been difficult to identify the genetic effects in high-yielding environments (1) where yield differences are accompanied by strong variations in the protein content of the grain and where a single genotype can produce grain with 8 to 18 per cent protein, depending upon the environment in which it is grown. Toft Viuf (15) has indicated that the nitrogen content of the modern Northwestern European cultivars of barley was about 20 percent less than in 1900 because of selection for higher yield, shorter and stiffer straw, and lower protein for malting purposes. In alfalfa and orchard grass, McLeod and Suzuki (16) indicated that potassium also increased total nitrogen and amino acid content, while the protein nitrogen fraction decreased. Potassium was suspected of playing the role of activator for a number of enzyme systems and of influencing nitrogen metabolism (16).

Inheritance of Protein Content and Composition

The consensus is that protein content and composition are quantitatively inherited characters, and therefore their genetic transfer is very complicated indeed. Protein content as well as the relative proportions of individual amino acids are affected by a large number of factors; they include water stress (17), day length (18), temperature (19), presence or absence of vernalization (20), and nutrition (21-24). In crosses involving high-and low-protein parents, the protein content of the progenies was generally equal to the middle parental value (11, 25, 26,). Transgressive segregation was observed and has been attributed to the presence of different genes in the parents (21, 27, 28). Seed protein in wheat was both quantitatively and highly heritable (27, 29). The numbers of genes controlling protein content have been found to vary from a single dominant gene (30), relatively few genes, (31) associated with at least five chromosomes (28), and even found on each of the twenty-one wheat chromosomes (20).

Heritability estimates for protein have been considered low (32), but Stuber *et al.* (13) obtained heritability as high as 0.82, which indicates that it was easy to make effective breeding progress. Haunold *et al.* (27) and Davis *et al.* (29) reported moderately high heritability esitmates of 0.65 and 0.67, respectively.

Correlation of Protein Content With Other Characters

There seem to be difficulties in transferring characters for high protein content from lines where it is linked to other characters.

Protein vs. Yield. Protein, like many quantitative inherited characters, is expressed differently in different environments. High-yield environments often result in low-protein percentage, while low-yield environments are often coupled with high-protein content of the grain (23). Bell *et al.*, (33) found that high yielding varieties have a low-protein content, while Schmidt *et al.*, (31) found that protein content was negatively correlated with yield whenever the soil nitrogen was low. When nitrogen in the soil was not the limiting factor, the correlation between soil nitrogen and protein content was low. The starch percentage was, however, negatively correlated with the amount of protein. Toft Viuf (15) found that, with high nitrogen content, the proportion of arginine, aspartic acid, glycine, alanine, and valine decreased, while proportions of glutamic acid, proline, and to a lesser extent, phenylalanine, were found to increase. The amounts of the other amino acids in the protein generally remained constant with the exception of the important amino acid, lysine, which increased linearly with increased nitrogen at low total nitrogen levels, but decreased at high nitrogen levels. For every variety, there existed a nitrogen threshold up to which increased protein was obtained in the grain independently of the yield level.

Investigators reporting a significant inverse relationship between yield and protein content have been numerous (27-30, 34). Haunold et al., (26) compared Atlas 66, a high-protein soft red winter wheat, with two hard red winter wheat varieties, Wichita and Comanche, during a three-year period. They found a significant inverse relationship between total grain yield and protein content of the grain. Atlas 66 produced grain with higher protein content, but it was significantly lower in yield and its protein production per hectare was lower than that of the other two varieties. Stroike et al. (9, 10) argued that protein content is not necessarily inversely related to yield. This mainly occurs in cases of availability of genotypes where the phenotypic expression of the high-protein trait is good. In a three-year experiment using high-protein lines derived from Atlas 66, the high-protein lines maintained two to three percent higher protein content across environments where they exhibited both lower and higher yields in comparison with control varieties. These results are supported by Schmidt (31), who found no negative correlation between yield of high-protein cultivars. Ackerberg (35) did not find a negative correlation between yield and protein percentage in oats, and Johnson et al. (36), using Atlas 66 in crosses with the hard red spring wheat Comanche, found selection 60306 slightly more productive and higher in protein than either parent. This indicates that it was possible to increase protein without yield loss, even if the yield increase over Comanche was not statistically significant. The genotypes they selected with high yield potential maintained a higher protein level than the lower protein checks.

Protein vs. Height. Height is another characteristic thought to have a negative correlation with protein content. Linkage between height and protein content, however, does not seem to be strong enough to prevent selection of tall or semidwarf genotypes with high grain protein. Johnson et al. (36) found a small but rather negative correlation with height, while Balla (25) found no correlation between height and protein content in the F2 generation of Bezostaya in high-protein cultivars Atlas 66 and Purdue 4930. McNeal et al. (37) found a positive correlation with height. The same interesting positive relationship is also found between straw length and protein content (15, 38). It was thought that a longer straw might be able to transport a greater proportion of the nitrogen to the grain where it can be converted to protein.

Protein vs. Disease Resistance. Johnson et al. (39) found a gene for high protein content in Atlas 66 closely associated with leaf-rust resistance. However, this has not been substantiated by any similar findings.

Suggested Approaches for Improved Plant Protein Screening

Because the environmental effect is large in comparison with the genotypic effect in protein inheritance studies, higher nitrogen applications remain the easiest and most effective procedure for increasing both grain protein content and grain yield. It is evident that cereal genotypes do exist in which a high-protein percentage in the grain can be achieved. The identification of those genotypes remains difficult, and the transfer of the high-protein trait is masked by the environment. Two possible screening approaches are available today; the first looks into the enzyme activity and the second concerns the dye-binding capacity of the proteins.

Enzyme Assays. To develop and select high-yielding and high-protein varieties, the level of activity of the enzyme, nitrate reductase, has been shown to be useful as a selection criterion (40). The level of activity of this enzyme is highly heritable (41) and varies widely within a species (42). Nitrate reductase enzyme activity is the rate-limiting step in the reduction of plant nitrates (43). Croy and Hageman (44) emphasized, however, that a genetic potential for high nitrate reductase activity is no guarantee of high protein production; other factors such as nitrate supply, transport efficiency, lodging, grain disease resistance, as well as other environmental factors, may exert decisive influence on the accumulation of protein in the grain. It seems reasonable to state that high-protein varieties should possess the genetic potential for high nitrate reductase activity, because the level of nitrate reductase is an index of the amount of reduced nitrogen available to the plant. Although it depends on the efficiency of the translocation system in the plant, Croy and Hageman added that an increased level of reduced nitrogen in the vegetative tissue should result in time in an increased deposition of protein in the grain. However, Johnson et al. (45) found that nitrate content of the leaves was not positively correlated with grain protein. They found a positive correlation between the input of reduced nitrogen and accumulated grain protein. This relationship holds only for some genotypes, because Monon, a low-protein soft red winter wheat with less enzyme activity, was able to accumulate more protein in the grain than Ponca, a relatively high-protein hard red winter wheat. However, they cautioned that if nitrate reductase activity is to be used as a selection criterion for the identification of high-and low-protein wheats, it should be measured when the plants are grown under conditions that would permit full expression of their genetic potential for high nitrate reductase. Another possibility is to screen seedlings under controlled environments; Warner (46) found that relative differences in nitrate reductase activity were similar for both field conditions and controlled environments. The protein content of the grain does not seem to be directly related to nitrogen uptake, but rather directly related to nitrogen translocation, and the two mechanisms appear to function separately in wheats (4, 45, 47).

Dye-binding Capacity Assay. The shortage of certain essential amino acids is characteristic of plant proteins in general and of cereal proteins in particular. The dye-binding capacity procedure is well suited for screening plant types for protein quality, mainly for basic amino acids, because it is a direct assay of unlinked-NH_2 radicals. Mossberg (48) believes that it should be complemented by determinations of total nitrogen and amino acids, as changes in the amounts of total protein bring about changes in the amino acid pattern (34). Dye-binding capacity assays have also been used to estimate protein quality. The main advantage of the dye-binding capacity procedure is that it is fast and inexpensive in screening large amounts of plant material.

Quality Testing at ICARDA

Breeding high-quality cereal varieties at ICARDA to meet consumer uses in the region relies heavily on classical and newly developed screening techniques in the cereal grain quality laboratory. Prior to release, genotypes are characterized for their efficiency of nitrogen uptake and plant utilization under field conditions. Both bread and durum wheats are used for bread-making in West Asia and North Africa. Durum is also used for various pasta products. Barley is used as food, feed, and for brewing. Quality tests in cereals depend on generation and availability of seed. The tests most commonly used at ICARDA for each of the cereal crops are listed in Table 3. These are also discussed in the paper by Williams in this volume.

Research on protein content in barley is routinely done at ICARDA on the most promising lines and cultivars. Five checks were used in the advanced yield trials; they are 2-rowed White Arabic, Minn126/CM67 and WI 2197, and 6-rowed cultivars, Beecher and 2762/Beecher-6L. Results indicated that the percentage of protein was negatively correlated with yield, (r = -0.79) while correlations between protein percentage and kernel weight were not significant (r = 0.20).

Similar correlations were obtained between yield, thousand kernel weight, and protein percentage in the 1980/81 Barley Yield Trial. The protein percentage was negatively correlated with yield (r = -0.57) but correlation with kernel weight was not significant. The results obtained on the checks from twelve advanced yield trials using four replications in each yield trial, and on the lines and cultivars entering in the Regional Barley Yield Trial from twenty-two locations in Western Asia and North Africa, indicate that in the germplasm pool available at ICARDA protein is negatively correlated with yield and thousand-kernel weight. Progress made in improving yield might have been obtained at the expense of nutritive value. Therefore, there is a need to add to the germplasm pool genotypes where yield and protein content are positively correlated.

Work on triticale was done to produce a cereal that combines yield potential and the grain use of wheat with a tolerance of rye to environmental stress and resistance to diseases. Triticale is just beginning to be accepted as a commercial crop in many areas in the world, and interest in its use as food is increasing. A large population of triticale genotypes has been analyzed for different quality characteristics in relation to yield. Four-hundred and fifty-six genotypes of triticale were investigated using 19 genotypes and five checks in each trial and with three replications. Plots were six rows in width and five metres long. The distance between rows was 30 cm. Notes were taken on agronomic characteristics such as height, flowering date, yield components, and yield. In the laboratory, test weight, thousand kernel weight, protein content, Pelshenke value and hardness (particle size index) were determined.

The results from Triticale can be summarized:

1. The correlation between yield and protein content was negative and highly significant ($r = -0.39$, $P < 0.001$).

2. The thousand-kernel weight, an important yield parameter, was positively correlated with the yield ($r = +0.28$, $P < 0.01$), but negatively correlated with the protein content ($r = -0.22$, $P < 0.05$).

3. It was possible to identify genotypes possessing high-yielding capacity, high thousand-kernel weight, and high protein content ($r = +0.28$, $P < 0.01$).

Conclusions

Cereals and cereal products are major components of the diets in West Asia and North Africa where they provide more than half the caloric requirements of the human population and a large portion of the required vitamins and minerals. The protein content of the major cereals, wheat and barley, is generally low and their protein quality is inadequate. Increases in protein content can be obtained through the exploitation of genetic diversity or, more easily, by increases in the nitrogen content of the soil. Genotypic variations for protein content are often masked by environmental effects.

In West Asia and North Africa cereals are often consumed in combination with legumes. Dried legumes are a good source of complementary proteins for cereal diets. Their high-protein content is often accompanied by higher levels of the limiting amino acids, lysine and tryptophan, and therefore they are a good supplement to cereal proteins.

If the trend toward decreasing food legume availability per capita continues, alternate sources of protein must be found for the Middle East and North Africa. Proteins should not have to come solely from cereals, and the idea of giving high priority to quality breeding in cereals is probably erroneous. Quality should rather come from diversity in agriculture, especially in the Middle East and North Africa where food legumes have traditionally been present in the diet. Couscous (Durum wheat) with chickpea and faba in North Africa, chickpea dishes in Syria, Lebanon and Jordan, and Foul (faba bean) dishes in Egypt and Sudan are examples.

Cereal breeders are always faced with a large number of morphological and/or physiological characteristics for which they should be breeding. They often have to make choices and decide to give priority to only a few factors. The priority is traditionally given to breeding high-yielding, disease-resistant cultivars adapted to certain agro-climatic conditions. Factors such as breeding for high protein content are secondary, while characteristics such as essential amino acid content constitute only a long-term objective. The market price for cereals in most developing countries is related exclusively to the crop's weight.

REFERENCES

1. V.A. Johnson, P.J. Mattern, D.A. Whited, and J.W. Schmidt, in New Approaches to Breeding Improved Plant Proteins, IAEA 29, Vienna, Sti/Pub. 212 (1969).
2. M.S. Swaminathan, A. Austin, A.K. Kaul, and M.S. Naik, in New Approaches to Breeding Improved Plant Proteins, IAEA 29, Vienna, Sti/Pub. 212 (1969).
3. E.T. Mertz, L.S. Bates, and O.E. Nelson, Science 145: 279 (1964).
4. O.E. Nelson, E.T. Mertz, and L.S. Bates, Science 150: 1469 (1965).
5. E.C. Miller, Kansas Agric. Exp. Station Tech. Bull. 47 (1939).
6. R.W. Thatcher, J. Amer. Soc. Agron. 7: 273 (1915).
7. H.A. Hageberg and K.E. Karlsson, in New Approaches to Breeding Improved Plant Proteins, IAEA 29, Vienna, Sti/Pub. 212 (1969).
8. L. Munck, Hereditas 52 (1964).
9. J.E. Stoike, V.A. Johnson, J.W. Schmidt, and P.J. Mattern, Nebraska Res. Bull. 145 (1971).
10. J.E. Stoike, V.A. Johnson, J.W. Schmidt, and P.J. Mattern, Nebraska Res. Bull. 248 (1972).
11. V.A. Johnson, P.J. Mattern, and J.E. Stoike, Proc. 4th Internat. Wheat Genetics Symposium, Columbia, Missouri, 547-556 (1973).
12. C.W. Stuber, J.A. Johnson, and J.W. Schmidt, Crop Sci. 2: 506 (1962).
13. C.W. Stuber, V.A. Johnson, and J.W. Schmidt, Crop Sci. 2: 286 (1962).
14. J. Hulse and E.M. Liang, International Development Research Centre, IDRC-021e Monograph (IDRC, Ottawa, Canada, 1973).
15. B. Toft Viuf, in New Approaches to Breeding Improved Plant Proteins, IAEA 29, Vienna, Sti/Pub. 212 (1969).
16. L.B. McLeod and M. Suzuki, Crop. Sci. 7: 599 (1967).
17. A.C. Chibnall, M.W. Ren, and J.W.H. Luzz, J. Sci. Food Agric. 14: 234 (1963).
18. F.C. Stewart, F. Crane, K. Millar, R.M. Zacharius, R. Rarson, and D. Margolis, Symposium Soc. Exp. Biol. 13: 148 (1959).
19. M.D. Wilding, M.A. Stahmann, and D. Smith, Plant Physiol. 35: 726 (1960).
20. P. Weinberger and C. Grodin, Canad. J. Biochem. 44: 1035 (1966).
21. C.A. Adams and R.W. Sheard, Canad. J. Plant Sci. 46: 671 (1966).
22. A.V. Baker and R. Bradfield, Agron. J. 55: 465 (1966).
23. L. Fowder, Ann. Rev. Plant Physiol. 18: 85 (1967).

24. L.W. Reed, V.L. Sheldon, and W.A. Albrecht, Agron. J. 52: 523 (1960).

25. L. Balla, Proc. 4th Internat. Wheat Genetics Symposium, Columbia, Missouri (1973).

26. A. Haunold, V.A. Johnson, and J.W. Schmidt, Agron. J. 54: 203 (1962).

27. A. Haunold, V.A. Johnson, and J.W. Schmidt, Agron. J. 54: 121 (1962).

28. C.R. Cowley and D.G. Wells, Agron. Abstr. 66: 51 (1974).

29. W.H. Davis, G.K. Middleton, and T.T. Hebert, Crop Sci. 1: 235 (1961).

30. C.R. Cowley and D.G. Wells, Crop Sci. 20: 55 (1980).

31. H. Schmidt, Z. Pflanzenz. 42: 117 (1958).

32. S. Barbacki, Rocz. Naukroe 99: 267 (1947).

33. G.D.H. Bell, Agric. Merch. 36: 69 (1957).

34. L. Munch, J. Swedish Seed Assoc. 78: 137 (1968).

35. A. Ackerberg, in New Approaches to Breeding Improved Plant Proteins, IAEA 29, Vienna, Sti/Pub. 212 (1969).

36. V.A. Johnson, D.A. Whited, P.J. Mattern, and J.W. Schmidt, Wheat Quality Conference Report, Crop Quality Council, Minneapolis, Minnesota (1968).

37. F.H. McNeal, M.A. Berg, P.L. Brown, C.F. McGuire, Agron. J. 63: 908 (1971).

38. G. Fishbeck, Z. Acker - U. Pflbau. 321 (1964).

39. V.A. Johnson, D.A. Whited, P.J. Mattern, and J.W. Schmidt, Proc. 3rd Internat. Wheat Genetics Symposium, Australian Academy of Science, Canberra, Australia (1968).

40. R.H. Hageman, E.R. Leng, and J.W. Dudley, Adv. Agron. 19: 45 (1967).

41. R.L. Warner, R.H. Hageman, J.W. Dudley, and R.J. Lambert, Proc. Nat. Acad. Sci. (U.S.) 62: 785 (1969).

42. J.F. Ziersel and R.H. Hageman, Crop Sci. 2: 512 (1962).

43. L. Beevers and R.H. Hageman, Ann. Rev. Plant Physiol. 20: 495 (1969).

44. L.I. Croy and R.H. Hageman, Crop Sci. 10: 280 (1970).

45. V.A. Johnson, P.J. Mattern, and J.W. Schmidt, Crop Sci. 7: 664 (1967).

46. R.L. Warner, Ph.D. Thesis, Dissertation Abstract No. 69 - 1480 (1968).

47. F.H. McNeal, M.A. Berg, and C.A. Watson, Agron. J. 58: 605 (1966).

48. R. Mossberg, in New Approaches to Breeding Improved Plant Proteins, IAEA 29, Vienna, Sti/Pub. 212 (1969).

TABLE 1. Changes in Cereals, Area, and Production

	Area (Million ha)			Production (Million tons)		
	1968	1977	1980	1968	1977	1980
Wheat	227.5	232.4	237.4	332.5	386.6	444.6
Rice	132.1	142.8	145.4	284.2	366.5	399.8
Maize	106.0	118.4	131.0	521.2	349.7	392.2
Barley	74.9	91.4	83.2	130.7	137.1	162.4
Sorghum & Millet	111.2	109.1	90.1	85.1	98.3	87.4
Oats	32.3	30.6	26.7	54.2	52.5	42.7
Rye	22.4	13.9	17.2	33.5	23.8	27.4
Total	706	738.6	731.0	1,171.4	1,450.4	1,555.6

Source: Production Yearbooks 1978, 1979, 1980 FAO, Rome

TABLE 2. World Wheat Production During the 3-Year Period 1979-81

Region/Country	Production (Million tons) 1979	1980	1981
Western Europe	60.3	69.6	64.4
Eastern Europe	23.2	29.4	26.9
USSR	90.2	98.2	88.0
North America	75.3	83.8	100.6
Mexico	2.3	2.8	3.2
South America	12.6	11.8	11.5
Asia	139.6	129.3	136.9
Africa	8.7	8.5	8.4
Oceania	16.5	11.2	16.9
World Total	428.7	444.7	456.8

Source: International Wheat Council, 1982

TABLE 3. Screening Tests Commonly Used to Assess Quality of Cereals

Test	Method	Value/Use
Bread wheat and Triticale		
1. Vitreous kernel count	Manual	Protein content, nutritive value
2. Thousand kernel weight	Manual or machine	Flour yield
3. Protein	N.I.R.S. (near Infrared Reflectance Spectroscopy) - Kjeldahl	Nutritive value
4. Wheat meal fermentation times	Pelshenke	Gluten strength, baking quality
5. Hardness	P.S.I. (Particle Size Index)	Gluten quality, bread-making
6. Milling	Buhler mill, Brabender	Milling quality
7. Mixograph	10 gm sample	Dough and bread quality
8. Farinograph	50 gm sample	Dough and bread quality
9. Moisture	Oven and/or moisture metre	Keeping quality of wheat
10. Baking	Simulated 2-layer bread baking	Industrial
11. Lysine content	Dye-binding capacity	Protein quality, nutritional value
Barley		
1. 1,000 kernel count	Manual	Malting, bread-making
2. Plump kernel count	Automatic shaker	Malting, germination
3. Protein	N.I.R.S. (near Infrared Reflectance Spectroscopy - Kjeldahl	Feed value, malting, nutritive value
4. Moisture	Oven - and Moisture meter	Bread making, malting
5. Diastatic activity	D.P. method	Brewing

TABLE 4. Yield, Thousand Kernel Weight and Protein

Entry	Prot.%	Weight per 1000 kernels (grams)	Yield kg/ha
1. Beecher	12.8	36.5	4242
2. Minn 126/CM67	14.3	45.4	3925
3. ER/Apm	12.5	39.8	5692
4. Api/CM67 CMB 72-60-500Y-502B-503Y-502B-0Y	14.3	25.1	4600
5. WI 2198	13.0	38.2	4621
6. CI8887/CI5761 SEA-13-20S-1S-0S	14.5	35.1	2983
7. CI8887/CI5761 SEA-13-34S-5S-0S	15.3	32.7	3025
8. Carina	14.3	29.5	3758
9. CN2/3/CI7772/Fun//Fun/Tch/4/Fun/5/Ki 11-11694-2B-Bulk-7N-4N	15.4	26.1	3742
10. M69.69/Apm-RL	11.9	29.3	4354
11. Ky 63-1294	15.01	27.2	4188
12. Api/CM67/Mzq CMB 73A-367-13B-1Y-0B	13.2	26.5	4954
13. Menuet	13.8	32.9	3892
14. CI7207/011i	13.1	28.1	3738
15. Fun/II45/PI36/Fun/3/Avt/Nor/92/Winn/ 4/Cer/2*Pro-6L	13.6	31.1	4275
16. Arizona 5908/Aths CYB 8-16A-1A-2A-0A	14.4	37.0	3908
17. Masurka	15.1	31.3	3504
18. M67.18/M14//5106 CMB 73A-448-1B-1Y-1B-1Y-0B	13.3	18.1	3500
19. Emir/Nordgard 265, Ca 3239	14.3	33.3	3525
20. SV 66344/Inis, Ca 12551	13.7	31.5	3788
Mean =	13.9	31.7	4011
S.D.	±0.98	±6.04	±639.99

Source: ICARDA, Regional Barley Yield Trial 1980-81.

BREEDING OF FOOD LEGUMES WITH PARTICULAR REFERENCE TO CHICKPEA AND LENTIL

K.B. SINGH AND W. ERSKINE

INTRODUCTION

Food legumes are important because of the high protein levels of their seeds, ranging from 18 - 30 percent. (See Tannous, Table 3). They provide a balanced diet to a large section of the world's population when consumed with cereals (1) because of their lysine content (See Tannous, Table 5). From 1975 to 1977 the proportion of animal to total protein consumed in the world was 34.6 percent, with the remaining 65.4 percent coming from plant sources (2). Of the plant protein consumed, approximately 70 percent was from cereals, and only 18 per cent from legumes (3). Food legumes are also important in the farming systems of the world because of their ability to fix atmospheric nitrogen, which plays a role in maintaining the fertility of the soil.

The production of the major food crops is shown in Table 1 (4). Soybean is not included because it is grown primarily as an oil crop; however, with production on 52,639.000 ha in 1980 (5) it is a most important crop.

Over the last quarter of a century the productivity of cereals has risen markedly; for example, the world average yield of wheat rose from 1,110 kg/ha during the period 1948-1952 to 1,760 kg/ha over the period 1975-1980. This is an increase of 59 percent. The corresponding increases for some legumes over the same period were only 13 percent (above 560 kg/ha) for lentils, and 24 percent (above 520 kg/ha) for chickpeas. The increase in the yield of cereals is the result of improved management practices and better cultivars.

Causes for the Low Yields of Legumes

An understanding of the factors limiting pulse productivity will help to formulate rational strategies for their improvement, and these are discussed briefly. Cultivars have a low genetic potential for high yield. They are also unable to respond to improved agronomic practices, such as early planting and increased inputs, or irrigation and fertilizer application to the same extent that cereals do. Consequently, farmers are loath to apply new management techniques. Losses from diseases and pests are high. Chemical control methods are uneconomical, and genetic control remains undeveloped.

The lack of mechanization for food legumes is turning the richer farmers, who can afford increased inputs, away from their cultivation when labour is either unavailable or not economical to use. Because food legumes enter little into world trade, they are given scant attention by policymakers. Consequently, the funds available for research to increase their productivity, extension, and farmer-incentives are low in comparison to those for cereals. Realizing the gaps in research on food legumes, the Consultative Group on International Agricultural Research (CGIAR) has been paying considerable attention to their development.

BREEDING METHODS

General Objectives

The major objective in breeding food legumes continues to be high yields. Gradually, breeding resistance to disease is gaining importance. For some crops, efforts are under way to breed for an improved plant type. The shortage of labour and increased cost of employment has forced plant breeders to develop cultivars that can be easily harvested mechanically. An increase in seed size has been an objective for many food legumes. There has been little conscious effort to develop cultivars with improved quality characteristics (6), but breeders have been monitoring the quality of their breeding lines in order to maintain existing standards. There now seems to be an increased awareness of the importance of selecting better quality legumes.

Breeding for wide adaptation has been receiving consideration in many crops. The development of lines tolerant to cold in crops like chickpeas and lentils, and chickpea lines tolerant to heat is one way to broaden the area of cultivation and increase yield. Breeding for resistance to insects has been neglected, mainly because of the unavailability of screening techniques and sources of resistance.

Production of Pure Lines

Large collections of germplasm have been assembled at the various international centres, but they are still underexploited. Further evaluation of this wide genetic base is required. To cite an example, the chickpea germplasm lines assembed at ICARDA were evaluated for Ascochyta blight and cold tolerance, and 22 resistant lines were identified. When these lines were evaluated internationally, a high-yielding and widely adapted line ILC 482 was identified. Clearly, national programmes with limited germplasm resources can benefit from the introduction of material "off the shelf" from either international or national germplasm collections for evaluation. Introduction followed by pure line selection is simple and may have great potential wherever resources are scarce.

The bulk-population method has been used by plant breeders for yield improvement *per se*. It is also useful in breeding lines resistant to stress conditions that occur irregularly, like late frosts.

The backcross method is generally adopted for the transfer of major genes to high-yielding cultivars. Resistance to disease and some qualitative characteristics, such as height, seed colour, etc. have been transferred to high-yielding lines.

The single-seed descent method, which is a modification of the pedigree system, has been advocated wherever greenhouse facilities permitting several generations a year are available. It has been used with varying degrees of success.

Population Improvement

Population improvement has played a vital role in some of the food legumes that are classified as often being cross-pollinated. Two food legumes, viz. faba bean (*Vicia faba* L.) and pigeon pea (*Cajanus cajan* L.), fall into this group. Various types of recurrent selection have been practiced in population improvement for different purposes. Inbred lines are drawn from the improved populations, and these are then used to produce synthetic cultivars.

Male sterile lines have been identified and utilized for population improvement. Cowpea (*Viga unguiculata L. Walp*) is a crop in which maximum exploitation of male sterility has taken place. Male sterility has been reported in chickpea and faba beans but has not yet been put to effective use. The International Crops Research Institute for the Semi-Arid Tropics (ICRISAT) has developed hybrid cultivars in pigeon pea by utilizing male sterility. The centre is about to release some hybrids to national programmes for evaluation.

Chickpea (*Cicer arietinum L.*)

Chickpea was grown on 9.3 million hectares during 1980 and ranked third in area harvested among the pulses. There are two types of chickpeas: *desi* (characterized by small, angular, and coloured seeds) and *kabuli* (characterized by large, ram-shaped, beige seeds). The *desi* type is characteristic of the Indian subcontinent and is also grown in Ethiopia and Iran, whereas the *kabuli* type is preferred in the Mediterranean region and in North and South America. ICRISAT, located in India, is mainly working for the improvement of the *desi* type, and ICARDA is exclusively directing its efforts to the improvement of the *kabuli* type. Several articles have been written on chickpea improvement by the scientists working at these centres (7-9). In this presentation, the results of recent advances made at ICARDA are discussed.

Development of Cultivars for Winter Sowing

Chickpea is cultivated during the spring season in the Mediterranean region. Prior to the establishment of ICARDA in 1977, two facts were apparent. First, chickpeas can tolerate the cold winter of the Mediterranean region at low to medium elevations. Second, Ascochyta blight disease, if not controlled, can completely destroy the crop. Blight-resistant lines have now been developed at Tel Hadya in Northern Syria and tested in many other countries through the Chickpea International Yield Trial-Winter (CIYT-W) and in on-farm trials.

The CIYT-W was initiated during 1979/80, and a summary of the results of the 1980/81 season is given in Table 2. The cultivar ILC 482, recorded, on average, the highest yield (2,402 kg/ha). A trial mean yield in excess of 3,000 kg/ha was observed at two locations, indicating the high yield potential of winter-sown chickpeas. The mean yield of CIYT-W was 60 percent higher than the equivalent trial sown in spring, emphasizing the potential impact of winter-sown chickpea in the Mediterranean region. The introduction of winter sowing means that the crop can be grown in drier areas than at present. Other advantages of winter sowing are a better plant stand and nodulation, and less damage from birds and insects; it does, however, necessitate weed control.

On-farm trials have been run by the Directorate of Agricultural Research, Ministry of Agricultural and Agrarian Reform, Syria and ICARDA for two seasons and the results are compiled in Table 3. The cultivar ILC 482, when sown during winter, produced more than double the yield of the local Syrian variety sown during the spring. This trial is being repeated for another year, and then ILC 482 will be considered for release by the Syrian government for cultivation in Syria. On-farm trials are also now being performed in Lebanon, Jordan, Morocco, and Tunisia.

Many progenies in advanced generations that were uniform, resistant to Ascochyta blight, and that had acceptable seed quality have been bulked, and their yields estimated for comparison with ILC 482. Many produced yields in excess of 3,000 kg/ha, exceeding ILC 482 (Table 4).

Resistance to Ascochyta Blight

The blight (*Ascochyta rabiei* (Pass) Lab.) is the most serious plant disease in the Mediterranean region. Resistance to this disease has been reported by various workers and has been reviewed (10). However, systematic work was lacking on this disease until research was started at ICARDA during 1978. A large-scale, reliable field screening technique has been developed, which involves sowing with spreader rows at frequent intervals, inoculation of the crop with diseased debris collected in the previous season, provision of sprinkler irrigation as frequently as required, and sprays of a spore suspension when needed (11). With the use of this technique, over nine-thousand lines have been screened in the past four years, and 22 *kabuli* and 131 *desi* resistant lines have been identified (Table 5).

The Chickpea International Ascochyta Blight Nursery has been in operation since 1978/79. Lines resistant to Ascochyta blight have been identified in countries of West Asia and North Africa through this nursery. Also six lines, namely, ILC 72, ILC 191, ILC 196, ILC 2380, ILC 2956, and ILC 3279, have shown resistance across locations and years. These lines, possessing broad spectrum resistance, are being fully utilized in the breeding programme.

Screening for Cold and Frost Tolerance

One of the major objectives in breeding cultivars for winter sowing is cold tolerance. The majority of the germplasm accessions have been screened for cold tolerance at Tel Hadya (North Syria), Terbol (Lebanon), and Hymana (near Ankara in Turkey) (12), and cold tolerant lines have been identified (12). Although variablility for cold tolerance among the accessions was noticed, chickpea plants in general were found to be more tolerant at the seedling stage than at the pre-flowering stage. During the 1981/82 season the cold conditions at Tel Hadya, with minimum temperatures below zero for about 15 days during January and February 1982, have provided a better opportunity for screening lines at the seedling stage. Three hundred *kabuli* accessions were evaluated for frost tolerance. Seven of these entries were highly resistant, and 50 were tolerant (Table 6). These lines will be used in the breeding programme after reconfirmation of their cold tolerance.

Desi x Kabuli Introgression

Both *desi* and *kabuli* types possess certain specific desirable genes that breeders have often attempted to transfer. The recovery of *kabuli* types from *desi* x *kabuli* introgression was reported to be small, but no precise estimate was available. The segregation pattern was examined in six crosses (Table 7) during 1979/80. The percentage of recovery of the *kabuli* types was only 5 per cent. In order to increase the recovery of *kabulis*, one backcross was made as: (*desi* x *kabuli*) x *kabuli* and studied in seven cross combinations during 1980/81. There was a 37 percent increased recovery of *kabulis* from this scheme (Table 8). This now poses such questions as whether some desirable genes are being transferred from *desis* to *kabulis* and whether grain yield can be improved through this introgression.

Lentils (*Lens culinaris* Med.)

The primary objective of lentil improvement is to increase the crop's productivity while maintaining the nutritional status of the grain. Lentil land races have a low yield potential, specific adaptation requirements, and are often unresponsive to improvements in husbandry, such as early sowing and phosphorus fertilizer application. They are susceptible to some insect pests, diseases, and parasitic weeds. In the Mediterranean region the *Sitona* spp. weevil and the parasitic weed *Orobanche crenata* are the major reducers of yield, whereas in South Asia and Northeast Africa, rust (*Uromyces fabae*) and both root rot and wilt are the most important limiting factors to full yield development. Many of the existing land races have a plant growth habit that is difficult to harvest mechanically.

The genetic resources and breeding aims and methods employed for this self-pollinated crop have been reviewed (13-15). Only some recent developments are discussed here.

Development of Cultivars for South Asia

Only *microsperma* lentils (seed size < 4.5 g/100 seeds) are cultivated in South Asia (Bangladesh, India, and Pakistan). Large-seeded *macrosperma* cultivars from West Asia and Europe are so late to flower in South Asia that they produce few or no pods. For example, Syrian local large (ILL 4400), a *macrosperma* type, flowered only three days after Giza 9 (ILL 784) from Egypt when they were grown in Northern Syria; whereas the difference in time to flower was 37 days in Pakistan (Table 9) where the photoperiod was less than 11 h. This precludes the use of *macrosperma* types even in hybridization.

This information on the adaptation of the crop is important in formulating a rational strategy for breeding. Thus, it is clear that selections for South Asia must be made under the appropriate environmental conditions of photoperiod and temperature. Accordingly, crosses are being made at ICARDA between South Asian material and both *macrosperma* genotypes and selections from Egypt and Ethiopia. The progeny of these crosses are distributed as a yield trial of bulk populations at the F3 generation, then selections are made between and within crosses by national programmes.

Development of Cold-Tolerant Cultivars

In the higher elevations of Afghanistan, Iran, and Turkey, lentil is commonly sown in the spring. However, the earlier planting of cultivars with winter hardiness results in higher yields. In cooperation with the Turkish Legume Program, a total of 3,592 germplasm accessions were screened for cold tolerance at Hymana, Ankara over the severe winter of 1979/80, when the temperature reached -26.8°C (16). A total of 238 accessions were undamaged by the cold, and these mostly came from either Chile, Greece, Iran, Syria, or Turkey. This material is now being tested for other characteristics in Turkey in order to exploit the cold-tolerant germplasm directly. Some of the selections are also being used as donors of genes for cold tolerance through hybridization. Tolerance to cold damage at the seedling stage is an example of a characteristic for which simple recurrent selection might be effectively practised if the hybridization technique in lentils is facilitated.

Resistance to Orobanche sp.

Parasitic weeds of the genus *Orobanche* are a major problem in lentil production in parts of West Asia and North Africa. Once an area is infested with *Orobanche* seed, which can remain viable in the soil for up to ten years, chemical treatment and crop husbandry cannot control it. Tolerant cultivars that have been found among other legumes (17) but were unknown in lentils present another means of *Orobanche* control. During the 1979/80 season 1,000 accessions of germplasm were screened for their reaction to *O. crenata* at Tel Hadya in heavily infested soil. There were highly significant differences in susceptibility to the weed, with 62 accessions having a maximum of only two emerged inflorescences of *Orobanche* per m^2. In the following season the most resistant entries were again planted in the infested soil. Genotypes ILL 3047 and 3112 from India were the most resistant to *O. crenata*, with an average of only 1.8 and 2.2 inflorescences of *Orobanche* per m^2 in comparison to 16.8 inflorescences per m^2 on the best local (Table 10). These Indian genotypes are now being used as sources of genes for reduced susceptibility to *Orobanche* infestation.

Development of Cultivars for Mechanical Harvesting

Lentils are still harvested by hand in the Middle East, but the high cost of harvest labour is driving some farmers from growing lentils. In North America, however, the crop is harvested mechanically. In view of the value attached to lentil straw as a livestock feed in West Asia, economic methods of harvesting both straw and grain must be found. The land races are both too short and prone to lodging to be easily harvested mechanically. Consequently a selection programme for tall, erect genotypes has been initiated.

Sources of increased height have been found in the germplasm (e.g. Laird-ILL 4349, ex Canada), but in view of their late maturity they are being recombined with earlier adapted selections. The mean plant height of bulk segregating populations in the F2 generations of crosses of this type was 35 $\pm$ 0.7 cm, with a mean of 118 $\pm$ 1.7 days to flower in comparison to a height of 31 cm ILL 4400 (Syrian Local Large) which took 116 days to flower at Tel Hadya in the 1980/81 season. Meanwhile, selection within germplasm accession has resulted in some tall and erect material that can be harvested mechanically, such as 78s 26002 (ILL 8) from Jordan. This selection consistently yielded more than the best check by a mean of 25 percent in three environments in Syria, and 18 percent more than the best local check in two environments in Lebanon.

REFERENCES

1. R. Bressani, "Legumes in Human Diets and How They Might Be Improved," in M. Milner, ed., Nutritional Improvement of Food Legumes by Breeding (Protein Advisory Group of the United Nations, New York, 1973).

2. K. Hoshiai, "Imbalance Situation of Essential Amino Acids in the World," Chem. Econ. Engineer. Rev. 13(9): 16 (1981).

3. M.E. Jalil and W.M. Tahir, "World Supplies of Plant Proteins," in J.W.G. Porter and B.A. Rolls, eds., Proteins in Human Nutrition (Academic Press, New York and London, 1973).

4. Food and Agriculture Organization, FAO Production Yearbook (FAO, Rome, 1972).

5. Food and Agriculture Organization, Production Yearbook (FAO, Rome, 1981).

6. J.H. Hulse, K.O. Rachie, and L.W. Billingsley, "Nutritional Standards and Methods of Evaluation for Food Legume Breeders" (Available from IDRC, Box 8500, Ottawa, Canada K1G 3H9).

7. K.B. Singh and A.N. Aukland, "Chickpea Breeding at ICRISAT," in Proceedings of the International Workshop on Grain Legumes, January 13-16, 1975, Hyderabad, A.P. India (Available from ICRISAT, Patancheru, A.P. 502324, India).

8. G.C. Hawtin, K.B. Singh, and M.C. Saxena, "Some Recent Developments in the Understanding and Improvement of Cicer and Lens," in R.J. Summerfield and A.H. Bunting, eds., Advances in Legume Science (Available from Royal Botanic Gardens, Kew, Richmond, Surrey TW9 3AE, U.K., 1978).

9. D.E. Byth, J.M. Green, and G.C. Hawtin, "ICRISAT/ICARDA Chickpea Breeding Strategies," in Proceedings of the International Workshop on Chickpea Improvement, 28 Feb. - 2 March, 1979, Hyderabad, A.P., India (Available from ICRISAT Patancheru, A.P. 502324, India, 1980).

10. Y.L. Nene, "A Review of Ascochyta Blight of Chickpea (Cicer arietinum L.)". Paper presented in the Workshop on Ascochyta Blight and Winter Sowing of Chickpeas, 4-7 May, 1981, ICARDA, Aleppo, Syria.

11. K.B. Singh, G.C. Hawtin, Y.L. Nene, and M.V. Reddy, "Resistance in Chickpea to Ascochyta rabiei," Plant Disease 65: 586 (1981).

12. K.B. Singh, M.C. Saxena, and H.E. Gridley, "Screening Chickpeas for Cold and Frost Tolerance," Paper presented in the Workshop on Ascochyta Blight and Winter Sowing of Chickpeas, 4-7 May, 1981, Aleppo, Syria.

13. G.C. Hawtin, "Strategies for the Genetic Improvement of Lentils, Broad Beans, and Chickpeas with Special Emphasis on Research at ICARDA," in G.C. Hawtin and G.J. Chancellor, eds., Food Legume Improvement and Development (Available from IDRC, Box 8500, Ottawa, Canada K1G 3H9).

14. F.J. Muehlbauer and A.E. Slinkard, "Genetics and Breeding Methodology," in C. Webb and G.C. Hawtin, eds., Lentils (Available from Commonwealth Agricultural Bureau, Farnham Royal, Slough SL2 3BN, U.K.).

15. M. Solh and W. Erskine, "Genetic Resources," in C. Webb and G.C. Hawtin, eds., Lentils (Available ibid.).

16. W. Erskine, K. Meyveci, and N. Izgin, "Screening a World Lentil Collection for Cold Tolerance," LENS 8: 5 (1981).

17. J.I. Cubero and A. Martinez, "The Genetics of Resistance of Faba beans to *Orobanche crenata*," FABIS 2: 19 (1980).

TABLE 1. Production of the Major Food Crops

	Production Metric Tons
Wheat	444,534
Rice	399,779
Maize	392,249
Sorghum	58,435
Millet	28,918
Total pulses	26,785

Source: Reference 4

TABLE 2. Performance of Selected Entries in Chickpea International Yield Trial-Winter During 1980/81

	CYPRUS		EGYPT		INDIA		LEBANON				SYRIA						TURKEY		JORDAN		GREECE		LIBYA			
	Nicosia		Ismailia		New Delhi		A.U.B.		Terbol		Jinderis		Lattakia		Tel-Hadya		Diyar-bakir		Marrow		Larissa		El-Safsaf		Mean	
Entry	Y	R	Y	R	Y	R	Y	R	Y	R	Y	R	Y	R	Y	R	Y	R	Y	R	Y	R	Y	R	Y	R
ILB 72[a]	218	20	861	18	1667	7	715	12	1781	12	2344	18	3268	7	2058	12	3005	12	1355	19	3302	14	1170	17	1813	16
202[a]	343	13	1035	15	1010	19	634	17	1793	10	2348	17	2889	10	2152	9	2647	18	1645	12	3010	18	1440	9	1746	19
249[b]	473	6	2167	1	1773	6	1226	1	2654	1	3762	3	3542	5	0	19	3662	1	1372	17	4070	1	1640	3	2386	2
482[b]	546	2	1792	2	1805	4	833	8	2354	2	4302	1	3406	6	2490	3	3641	2	2118	4	4063	2	1478	7	2402	1
484[b]	499	5	1306	8	1669	8	923	6	1929	7	4011	2	4257	1	3118	1	3134	7	2154	3	3354	13	1939	1	2358	3
3279[a]	224	19	917	16	1286	15	619	18	1988	5	2777	12	3706	3	2488	4	2783	17	1954	6	3164	17	942	18	1904	10
Local check	385	11	1160	14	2635	1	584	19	1626	17	3473	4	0	20	0	19	2583	19	1418	16	1169	20	-	-	1879	12
Location mean	394		1244		1560		807		1864		2913		2826		2137		3030		1731		3359		1399			
C.V. %	28.71		33.18		26.28		25.97		9.45		21.18		14.88		10.49		7.43		30.44		13.02		18.18			
L.S.D. %	159.93		584.00		579.88		296.32		249.00		872.57		594.70		320.47		318.16		745.05		618.67		359.60			

a = Tall type; b = Conventional type; Y = Yield in kg/ha; R = Rank

TABLE 3. Mean Performance of ILC 482 and Syrian Local During Winter and Spring at Farmers' Fields and Experiment Stations in Syria

Year	WINTER		SPRING	
	ILC 482	Syr. Local	ILC 482	Syr. Local
1979/80	1839[a]	988	-	973
1980/81	1724[b]	479	983	798
Mean	1782	734	983	886

a = Average of 18 locations; b = Average of 21 locations

TABLE 4. Performance of the Best 10 Bulked Blight-Resistant Progenies at Tel Hadya During the Winter of 1980/81

Pedigree	Yield kg/ha	% increase over ILC 482	Disease reaction[a] Veg.	Pod
ILC 51 x ILC 200	3600	93	3	2
ILC 618 x ILC 194	3293	66	3	3
ILC 523 x ILC 183	3333	86	3	2
ILC 1929 x ILC 200	3328	7	3	3
ILC 1929 x ILC 200	4848	30	5	5
ILC 72 x ILC 897	3471	100	3	3
ILC 72 x ILC 897	3977	17	3	3
ILC 72 x ILC 897	3502	38	3	3
ILC 201 x ILC 571	3302	31	3	3
ILC 202 x ILC 893	3373	23	3	3
Average	3603	40		

a = Disease reaction: 1 = free; 9 = killed

TABLE 5. Summary of the Screening of Chickpea, Kabuli and Desi Germplasm Lines for Resistance to Ascochyta Blight at Tel Hadya, ICARDA, Syria

Disease Rating	Kabuli		Desi	
	No. of entries	% of total entries	No. of entries	% of total entries
1	0	0.00	0	0.00
2	0	0.00	13	0.22
3	18	0.53	118	1.97
4	4	0.12	524	8.72
5	43	1.28	253	4.21
6	17	0.53	76	1.27
7	859	25.50	246	4.10
8	14	0.42	20	0.33
9	2412	71.63	4755	79.18
Total	3367	100.0	6005	100.00

1 = Highly resistant; 5 = Tolerant; 9 = Highly susceptible

TABLE 6. Evaluation of _Kabuli_ Chickpeas for Frost Tolerance at Tel Hadya During 1981/82

Frost Rating 1-9 scale	No. of Entries	% of Total
1	7	2.0
2	15	5.0
3	35	11.7
4	56	18.7
5	63	21.0
6	51	17.0
7	45	15.0
8	25	8.3
9	3	1.0
Total	300	100.0

1 = Highly resistant (free); 5 = Intermediate; 9 = Highly susceptible (killed)

TABLE 7. Classification (%) of F2 Plants into Six Classes, Based on their F_3 Seed Characteristics, from Six *Kabuli* x *Desi* Crosses

		Seed Classification (%)						Total of F2 Plants Classified
		Kabuli		Intermediate		Desi		
		White	Dark	White	Dark	White	Dark	
X79TH	4	7	8	16	33	11	23	383
	62	5	14	13	44	8	15	648
	85	4	16	11	29	10	30	1488
	115	2	3	11	53	7	25	847
	138	9	11	23	26	15	16	1113
	148	5	6	14	41	7	28	832
Mean		5	10	15	36	10	24	

Source: Unpublished data from Chickpea Breeding Sub-program at ICARDA

TABLE 8. Recovery of the Kabulis from Three-Way Crosses (Kabuli x Desi) x Kabuli in F_2 Generation During 1980/81 at Tel Hadya

Cross	Seed Classification						Total
	Kabuli		Intermediate		Desi		
	White	Dark	White	Dark	White	Dark	
(ILC 118 x NEC 1813) x ILC 215	145	13	50	28	27	6	269
(ILC 16 x NEC 1096) x ILC 248	39	34	27	47	1	-	148
(ILC 868 x NEC 1813) x ILC 183	302	10	149	180	41	20	702
(ILC 1919 x ICC 5127) x ILC 493	597	-	430	182	55	29	1293
(ILC 1403 x NEC 1163) x ILC 215	78	-	43	90	18	35	264
(ILC 263 x NEC 1813) x ILC 249	72	1	21	6	17	-	117
(ILC 265 x NEC 798) x ILC 190	120	2	263	149	74	227	835
Total	1353	60	983	682	233	317	3628
Mean (%)	37	2	27	19	6	9	100

TABLE 9. Time to 50% of Plants Flowering in Two Contrasting Environments*

Particulars	Locations: Islamabad, Pakistan	Locations: Tel Hadya, Syria
Latitude (°N)	33	37
Photoperiod**	10.9	12.2
Mean temperature (°C)		
Maximum	19	16
Minimum	6	6
Mean time to 50% flowering (d)		
Cultivar - Giza 9 (ILL 784)	108	96
Cultivar - Syrian local (ILL 4400)	145	99

*Data from Lentil Adaptation Trial 1979/80
**Photoperiod includes twilight and is at one week prior to flowering
Temperature is the average over the month prior to flowering

TABLE 10. Average Number of Inflorescemces of *Orobanche crenata* per sq m on Selected Lentil Accessions in the 1980/81 Season

Accession Number	Number of Inflorescences/sq m
ILL 3047	1.8
ILL 3112	2.2
ILL 4400 (Syrian local large)	19.8
ILL 4401 (Syrian local small)	16.8
L.S.D. 5%	7.2

DISCUSSION

SESSION IV - GENETIC IMPROVEMENT AND NUTRITION

GEOFFRY C. HAWTIN

I would like to begin my comments by taking another look at the food legumes. Several participants at this workshop have pointed out that they are comparatively unimportant in the diets in most countries of the ICARDA region. We have been shown figures indicating that their average contribution to dietary protein is only in the order of about 10 percent. One may well ask, why the interest in food legumes?

Of course a major reason for the interest is the desire to increase the protein available in human diets; an objective that, as we heard yesterday, has once again become respectable following the recently published re-evaluation of human protein requirements. It must also be remembered that the average figures quoted may well belie the true value of food legumes to certain, particularly the poorer, sections of the population, and in certain countries. However, I would be surprised if food legumes ever contributed more than 20 percent of dietary protein even among the highest-consuming families in the Middle East. I would be interested to hear if any of the participants here have data on any communities in the region that do, in fact, rely on food legumes for a significant proportion of their protein intake.

Food legumes are well-known and popular items in the diet, with dishes such as hommus bi taheeni, foul, and falafel being famous. Again, we must ask the question: If food legumes are both popular and nutritious, why do they account for such a small proportion of the diet?

I think that Singh has provided us with at least part of the answer; it is a question of productivity. Food legume yields are very low and if we are to make any impact on diets in the region it is imperative that the first priority be given to increasing and stabilizing yields, and thereby reducing prices to a level where more people can afford to buy them. This need to increase productivity has, I believe quite rightly, already been stressed by many participants at this workshop.

In this regard, many countries in the region have very ambitious plans for increasing legume production; some to the extent of calling for more than doubling production within a five-year period. This, however, is to be achieved largely by replacing fallow in the medium and higher rainfall zones, but increasing productivity is also an important objective.

The emphasis on legumes has been fostered by the recognition not only of their dietary value, but also the role they play in maintaining, or even improving, soil fertility through their ability to fix atmospheric nitrogen, and their importance in increasing agricultural diversification.

If the objectives of these plans are realized, and productivity is dramatically increased, one can imagine a situation in which overproduction could lead to prices falling to the extent that the crop would only be profitable in the more favourable, higher-yielding environments; thus the majority of farmers in the poorer areas could be denied the benefits of having food legumes as an economically viable option in their rotations. This certainly would be an undesirable consequence of increased productivity, even if prices were to fall sufficiently to stimulate some increased consumption. Of course, demographic expansion alone is expected to result in a substantial increase in demand, but I believe that it is also highly desirable to look for other ways of stimulating this increase. We should consider, for instance, exporting to other regions, especially Europe; this in turn may affect the quality characteristics required in the crop, as, for example, very large seed size in chickpeas.

Another way would be to incorporate more food legumes into animal feeds; again, this could have considerable consequences for quality requirements, and hence breeding objectives, especially if premium prices were to be paid for good quality, i.e., high protein, high methionine, high digestibility and low antinutritional factors.

There may be other ways to increase demand through considering some of the secondary causes of low consumption. One may be the well-known problem of flatulence, with physical discomfort setting an upper limit to an individual's consumption. Legumes, the "poor man's meat", require a very long cooking time; this being both inconvenient and expensive in fuel. Convenience preparations such as canning, freezing, freeze-drying and fast-cooking treatments may play a much more important role in the future and we need, even today, to consider the quality requirements for such preparations. Plant-breeding is a very long process; if we set a breeding objective today and start making crosses this season, it will be fully ten years before any cultivar originating from this effort will be grown commercially on farmers' fields. An objective set today may be substantially less important ten years, hence and new problems, not considered today, may have arisen. A plant breeder has to crystal-ball gaze, and I think a workshop such as this provides a good opportunity to do so.

Accepting the very great importance, both from an agricultural and a nutritional point of view, of increasing and stabilizing yields, I think we should give some attention to discussing exactly what quality objectives should be considered by breeders. Bressani has indicated a large range of different factors that could be taken into account. A plant-breeder could not possibly consider them all. Several purely technical, rather than nutritional, considerations may affect our choice of objectives. It may be considered very desirable nutritionally to breed for a particular characteristic, but unless there is enough genetic variability available, the task may be impossible. In addition, it is normally necessary, in a breeding programme, to screen hundreds, if not thousands, of samples, often in a short period of time and on limited seed quantities. Unless an adequate screening technique is available, it may prove too expensive to make the genetic advance desired.

When considering breeding objectives for seed quality, I believe we can broadly distinguish three groups of factors:

1. First, there are factors that may affect nutritive value, such as total protein quantity and quality. Such factors may be considered high priority nutritionally, but may be of very limited value commercially. Much effort could go into raising the quantity of protein in a legume seed, yet in the absence of a premium pricing system for protein, which does not exist anywhere in the world for legumes for human consumption, then the cultivar concerned will never be adopted by farmers unless it also has high yield or other commercially important attributes. I believe the positive improvement of such factors should, in

general, receive a low priority in breeding programmes. Other factors in this same category would include digestibility, trypsin inhibitors, phytohemagglutinins, and flatulence factors.

2. A second group of factors that are more important from a breeding standpoint are those considered important by the consumer, and hence are likely to affect the level of consumption and, generally, also the price. Indeed, these factors may be of such importance that unacceptable characteristics may result in complete rejection by the consumer. One example of such a factor is cooking time. Among the lentils, for example, types known to have good cooking characteristics may fetch a premium price, and thus there is a strong incentive for farmers to grow these types. In breeding for short cooking time, the possibility of a concomitant increase in susceptility to storage insects should be considered. There is strong, admittedly mainly anecdotal, evidence to suggest a relationship between these factors. Other factors that come within this group of consumer-oriented objectives are seed colour, size, and shape. Hulling percentage in the case of lentils may also be considered in this group.

The case of polyphenols is interesting. Although of nutritional significance, their influence on seed colour may require that breeding for their presence of absence be determined primarily by consumer colour preferences rather than nutritional considerations. We know that in many legumes, e.g., faba beans, it would be comparatively easy to breed polyphenol-free types. Such an objective could be considered important nutritionally, especially in those countries where light-seeded types are well accepted. However, there is a fair amount of evidence to suggest that polyphenols in the seed coat play a role in disease and pest resistance; polyphenol-free types frequently appear to be more susceptible. In this case the breeder might have to decide between a nutritional objective, or maintaining levels of resistance to pests or diseases.

3. Finally, there are those factors that relate to human health. In this respect the most important one, with regard to ICARDA's crops, is the relationship between faba beans and favism. This disease, a hemolytic syndrome, occurs in genetically susceptible individuals as a result of consuming faba beans. The disease is well-known and widespread through most of the ICARDA region and can be fatal in children. I strongly suggest that ways of reducing or eliminating the factors in faba beans thought to be responsible for favism (vicine, convicine, and possibly DOPA) should be given a high priority in research and breeding programmes.

Thus, I would conclude that factors that affect nutritive value only, but have little effect on consumption or prices, should only be monitored by breeders to ensure that they do not fall to unacceptable levels. Factors for which there are strong consumer preferences must certainly be considered by breeders, as should factors affecting human health.

On this last point, and because of the importance of favism, I would like Leila Hussein, who has been working on some aspects of the problem in Egypt, to say a few words.

Hussein: Favism is a disease characterized by hemolytic anemia that occurs when individuals who are deficient in Glucose-6-Phosphate Dehydrogenase (G6PD) consume faba beans. This enzyme deficiency, which is genetically controlled in humans, is common in populations in the Mediterranean area. The deficiency is believed to have a selective advantage, in humans, as a defense mechanism to malaria. In susceptible individuals the level of glutathione in the erythrocytes is also reduced.

Three different compounds present in faba beans have been implicated as playing a causative role in the disease. Two of these are glycosides known as vicine and convicine, and the third is an amino acid derivative known as dihydroxyphenylalanine (DOPA). These are present only in the cotyledons of the beans, the hulls (testae) being essentially free. We looked at these three different compounds in different cultivars of faba beans grown in Egypt and Sudan. The three compounds can be quantified separately, and in a short period of time (15 minutes per sample) using reverse phase high performance liquid chromatography (HPLC). Our preliminary studies have shown differences between cultivars in the levels of these compounds. The cultivar known as Triple White was found to have the lowest levels of vicine, convicine, and DOPA. It should be possible to breed cultivars that are free, or have only very low levels, of these factors.

We have looked at the effect of different home cooking practices on the levels of the three compounds. We found that germinating the beans until the sprout appeared had a positive effect in lowering the levels of these compounds. Such sprouting was a common practice in Egypt in the 1950s in the preparation of a dish known as foul nebit. This dish is still popular today, especially in the rural areas. In our trials, vicine concentration was reduced from 0.77 to 0.46 per cent in the preparation of foul nebit. The consumption of this dish should be encouraged. In the process of boiling faba beans, much of the vicine and convicine is eliminated in the stewing liquor, and the concentration remaining in the beans is substantially reduced.

In addition to the above work, we have also studied the relationship between income and the form in which faba beans are consumed, and we have compared consumption in urban and rural areas. We are now undertaking research into the mechanisms of hemolysis induced by vicine and convicine.

Pellett: I would like to comment on the question of protein and legume consumption that was raised earlier. I have data here from food balance sheets. Although these data have limitations, world figures show that about eight per cent of the protein comes from legumes. In the developed countries legumes contribute as little as two percent. In the Middle East, Saudi Arabia receives only three percent of its protein from legumes, while Syria obtains as much as 11 percent. These are average data for each country, and it is likely that the poorer segment of the population would consume larger porportions of legumes.

Scrimshaw: If you had a corn and bean diet in which the beans were 10 percent of the diet in dry volume, and that is all you had, you would have 25 percent of your nitrogen coming from the beans. This would be markedly reduced by the digestibility factor that Bressani indicated was something less than 20 percent. If you had a rice and bean diet with beans as 10 percent of the diet then the nitrogen provided from beans would be over 30 percent. If you were dealing with soy you would not have such a reduction because of the digestibility factor. These figures do not show the reality, only the potential. Nevertheless, they do emphasize the importance of the digestibility factor.

If you feed a rat 10 percent legume protein, the deficiency of methionine shows up very sharply, and if you add methionine there is an improvement. If you do this with humans, adults or children, at deficient levels, they have a strongly negative nitrogen balance and added methionine increases retention. But if you provide protein at required levels, the methionine deficiency is not so apparent. Adding methionine to soy provided at required levels to adults, children or infants, has no effect on nitrogen balance. It is easy to overemphasize the effect of methionine in human diets from looking at rat experiments or studies in humans when testing is done in the conventional manner of feeding at a deficient level.

Parpia: The patterns of consumption of beans or grain legumes vary a great deal in different parts of the world. In Latin America, the retention of shape of frijoles is rather important, but where certain types of pastry products are consumed, for example quesafillas, cooking time can be substantially reduced by flaking. This work has been done aleady at CFTRI and there are several small companies now manufacturing flaked grain legumes that are almost instant products for consumption.

The second point in this respect is that there is a traditional practice of adding a certain amount of carbonate, which reduces cooking time substantially. However, I do not know what effect that alkalinity has on amino acid composition, and this needs to be studied more carefully. While the flatus factor is important, there are varieties of legumes known to cause very little. An example is Phaseolus aureus (mung bean), which has not been mentioned at all. This crop has a long growing season and can be cultivated in many countries between two seasonal crops. Therefore, it can be a very good additional food source.

Lastly, I would say we have not sufficiently discussed the fibre content of grain legumes. This is very important, and already some studies have attributed a reduction of blood cholesterol to this factor. We should therefore look more broadly at the nutritional make-up of grain legumes. The cooking time factor should be given greater attention becuase in many villages there is a shortage of fuel caused by deforestation.

Alderman: I would like to point out possible interfaces among the different scientists here. Plant breeders seem to have potential breakthroughs in the case of chickpeas, and maybe now the economists and nutritionists can do some ex-ante assessments of impact rather than their traditional ex-post studies. We have discussed the production potential for chickpeas, but if production goes up, will exports increase? If this happens prices may not be reduced. How will this affect changes in income or in labour requirements at different times of year? What will happen to other crops and animals in the farming system? Many questions arise concerning the changes in the form and availability of the crop that would occur should any slight change be made in its cultivation.

Similarly, for the nutritionsits, we must ask how increased chickpea availability would fit into the diet. It would also be interesting to look at different income groups and different age groups. Are we talking about foods that are primarily eaten by adults or children? Obviously, the nutritional impact would be quite different. The digestibility and fiber content would have a big impact on whether it is a useful product for a young child as part of a weaning formula or whether it would be better for slightly older children. There are a number of questions to which I will not propose any answers, but rather suggest that this is a chance for the different disciplines to come together to use something that the plant breeders have introduced.

Nygaard: ICARDA has not yet answered all those questions, but we are working on them. Let me mention one area that we think has promise as an example of an ex-ante contribution by economists. We have divided the effects of introducing winter planting of chickpea into two areas. One will be the area where chickpeas are already grown, but the new variety and an earlier planting date will be introduced. The other will be an area where chickpeas have not been grown, but could be using the new variety because it can take advantage of the extra moisture available in winter. To illustrate this first case, we are doing some partial budgets and measuring the impact of wage rates and increased labour demand. For example, if chickpeas are planted earlier there is more competition for labour because wheat, barley, and other crops are also planted at this time.

One of the advantages of the traditional practice of late planting is that it is at a rather slack time in the labour season.

What we cannot say much about yet is how the farm families will respond to this new opportunity. We believe that the answer to many of these questions will come in our testing of the new variety on farmers' fields. This is a new dimension to the Farming Systems Program's research activities. We have shown that planting winter chickpeas is technically feasible from an experimental standpoint and that it is economically feasible as well. The next step is to test the new technique on the farmers' fields. We find it useful to differentiate between scientist-managed tests, scientist/farmer-managed tests, and farmer-managed tests. Until this year, we have not had enough seed of the new variety to have significant farmer or joint-managed tests on farmers' fields. This year we do, and tests are in progress. These farmers will be monitored, visited, questioned and listened to, so we can better understand what the effect will be of their adopting our recommendations. Perhaps we can start looking at issues of home consumption, storage, and the impact on the diet, and at labour use as well.

Alderman: Could you make a guess about the potential differential rate of adoption? This is such a new way of growing the plant that you may see different attitudes toward risk, and this may affect who is going to take the first step. There could be an impact on income distribution.

Nygaard: It is not such a different way of growing the crop. The date of planting is earlier, but other management practices are the same. Therefore, we feel there should not be constraints on adoption in that sense. One exception is weed control. Earlier planting could cause a serious weed problem that does not exist now, and this has to be looked at.

Alderman: Farmers are not accustomed to planting their crop so early in the year, and they may expect it to be devastated by diseases if they plant early. This is an important change.

Nygaard: I believe a more important danger is that there may be a fast rate of adoption, a tremendous influx of chickpeas on the market, and a substantial drop in prices that could wipe out the technological gain.

Gerhart: What proportion of the chickpea crop is marketed now? Is it largely subsistence? If so, the farmers could reduce the area planted.

Nygaard: Most of the chickpeas produced are marketed.

Srivastava: There are two points I would like to make. Bressani gave us a list of what plant breeders could do. It is proper that we should look at all the factors, but we also have to set our priorities. Let us take the example of food legumes. Even if there were more chickpeas available, the population would not consume more than a certain quantity because of flatulence. Perhaps efforts should be in other directions.

I would like to turn to cereals, which in this area, provide not 10 percent of the protein consumed, but 50-60 percent, according to the information I have, as well as a fairly large portion of energy. For the region as a whole, about 80 to 90 percent of its arable area is rainfed. At the current level of technology, faba beans and chickpeas cannot be grown under low rainfed conditions. There is no other crop that can replace barley at present, and barley does provide protein and energy. I would therefore like to discuss more immediate problems instead of reiterating how food legumes will satisfy nutritional needs in ten years. I would like to know how the current crops are nutritionally deficient. Is there some kind of combination of wheat, barley, and chickpea that can solve dietary deficiency immediately?

We talked about increased yield and protein content but have not resolved the issue. Is there definitely a negative correlation between them? I do not believe we have made enough of an effort to find out. There may be some way to improve both. Mekni mentioned that growing a cereal with nitrogen fertilizer will increase both nitrogen content and yield. We must look into lysine content and protein balance. At ICARDA we are doing quality-testing in order to determine the effects of some environmental factors, such as level of fertilizer use and moisture availability.

Finally, I would like to pose a challenge to the economists. The plant breeders will work on improving the quality of the grain if the economists will try to convince the policymakers to buy grain on the basis of quality and not by weight. The price of wheat should reflect the protein content so that, although the wheat may be of lower weight, the farmer will not suffer.

<u>Miladi:</u> I think there is some confusion here. In this region there is no protein deficiency and the diet is well balanced. We do not need to worry about protein, lysine or methionine, but need an increase in production. This is what the nutritionists are telling the agricultural scientists. Just increase production. We have had a good diet in this region for centuries. The food habits that have been established, for example <u>couscous</u> and the preservation of wheat and the mixing of cereals and legumes, were developed centuries ago by our forebears.

It is very seldom that one finds malnutrition or even undernutrition among the adult population. This is because food is very important in our culture: when a person dies, the relatives and friends eat; when a woman gives birth, we eat; and when you are a guest, you have to eat out of respect. Even when a person kills another person, the families slaughter an animal and eat it. The nutritional problem we are facing is one of the preschool child and the influence of other cultures on our diet. To this end chickpea and lentils are being added to infant weaning formula in Tunisia, Algeria and Egypt.

Finally, let me remind you that there are limitations to the Food Balance Sheet and we cannot be sure of these production and consumption figures, yet they are being used or possibly misused by governments.

<u>Mekni:</u> I would like to point to one obvious fact: areas planted with legumes are decreasing and areas under cereal cultivation are increasing in this region. Regardless of food habits, if you intend to maintain the same nutritional balance, you have to keep the diet the same. Thus, the food sources mentioned either have to be produced locally or imported. To compare legumes and cereals, we should consider the fact that by increasing yields in cereals we can obtain more protein per unit area than we could with legumes. How are we going to solve the problem of decreasing legume cultivation?

Another point that should be considered is that many cereals can be turned into other forms of proteins. We know that barley in this area is grazed at least part of the season, and I do not see why a higher protein barley would not result in higher yields of animal protein.

<u>Williams:</u> As a grain technologist, I often find myself caught between plant breeders and nutritionists. We have been emphasizing breeding in this session, but really the progress made in chickpea production was due to agronomy and hus-

bandry achievements rather than a breeding achievement. If plant breeders are lucky, they will achieve a 5 percent increase in yield with a new line, whereas an improvement in husbandry will bring about a 30 to 50, even a 100 percent increase in yield, and it will achieve this over a much shorter period of time. What are the influences of some of these cultural practices? For example, Srivastava questioned the negative relation between yield and protein content from a breeder's perspective. An agronomist can increase yield with fertilizer applications and often the protein content goes up at the same time.

Singh: What Williams said may hold true for other crops, but it is not true for chickpeas. It is variety that has played the most significant role. As you saw in my slide presentation, the Syrian "local" chickpea was completely destroyed by cold, but the new variety survived. I do not deny that other factors are important, too. For example, this year we have introduced spacing as an additional variable in our on-farm trials. Saxena has demonstrated that with closer spacing, yield increases of anywhere from 15 to 25 percent could be achieved. In contrast, fertilizer use has not caused an increase in yield in either the winter or spring chickpea crop.

Williams: This is not a criticism of breeders because there is no question that when you develop an improved variety it will respond better to improved cultural practices. It is just a question of the integration of the two, and I think we probably should give more emphasis to agronomy and farming practices in these developing regions. It is much more difficult to do.

Scrimshaw: I am going to say something that will seem contradictory at the start, and that is that one should not pay too much attention to the Food Balance Sheets. After all, they are an effort to determine total food availability and divide it by the number of people. It does not tell us anything about distribution, and in the case of protein, people can and do eat much more protein than they need if they can afford it. That leaves less protein for the poorer people. Therefore, to conclude there is plenty of protein from the Food Balance Sheets is false.

Having said that, however, I would suggest that if one looks at most of the diets in the region, Miladi is quite right. The percentage of available protein-calories is well above this ten percent figure that I indicated, or eleven percent if you make corrections for quality in the diet. It is not necessary to emphasize more protein in the ordinary diet. In addition, the higher protein requirements should not set off a wave of exaggeration of the need for protein in the diet. However, legumes are an important source of complementary protein for the poorest segments of a population who depend primarily on cereals and who have virtually no access to animal protein at all. Under these circumstances, if the production of legumes relative to cereals goes down and the price goes up, these people will suffer. Among the poorest of the poor, those most vulnerable, such as growing children and pregnant or lactating women, will suffer. We are not saying that you need more protein in the ordinary diet, but legumes must be available to the very poor who do not have access to animal protein.

Salameh: I would like to refer to Bressani's paper and to what Scrimshaw just said about animal protein. I see a large gap between breeding results of the types referred to by Bressani and the efforts of government to put those results into practice and enact policies. Whose responsibility do you think it is to start filling this gap? Is it the job of industry, of health ministries or of the universities? I think research centers such as ICARDA have a duty in this respect.

Bressani: Are you referring to the transfer of technology?

Salameh: Yes, because we are in need of animal protein.

Bressani: Well, somebody said that there is no need for animal protein; there is no lack of it.

Pellett: May I answer that question? I think you are asking about the great importance of complementary proteins in meeting protein needs within society. This is true. However, in the Middle East, it is not something that needs government intervention. The normal diet in this region tends to produce a mixture of proteins that is better in protein quality than any of the components alone. The dietary practice here already makes that complementation. Certainly, however, major changes in patterns of consumption could lead to negative effects.

Salameh: We do feel that eating habits are deteriorating and uses of bulgur and legumes are disappearing from the diet.

Miladi: I do not think our traditional diet is deteriorating. I do not think there is any house in Tunisia where couscous will not be consumed every week. I do not think anyone in Egypt will not eat faba beans or tameya. In Syria, one always eats hommus and moutabil. Our diet is not deteriorating; but it may be changing.

Hawtin: I think this point perhaps does need a bit more clarification because we have had figures to indicate increasing cereal production, and decreasing legume production, at least relative to population. If that is not leading to a poorer diet, the difference is being made up by imports in some way. How would you explain this?

Salameh: The percentage of animal protein out of the total protein is about 15 percent. Do you agree with this percentage? Some nutritionists say it should be over thirty percent. If this is true then we are in need of animal protein.

Pellett: I do not think there is anybody in the field of scientific nutrition who would say that there is an absolute need for animal protein. There are certainly higher levels of several vitamins and minerals commonly associated with animal proteins than with vegetable proteins as well as generally higher levels of essential amino acids, but you can meet your ordinary protein needs from mixtures of vegetable proteins very adequately. If that were not true, vegetarians would not survive at all and vegetarians generally survive very well indeed. We can thus meet protein needs by complementation.

Over the centuries the Middle East has evolved a dietary pattern that is extremely effective in increasing the amount of utilizable protein from wheat, which is low in lysine, by supplementing it with legumes, which have up to four times the lysine of wheat. This combination can meet the protein needs for adults and even approaches the protein requirements for children.

Srivastava: I disagree with Miladi's statement that the food habits of the Middle East have not changed for the worse. In Syria, for example, meat prices have risen from 20 Syrian lira four years ago for a kilo of lamb to 50 SL today. Whole wheat flour used to be consumed, and now 85 percent of the bran has been removed before the wheat is eaten. The per capita availability of legumes has gone down. These changes must be affecting the dietary habits somehow. Those who can afford to do so are probably eating better, but when it comes to the lower income groups, I believe that habits have been forced to change.

Myntti: I am a little bit confused because I am hearing from nutritionists that the diet, as far as protein is concerned, is adequate. On the other hand, anemia is a very serious problem among the children and women in the Middle East. Others are saying that legumes have the problem of low protein digestibility. Can one of you speak to these contradictions and tell us what sort of research is needed?

Scrimshaw: I think first we have to separate the issue of protein and iron. I would like to pose a question to the plant breeders in general as to what they think they might be able to do to increase the very low availability if iron from plant sources. We do not know fully why iron is so poorly available. We do know that the presence of oxalate, phytate and crude fibre all interface with iron availability. Thus, for populations that do not have access to the iron in hemoglobin that is obtained from red meat, it is very difficult to get iron from predominantly vegetable diets, particlarly when there is a reason for increased iron loss such as is associated with hookworm, schistosomiasis or malaria. There can be real problems of iron availability.

The protein problem is a separate issue. If you look at diets around the world, they appear to have sufficient available protein. But when you look at the distribution within populations, you find that protein is unevenly distributed, and for the group at the lower end of the economic scale, protein is limiting or at least borderline. It is those whom we do not expect to be able to protect by making animal protein available because it would be impractical in many countries. We would like to prevent or remedy the situation by keeping the price of legumes down and the availability up.

Mansour: As a nutritionist, I am not comfortable hearing that our diet in the region is not deteriorating. I think we have to be cautious, because if we look at the lowest percentile or the population, diets are not adequate. There is evidence from the last food consumption survey in Tunisia that the diet of the lowest 30 percent of the population has not improved in the past five years. With regard to nutrition-related health matters, we cannot say that our diets in the area are not deteriortaing.

The second point is that there is a problem of protein for this segment of the population where both energy and protein intakes are low. One of the solutions is to increase the production of legumes that supplement cereals very well. I wish to leave the impression that I am concerned about the diets for that 30 percent of the population who are poor.

Pellett: We also have to remember the interaction of food, nutrition, and all the other aspects of health, such as infectious diseases. While we can make observations about diet, it is impossible to make a statement about overall improvement without considering health factors. The lack of a clean water supply can produce malnutrition in the presence of an adequate diet.

Parpia: I would like to reinject a certain amount of interdisciplinary consideration. If a crop we breed is very high-yielding but is not easily acceptable, then there may be a technology to make it acceptable. I do not think we have considered this factor in our discussions. Technology can make products safer and better. It might even reduce the energy required to cook these foods. We have to be careful, however, not to get into a situation where the marketing costs and margins increase greatly, because I know of examples where margins have gone up from 30 to 100 percent.

One of the largest surplus proteins that goes into animal feed today is groundnut protein. It has been possible to make it aflatoxin-free, and to use it as a substitute for milk and as a milk extender. This has been done very successfully, and today commercial and semi-commercial plants are in operation. In addition we must also consider cereal-legume mixtures, but since I am going to discuss this in the last session I only raise the issue here. We should therefore try to identify such interdisciplinary research where the breeder, the technologist, and the nutritionist can work together to develop a product of the desired type. We can use the flexibility of a breeder to produce a high-yielding crop that can then be processed into a better product from a technical and nutritional point of view.

Hawtin: I think the points you have made are valid, but since this session is entitled "genetic improvement and nutrition", I would like to return to this subject. Does anyone have any comments particularly related to genetic improvement?

Saxena: I would like to return to the question of digestibility of protein in food legumes. I know, for example in the case of soy protein, that the digestibility definitely improves with heat treatment. Does the same thing hold true for other food legumes? If digestibility is important, as Bressani indicated, breeders should be paying attention to this, but we need a rapid method for evaluation. We cannot run large-scale biological trials for this therefore tests are needed to screen large amounts of germplasm.

Bressani: I agree. Among food legumes the three that have relatively high protein digestibility are soy bean, chickpea and peanuts. Other legumes, including lentils and *Phaseolus* varieties and pigeon peas, have low digestibilities but we do not know the reason for this. Even worse, when these are put in a mixed diet, the overall digestibility seems to drop towards that of the food legumes. We are therefore trying to find out what factors are causing this low digestibility. This is one of the reasons why we have been studying the role of polyphenols. Polyphenolic compounds in human studies have been found to account for only about 8 to 10 percent of the negative digestibility factors so they may not be that important. With respect to rapid tests for detecting this, there is a multiple-enzyme test where a change in pH is measured which offers results in 15 minutes and this correlates very highly with animal and human data.

Finally, I do not think there is a need to select for higher protein concentration in food legumes, because the levels we have found are sufficient. I would try to correct for protein digestibility first and then work on higher protein concentration.

Hussein: After the inactivation of trypsin inhibitors that are present in *Phaseolus vulgaris*, most of the amino acids are still not digested and are all excreted in the faeces. As you know, *Phaseolus vulgaris* is one of the leguminous seeds that is highest in trypsin inhibitor content. So if you can select cultivars that are low in trypsin inhibitors, that would affect digestibility positively.

Bressani: I am not sure whether I agree with that. Trypsin inhibitors are very rich sources of sulfur amino acids. We know that if the beans are cooked under good conditions of moisture and heat, the trypsin inhibitors disappear completely. Also, the *Phaseolus vulgaris* trypsin inhibitor is different from the soy bean trypsin inhibitor, and soy beans have much higher levels of trypsin inhibitors that are destroyed during processing. In a recent meeting in Ottawa to determine nutritional priorities, it was decided not to try to eliminate trypsin inhibitors because correct processing gets rid of the problem. Hemaglutinin compounds are not a problem either because they are also destroyed.

The reasons for low digestibility is that the globulin fraction in Phaseolus vulgaris is not easily digested by the normal enzyme systems of animals or humans, and it is this fraction that is responsible for the problem.

I want to come back to another question about iron deficiency anemia and Phaseolus vulgaris. There were some studies carried out in Venezuela suggesting that the availability of iron from beans is relatively high. In a recent survey that we carried out in Guatemala on the home preparation of beans and on the distribution of the beans and broth within the family, we found that mothers begin to give infants a broth with corn at two months of age. When asked why they do this, they replied that it is ".....good for blood production to control anemia". They have known this for many years and this is something that we have to respect. One of the reasons we are selecting for a variety with a short cooking-time and complete destruction of the inhibitors, and that will allow the solids from the cotyledons to pass into the liquid, is because we want a higher concentration of solids in the cooking liquor -- like a thick soup. Mothers should give this more nutritious broth to children when they are very young.

Karrar: It seems to me that as nutritionists we are concentrating on protein-energy deficiency and are neglecting the micro-nutrients. Scrimshaw pointed this out very clearly in his presentation and breeders should pay attention to that. Bressani said that supplementation of corn-bean based diets with minerals will produce a weight gain as good as when you add lysine and methionine. In the Sudan there are millets that have been found to contain goitrogens, so we need to concentrate on micro-nutrients and on these toxins instead of protein and energy, which many speakers have shown not to be deficient in this region. Can we breed cultivars with higher amounts of zinc and copper, and do we know the effect of these minerals? Can these be added to the fertilizers?

Alderman: I have a technical question about iron. What is the role of tannins in inhibiting the absorption of iron? Is tannin something that is related to consumer desirability? Could you kill two birds with one stone if you could reduce the tannins?

Bressani: Tannins bind iron, and as a matter of fact, the method of measuring tannins involves the use of ferric chloride. When we do our balance study of tannins in the cooked beans and compare the amount of tannins in the broth, we find that the broth will have something like 25 to 30 percent tannins, but these are probably already bound to protein because they are reactive to protein groups. We suspect that mothers would feed this type of broth to their children because tannins have the capacity to bind proteins, which is a useful cure for diarrhea. We hope to get some information from the survey that I just mentioned on the possible role of tannins.

With respect to acceptability, in Latin America, people will not consume white beans. They do not like them. They say they have no flavour, so they prefer black or red. Therefore, I think there is an association between tannin concentration and acceptability of beans.

Alderman: Do white beans have more tannin or less?

Bressani: The white beans have extremely low levels of tannins. They are preferred in North America, but white beans are not even produced in Latin America because people do not like them.

Nordblom: I would like to mention something about animal nutrition that has received almost no coverage yet in the conference. In the specific case of sheep nutrition in Syria, and this has relevance to cereal and legume breeders, the sheep systems are based on grazing the native forage in the steppe areas for part of the year, grazing on crop residues later in the season, and being fed crop residues during the winter. Most of the crop, both grain and straw, is used by the animals, and thus the connection with human nutrition is only through the animal. Barley plays an extremely important role in in these systems so maybe we should be looking at the quantity and quality of the grain and the residues.

El-Sayed: Mekni said there was a negative correlation between yield and height and a negative correlation between protein and yield. Although this is generally true, it may not always be true. There is always genetic variability available that the plant breeder can use.

Hawtin: I detect a bewildering array of advice coming from all quarters to plant breeders during the course of this discussion to the extent that, as a plant breeder, I do not know where to begin. Let me throw the ball to the nutritionists, to try and sum up a little bit. What are the priorities that they would like to see ICARDA breeders do for nutritional aspects of their work? We all accept that increased production is one, but what about nutritional goals?

Pellett: I will try by summing up what other people have said. The important thing to remember is that, in most of the industrialized countries, we do not depend on animal foods only for protein but also for a wide range of vitamins and minerals. If in the developing parts of the world, people are dependent on diets that do not contain adequate amounts of animal protein we must find some other way for them to get iron and other micronutrients in order to meet their requirements.

Hawtin: Your advice to a breeder would be to monitor levels of vitamins and iron, or to raise the level of iron in lentils?

Pellett: The trouble is, it is not as simple as that. It is not only the total amount present, it is also their availability. This means one has to test for bioavailability as well. This is an extremely tall order.

Pinstrup-Andersen: I am not a nutritionist but can I give advice anyway? It seems to me that, even though we all agree that we should produce more protein and energy, the issue we should add to is the need to produce more of the kinds of food that poor and malnourished people have access to, and higher yields for the food that is produced by this same group. What that frequently implies on the production side is to produce a technology that is suited for something less than optimal environmental conditions. We should add that to our objectives.

Scrimshaw: This may be anticipating tomorrow's discussion, but preoccupation with a single crop when the diet must be made up of many crops in order to be nutritious is where mistakes have been made in the past. As Pinstrup-Andersen has pointed out, a programme that is not able to respond to nutrition education efforts to increase lentil consumption or a programme that does not look at farming systems so that the families have some fruits and vegetables as well as cereals and legumes, is not doing its full job.

Williams: I am going to ask Bressani to clear up one point for me. With respect to Nygaard's question in Session II, I would like to change my answer from that session and say yes, I have learned something new, and that is this business about protein digestibility. I would like to learn more about it. Perhaps we can detect improved lines of legumes on this basis. Can you tell me anything that is correlated to cooking time or hardness, for example?

Bressani: The problem of protein digestibility occurs in a food legume that has been recently harvested. It is aggravated by the process of hardening because then there is less water absorption, and it is difficult to hydrolyse the carbohydrate fraction in the bean. We have conducted some experiments with human subjects, feeding them up to 0.7 grams of protein per kilogram body weight per day just from legumes and they have a difficult time digesting this amount of material. We also ran tests on the faeces from these subjects to compare levels of protein between the food and faeces. We found some protein in the faecal material had been broken down by digestive enzymes. We are also trying to isolate the globulin fractions. There are G1 and G2 types and we do not know whether to feed them together or apart. There is some work from Venezuela showing that the globulin fractions are the ones most resistant to proteolytic enzymes. Of course, we realize that it is difficult for plant breeders to conduct digestibility tests on humans, so we have been working on faster testing methods. We have been working on an *in vitro* multiple enzyme procedure that use pH changes and shows results in 15 minutes.

Nygaard: Hawtin asked for comments on priorities. What I would like to ask is not what should your objectives be, but what priorities do you give to them. This stems from experiences economists have had in optimizing decision-making when, if your objective is to maximize profit, the calculus is rather simple and one can determine an optimum solution. To maximize profit and minimize risk simultaneously makes the mathematics much more complex, but a solution can still be derived. If other objectives are added, such as assuring a certain cash flow at a certain time, then the calculus becomes very difficult and the applicability to real problems becomes almost impossible. There are usually five or six objectives in most breeding programmes. I would submit that, in an optimization framework, so many objectives are impossible to handle. In the second session, Pinstrup-Andersen encouraged us to add a nutrition objective to development projects. I think everybody agrees, but what does adding this to the list mean in terms of doing things differently? If we could convince the breeders today to make protein content an important objective, how would that change your breeding strategy? Or does this not worry the breeders?

Bressani: At the beginning of my talk, I pointed out a number of factors that could be selected to improve food legumes. It is important to realize that the factors we select are crop-specific, and how the food is used is important to consider. For example, there are tremendous differences in food legume preparation between India and Latin America, and we do not expect to use their technology for our purposes. For example, for faba beans, it is necessary to screen for the factor that induces favism. If I had to determine a general course of action, I would choose two things. The first is this problem of cooking time and I think this is very important. If people do not consume more legumes in the world, it is because of the difficulty of obtaining fuel. Second, I would try for higher digestibility.

Hawtin: To close the session, I would like to thank everyone who has participated. I look forward to the working session, when perhaps we can pull together some of these divergent views into a set of recommendations.

SECTION V

FOOD PRODUCTION VERSUS NUTRITION

THE GREEN REVOLUTION: ACHIEVEMENTS AND IMPLICATIONS

KUTLU SOMEL

INTRODUCTION

The meaning of the term "green revolution" does not need to be reiterated. As a label it was colourful, but scientifically it was a misnomer. According to Ruttan and Binswanger, "It [the green revolution] is more accurately viewed as part of the continuing evolution of more intensive systems of agricultural production, based on advances in biological and chemical technology" (1). As such, "the green evolution" may have been a more appropriate term. As the late R.G. Anderson put it: "Firstly, the term was invented by the press not the scientists. Secondly, it was never meant to be anything but an attempt to provide breathing space in which to bring population into balance with the resources" (2). Hopper's comments about India can be generalized to give us an idea about the size of this breathing space:"....The Green Revolution seems to be a one-time event that shifted [India's] production curve upward... This will be the case if the ingredients of its beginning are neglected in the future" (3). According to Hopper, the green revolution stood on three legs: (i) viable technologies; (ii) effective incentives to make these technologies economically interesting to the producers; and (iii) a well-lubricated infrastructure to allow the technologies to become operational on farmers' fields.

The purpose of this paper is two-fold:

- To discuss some of the more acute discomforts felt while standing on those three legs, and,
- To conjecture that future endeavour in agricultural research and development will be a harder task (if not Herculean), and similes to centipedes may be inadequate in expressing the necessary number of legs required.

The basic mandate for, and hence the goal of, the scientists involved in the green revolution was simply to achieve rapid increases in food crop production (4). Without a doubt this was achieved. Most analyses substantiate significant shifts in production. At this juncture, it is not very useful to go into the counterfactual discussion of what would have happened if the production increases provided by the green revolution had not occurred, even though this would give us a real idea about the opportunity cost of the green revolution.

Between 1954 and 1970, food aid to the developing countries totalled 25 billion US dollars. Nearly 80 percent of this emanated from North America and less than 20 percent was in the form of donations (2). Policy reversals, especially in North America, would probably not have allowed this trend to continue in the same magnitude. Hence, the green revolution did fill an important gap. True, food imports were replaced by energy imports, fertilizer, etc., but there was an advantage in that national agricultural productive capacities were mobilized. This mobilization produced irreversible changes in agriculture. Looking back at the production achievements of the last two or three decades, agents of agricultural change can be proud that overall food production has kept ahead of population growth (much to the chagrin of neo-Malthusians). These increases have not only satisfied what Yotopoulos calls "hold-the-line" minimum requirements, but also the "affluence" requirements generated in the developed countries and by increasing incomes in general (5).

Again, without a doubt these achievements have not been without cost. Controversies have surrounded several generations of effects presumed to have been caused by or exacerbated by the green revolution. These controversies have centered upon issues in three interacting spheres; the socio-politico-economic, the environmental, and the technological.

The tendency has been to analyse problems of the green revolution in one or the other sphere, as I will try to exemplify. Getting a bit ahead of myself, I would like to emphasize that we should anticipate problems of agricultural technological change in the future to be more and more spread over these three spheres, affecting the interactions among them. In other words, problems belonging uniquely to one sphere will become less common. Consequently, the challenges that we shall face will become increasingly more complex.

I neither intend to look into all the problems of the green revolution nor do I have the capacity to do so. What I would like to do is to look at four issues around which some stormy controversies have arisen. These are:

--The ecological impact of the green revolution.

-- Employment and mechanization effects.

-- Income distribution effects.

-- Nutritional impact.

In my discussions I have no intention of giving credibility to the entrenched and intractable positions on all sides of the controversies, dug with dogmatically preconceived and/or theoretically misconceived perceptions. I will try to present both the pros and cons. After all, our intention is not to canonize or condemn the green revolution, but to learn from the experience.

ECOLOGY AND THE GREEN REVOLUTION

Harris classifies agricultural systems according to (i) the type of energy they depend on, and (ii) the diversity of plants and animals that they incorporate (6). Two dichotomies typically characterize each point of classification:

(i) the internal combustion engine with combustible fuels vs. human or animal labour.

(ii) neotechnic agriculture with low diversity vs. paleotechnic agriculture with greater biotic diversity.

Of course, this classification is relative at given points in time and space. Holdgate claims that currently in world agriculture there are under 100 plant species and under 50 animals in use, and furthermore, that any particular system depends on only a few of those.

From an ecological point of view, agricultural development is tantamount to a transition from ecosystem manipulation to ecosystem transformation. This transformation to more modern agriculture produces three significant effects:

a. Modification of wild plant and animal communities resulting in lower ecological diversity.

b. Direct or indirect alteration of hydrological systems.

c. Elimination of valuable varietal diversity and a lowering of an agriculural system's ability to withstand environmental stresses such as disease and drought. (To put it another way, substantial costs are involved in the efforts to counteract these effects.)

How does the green revolution stand up to these criteria? I claim that it was among those cases of technological change with relatively more consciousness of, and consideration for, ecological issues. For example, in 1941 in Mexico, consideration for technological change involved an ecological insight of significance -- that of plant breeding for disease resistance (7). Germplasm maintenance is an integral part of agricultural research even though diversity in production at a given time is lower. However, intertemporal diversity has increased, thanks to improvements in and turnover of material in anticipation of problems. This does not mean that there have not been adverse effects. For example, the heavy dependence of green revolution technologies on irrigation has compounded problems of salinity. Incentives to expand production areas have accelerated deforestation with severe effects. Holdgate quotes Likens and co-writers as stating that they "....recorded in the Hubbard Brook catchment a net loss of 65-90 tonnes of nutrient salts per year of run-off from cut forest as against 4.5-6 tonnes per year from uncut woodland" (8).

To summarize this section, I would like to put forth a counter-factual defense for the green revolution vis-a-vis ecology. Without the green revolution, the effects on the environment would probably have been devastating. In the first instance, equivalent production increases could only have been achieved with considerably more pressure on the environment. Increased yields achieved by green revolution technologies probably reduced significantly the magnitudes involved in the tradeoffs between the environment and production requirements. Increased fertilizer use, by increasing the fertility of the soils, reduced the pressures for land expansion. Furthermore, lessons from adverse experiences caused research to be undertaken to reverse these negative effects. Improved drainage, better management practices, and the incorporation of drought and disease resistance in varieties are examples. In the balance therefore, the green revolution has fared quite well in the inevitable ecosystem transformation required for agricultural development.

EMPLOYMENT AND MECHANIZATION EFFECTS

I start with two propositions, both open for debate:

a. Mechanization was in some cases necessary, but never sufficient for the achievements of the green revolution.

b. Mechanization is an independent process that is (or should be) based on the relative factor scarcities of an economy.

These are strong statements that require caveats in anticipation of some preliminary criticisms. As far as the first statement is concerned, mechanization probably enhanced the technical efficiency of green revolution technologies by fostering more timely and precise practices. For the second statement, what should be and what is are two different things. I am sure that a survey confined to the recent past 20 to 30 years would not produce many cases where mechanization was a result of responses to actual relative factor scarcities. In most cases, mechanization came about through distorted agricultural policies that artificially altered relative prices to the advantage of capital equipment (9). I suspect several factors caused these policies. Two of the more important ones are pressures from multinational firms in search of new markets, and the Western and elitist bias in agricultural training in the developing countries.

The moral of the story is that mechanization is a process that has occurred independently of the green revolution and in some cases has even predated it. Consequently, it is hardly justifiable to attribute all the effects of mechanization on employment to the green revolution. Furthermore, the popular claims that each tractor displaces so many workers are rather simplistic (10). The transformation processes that evolve around or involve mechanization are considerably more complex. There are buffer mechanisms within agriculture that absorb the labour displacement effects of mechanization (11). The general impression, however, is that the elasticity of substitution between capital and labour in agriculture is not less than one in general. Most studies specify a Cobb-Douglas production function that has a unitary elasticity of substitution. CES or translog specifications usually produce values of elasticity of substitution between capital and labour that are larger than 1. This implies that government policies that reduce the relative price of capital cause a more than proportionate reduction in the share of labour in output.

Let us review some experiences with the green revolution as far as employment and mechanization are concerned.

a. First, mechanization has a more significant displacement effect on animal power than on human labour (12,13).

b. At a given level of mechanization, the green revolution has an employment-increasing effect, particularly for skilled labour. This is because of possibilities for increased cropping intensities, higher labour requirements for irrigation, fertilizer application, and similar activities (12,14-17).

c. With mechanization, the employment effects of the green revolution are not easy to determine but are usually negative. Furthermore, the mechanization of some agricultural activities, such as harvesting and threshing, have a more serious effect on employment (14,16).

d. The green revolution facilitated the development of custom services, and this allowed the small farmers to benefit from technological changes. However, at the same time a form of capitalist sharecropper evolved. These tractor-owning sharecroppers enabled the small farmers to leave their farms without losing the land. In other words, small landowners became absentee landlords, and as they invariably migrated to the cities, they contributed to urban unemployment or filled the ranks of the marginally unempoyed (11,16,18,19).

Overall, mechanization and employment effects of the green revolution do not appear to be unequivocal. There are location-specific experiences influenced by the particular policies in that environment.

INCOME DISTRIBUTION EFFECTS

The income distribution effects of the green revolution have been analysed exhaustively in four dimensions:

a. Differential effects according to farm-size,

b. Interregional differential effects,

c. Intercrop differential effects, and,

d. Rural-urban (or producer-consumer) differential effects.

Let us look at each separately.

Farm Size Effects. Farm-size effects have usually been expressed in terms of farmers with larger landholdings benefiting more from the green revolution than those with small farms. While this is clearly acknowledged in some cases (2), it has been frequently criticized by those who claim that the green revolution technologies are scale-neutral (20).

Certain observations are worth noting in this respect:

i) While there is substantial evidence of the large farm bias of the green revolution, there are exceptions to the rule where small farmers have also benefited equally or more from projects (21,22).

ii) Equal per unit area benefits naturally imply larger total benefits to the large farms, but this is more a reflection of inequalities in land distribution. In particular and rare cases where new land is opened up and its owners reap the benefits of technological change, one can claim green revolution technologies to be directly responsible for producing inequalities (23). It may in fact be too harsh to hold it directly responsible since the example in this reference is actually a case where inequalities in education and information were exploited to get land in order to reap the benefits of the green revolution.

iii) The inequalities that cause large landholding farmers to reap more benefits may arise because of the gradual processes of diffusion. Such benefits are transitory (24). A study by Shingi et al. clearly illustrates that, not only have the laggards of the past caught up, but the leaders and early adopters of new technologies are clearly no longer any better off than the rest of the farmers (25).

iv) On the other hand, inequalities caused by differences in access to inputs are not transitory. Such differences arise because of inadequate infrastructure, financial economies of scale, and biased government policies (26). These factors cause imperfections in input and factor markets that, in turn, cause input and factor utilization differences. Binswanger and Ryan argue for increased efficiency in markets to eliminate inequalities under those circumstances, as opposed to developing different technologies for small and large farms (24).

v) In some cases, the distribution of income is so skewed already that the green revolution does not have any effect one way or another (27).

As far as inequalities with respect to farm size are concerned, the green revolution may not be the culprit or the prime suspect. However, it has in general done very little to release or reduce the effects of existing inequalities.

Interregional Effects. Interregional disparities really arose from the immediacy of increased production requirements. The probability of success was higher in areas with an already advanced agriculture, better infrastructure and, above all, irrigation facilities, and these areas were the first to receive attention. Subsequently, emphasis in technological advances shifted to high and stable rainfall areas. Recently, the priorities appear to have reached lower and more variable rainfall zones. Thus, we have an example where the green revolution has directly caused an increase in inequalities among regions.

Intercrop Effects. Intercrop differentials in technological change have not originated with the green revolution. Research on products of the colonial and enclave production systems, such as sugar cane, cocoa, rubber, cotton, etc., beat the green revolution by a wide temporal margin. However, the green revolution itself has also suffered from disproportionate emphasis on a few crops such as wheat, rice, and maize. The focus on poor people's crops such as roots, tubers, and pulses is relatively recent. This may be because wheat, rice, and maize are the most important crops in terms of production in the world, and in specific areas their respective relative importance increases.

In areas where it has been possible to substitute production and consumption of these major corps for other basic staples, intercrop differentials may not have caused serious income distribution problems. However, in areas where this has not been possible, producers and consumers of alternative products have been cut off from the benefits of the green revolution (28).

Rural-Urban Effects. It is often claimed that the green revolution has an urban-consumer bias. This claim is based on two assumptions. The first is that the demand for the commodities being influenced by the green revolution, usually basic staples, is inelastic. Hence, production increases that shift the supply curve cause significant price decreases that benefit urban consumers. The second assumption is that there are no interventions in these markets.

The first assumption is generally justifiable even though there may be exceptions. In some cases, the green revolution may have brought about changes in preferences, for example, from rice to wheat, or from one variety of rice to another. Under those circumstances, the commodity towards which preferences are shifting may not have an inelastic demand, and this will cause producers of such products to get a higher share of the benefits.

The second assumption of competitive markets is more problematic. Invariably, in developing countries there are effective oligopolistic public purchasing institutions in staple commodity markets. These agencies may be protecting the producers or the consumers, the urban or the rural populace. It may even be protecting both, even though those who finally pay the costs of this protection in one way or another may be the same as those who are being protected. The improbability of having the incidence of costs accrue directly to those who benefit also has adverse income distribution implications. The usual case is for both outputs and inputs to be subsidized on the production side as part of an incentive scheme while subsidizing consumers as part of a welfare scheme. The perversities of such policies create price distortions that make it very difficult to generalize who benefits and to what degree, and to what extent the green revolution is responsible. Apart from claiming that the green revolution has enabled a larger output to be available, it is difficult to make general statements. it is necessary to look into individual cases to evaluate income distribution effects.

To summarize, the green revolution does not appear to have such a good record on the question of income distribution. Directly or indirectly, it has caused or increased inequalities.

THE GREEN REVOLUTION AND NUTRITION

It is true that the green revolution has increased the amount of food produced. However, whether this food has been accessible, especially to those who need it more, is not clear. Nutritional problems emanate more from income distribution inequalities than from any other factor, as discussed in the previous section. The green revolution thus has contributed to nutritional problems to the extent that it has influenced inequalities in income distribution. This effect is probably site-specific. Unfortunately, I could not find any micro studies that analyse the nutritional impact of the green revolution, but general statements abound in the literature. For example, Dantwala states that "... the price restraining effect of higher food grain production.. has relieved to some extent the burden of poverty" (29).

Studies that specifically bring together the income distribution and nutrition dimensions of the green revolution are hard to find. An exception to this is Bowonder, who looks at the developments in India. However, Bowonder emphasizes expenditures on cereals and pulses rather than actual caloric and protein intakes. Despite this, the conclusion reached is, "The lowest income level of the population has suffered from protein: calorie malnutrition due to the constraint intake of cereals with decreasing consumption of pulses" (30). This is attributed to the price increases in pulses because of their reduced availability with the advent of the green revolution emphasis on grain production.

I would like now to provide a short review of a related controversy surrounding the nutritional impact of the green revolution. This is the discussion of the foodgrain-pulse balance, or the calorie-protein balance, in India. Unfortunately, the discussion is confined to national averages and hence avoids (but does not ignore) the problems of inequalities in access to food.

In India during the process of the green revolution, the wheat area increased while the land area allocated to produce mostly poor people's foods, such as millet, pulses and barley, declined (28). As the green revolution had less effect upon these foods, declines in their availability forced people to turn to the more expensive alternative of wheat (30). While Namboodiri and Choksi claim that, as wheat is a cheaper food the nutritional status of the poor may have improved, Ryan and Asokan indicate that protein from wheat is (slightly) more expensive than that from gram (31,32). Hence, whether the nutritional status of the poor has improved or not is still somewhat a mystery. What is unequivocally clear is that the increase in wheat production has more than made up for the losses in protein availability caused by reductions in the area devoted to production of pulses (30-32). However, this refers to the total amount of proteins, not to specific amino acids (31).

This achievement of the green revolution has led to conclusions that really merit serious discussion. Ryan claims that "...the implication....for crop breeding strategies in (semiarid tropical) India is that, to the extent that the attainment of improved yield potentials in improved cultivars is made more difficult by trying to include increased protein content and quality attributes, priority should be given to yield and yield stability" (33). Given the trade-offs between yield and protein quality and quantity (even though there does not appear to be consensus on these trade-offs), Ryan's statement can be accepted to some extent. However, given our ignorance on the effects of the green revolution on the nutritional status of the poor, the following claim by Ryan and Asokan appears to be an overstatement: "....a predominantly yield-oriented strategy is more appropriate than improvement of grain protein percentage and other cryptic qualities in breeding improved foodgrain varieties of the people living in the semiarid tropics, particularly for people regarded as nutritionally vulnerable" (32).

To reiterate, the green revolution has increased the size of the pie, but whether those who need it more have a larger share of the pie is not clear, nor is it known whether the nutrition of these people has improved.

I have discussed four issues related to the green revolution: the environmental impact, employment and mechanization, income distribution, and nutrition. A closer examination will indicate that the first three issues also impinge on nutrition, which is the main topic of this workshop. Environmental deterioration, substitution of capital for labour in production, and income distribution inequalities all adversely influence access to sources of nutrition, especially for those who have less control over the processes of change that result in these negative effects (34).

Thus, it is necessary to take stock of the fact that the green revolution has achieved much, but that first, this has not been without cost, second, some of these costs were not anticipated, and third, the costs have not been borne equally by all those who have been influenced by the green revolution. With this stock-taking we can now turn to the future.

IMPLICATIONS FOR THE FUTURE

The past has not been without its problems, however, I am sure that it will be remembered fondly as the future holds no promise of being simple. Higher sensitivities will be required in the face of issues that will get increasingly more complex. In the past, for example, it was not unusual for economists --both trained and self-made ones -- and other scientists to judge the chances of success of some green revolution technology by asking how many kilos of wheat could be produced per kilo of fertilizer or by comparing the relative price of wheat to fertilizer. (This rule of thumb suffered from one basic error: it assumed that all other inputs were free.) Such instant devices of evaluation will not be available in the future.

Ruttan warns that previous achievements of the International Agricultural Research Centers should not be expected to be duplicated and that we should anticipate that:

-- Further gains will be harder to achieve,

-- Problems with effective demand for increased production, and,

-- Higher skills will be required for further technological change (35).

It is worthwhile to go into more detail to look at these challenges.

As mentioned previously, the green revolution, with its objective of food production, gave first priority to irrigated areas followed by attention to areas with relatively higher and/or more stable rainfall. Next in priority were areas with lower and/or more variable rainfall. In these lower rainfall areas we face several problems:

a. Production here is riskier compared to that in irrigated and high rainfall areas. This makes the costs of technological change considerably higher. Furthermore, technology support systems and administrative capacities in these areas are not well developed.

b. Producers in such areas are more disadvantaged. This makes adoption of new technology more difficult and hence diffusion slower.

c. Lessons of agricultural development from irrigated and high rainfall areas cannote be generalized to lower rainfall areas _a priori_ (36). This, in some respects, implies more expensive location-specific research.

d. The environment and the ecological balances in such areas are in a more tenuous and precarious situation. This means that social costs of technological change will be more important than before. The continuation of present trends and practices will have irreversible adverse effects on the environment. This produces an interesting dilemma: research directed at these areas may reduce such social costs; however, the impoverished producers who are sensitive to private costs may not be interested in changes that do not recognize these costs. An example is the overgrazing of marginal areas. Currently, the private cost of this practice is quite low, even though the social costs of long-term effects are possibly quite high. Their prevention may involve policies unattractive to sheep owners, and may even increase their private costs.

Clearly, all these obstacles will be hard to eliminate. However, with a little foresight, headway is possible in agricultural research. The typical approach in agricultural research has been to strive for package technologies. We now have sufficient evidence that producers do not adopt technologies in packages, but, because of cost and risk considerations, adopt components of these packages (37). This will be especially true for the impoverished producers of drier rainfed areas. Consequently, we should start emphasizing agricultural research that identifies payoffs from components rather than from adoption of complete packages. Subsequent extension oriented toward a priority list of components to promote stepwise adoption will allow greater chances of adoption and quicker diffusion of the technology.

Due to the delicate ecological balances involved, neotechnic, low biotic diversity (6) may not be that desirable. According to Koppel, "....breeding for generalized environments will be only a limited possibility. If reducing variability in agricultural environments through physical modification is not crucial, increasing productivity in a manner consistent with ecosystem stability and resilience will require fresh research strategies (36). Without a doubt, such strategies will be considerably more expensive than those used in the past.

On-station research will have to be more sensitive to applicability on farmers' fields. According to the methodology developed at the International Rice Research Institute, the difference in yields at the experiment station and on-farm trials is called Yield Gap 1, and the difference in yields between on-farm trials and the farmers' fields is called Yield Gap 2. A large Yield Gap 2 shows the potential of the technology on farmers' fields, while a large Yield Gap 1 is indicative of the irrelevance of experiment station research for the producers (38).

Adverse effects of income distribution inequalities will increase. As incomes increase, and as consumption patterns change with increased income, the rich will increasingly crowd out the poor. This will result in a lowering of the effective demand by the poor for food simply because their budget constraints become more and more binding, while the rich bid up the price of food.

Food production will also become problematic with a higher incidence of crises unless serious and conscientious measures are taken (36,39). The recent work by FAO on projections for the year 2000 provides interesting insights into these measures. Two scenarios are constructed, each based on a different set of assumptions about changes in food production, population growth, etc. Their more conservative scenario B aims at a 3.1 percent growth rate in agricultural production and at increasing the level of average calorie consumption per capita per day from 2180 in 1975 to 2500 in 2000 for 90 developing countries. The magnitude of investments necessary to achieve these targets totals 1,386 billion US dollars (in 1975 values) for the period 1980-2000.

If successful, it is estimated that such policies will have reduced the number of seriously undernourished people in 86 developing countries from 436 million in 1975 to 390 million people in the year 2000. "...to reduce the incidence of undernutrition to very low levels, say one percent of the population in developing countries, would take an economic growth rate of over 10 percent annually in each year up to year 2000" (39). Very high growth rates are required for improvements in income distribution, too.

Ruttan, referring to the earlier phases of the green revolution, indicates that "(It) shifted attention from the earlier architects of development, planners, economists and other social scientists - to geneticists, plant breeders and agronomists" (20). Today, however, as Pereira states, "...agricultural technologies have already been developed to the stage at which the historical dominance of biological and physical constraints on production has now given place to political, social and economic constraints. Although many scientific and technical problems remain to be solved, their scale is now minor in comparison with that of the 'social engineering' required" (40).

The pendulum has swung to an intermediate position. Now, more than ever, there is a critical need for the multidisciplinary approach and interdisciplinary cooperation in agricultural research and development. Only such a merger of disciplines can provide the perspectives necessary for the analyses of technologies. Without such evaluating procedures as technology assessment (41-43), estimation of payoff matrices (42), or _ex ante_ research resource allocation criteria (24), most technological research will be relatively ineffectual. Using these tools, we will not only make an effort to determine the costs and benefits of our research results, but also will try to differentiate between groups of beneficiaries. These procedures of "constrained optimization" will allow us to be more effective, but they can be undertaken only in an interdisciplinary manner involving scientists trained in the technical, biological, and social sciences. We can no longer afford to confine ourselves to what happens in the experiment fields.

Recall the plaintive protest of Wolf Ladejinsky after a field trip in India in 1969: "When all is said and done, it is not the fault of the new technology that the credit service does not serve those for whom it was originally intended; that the extension service is not living up to expectations; that the _panchayats_ are essentially political rather than development bodies; that security of tenure is the luxury of the few; that rentals are exorbitant; that ceilings on land are merely notional; that for the greater part tenurial legislation is deliberately miscarried; or wage scales are hardly sufficient to keep body and soul together" (44).

Neither technology nor we, its scientists, are responsible for these things. But, we cannot shun the responsibility of being conscious of them. As scientists involved in technological change in agriculture, we can no longer afford that luxury because we now know that this is where the heart of the matter is.

REFERENCES

1. V.W. Ruttan and H.P. Binswanger, "Induced Innovation and the Green Revolution," in H.P. Binswanger and V.W. Ruttan (written with Uri Ben Zion and others), Induced Innovation: Technology, Institutions, and Development (Johns Hopkins University Press, Baltimore, Maryland, 1978).

2. R.G. Anderson, A Second Look at the Green Revolution, Klinck Lecture of the Agricultural Institue of Canada, 1974. Translations and Reprints No. 21 (CIMMYT, Londres, Mexico, 1974).

3. W.D. Hopper, "A Perspective on India's Food Production," Fertilizer News 21:21 (1976).

4. K.A. Dahlberg, Beyond the Green Revolution: The Ecology and Politics of Global Agricultural Development (Plenum Press, New York, 1979).

5. P.A. Yotopoulos, "The Population Problem and the Development Solution," Food Res. Institute Stud. 16:1 (1977).

6. D.R. Harris, "The Environmental Impact of Traditional and Modern Agricultural Systems," in J.C. Hawkes, ed., Conservation and Agriculture (Duckworth, London, 1978).

7. M.W. Holdgate, "The Balance between Food Production and Conservation," in J.C. Hawkes, ed., Conservation and Agriculture (Duckworth, London, 1978).

8. S.D. Biggs and E.J. Clay, "Sources of Innovation in Agricultural Technology," World Development 9:322 (1981).

9. R. Dumont and N. Cohen, The Growth of Hunger: A New Politics of Agriculture (Marion Boyars, Inc., London, 1980).

10. C.A. Baanante and S. Sihu, "Input Substitution and Agricultural Research," IJAE 35:28 (1980).

11. I. Tekeli, Dependent Urbanization: The Transformation Process in Rural and Urban Areas, Chamber of Architects, Publication No. 18, Ankara, Turkey (1977), in Turkish.

12. R.T.R. Naidu, "Trends in Farm Mechanization during the Post-Green Revolution Period and Associated Variables - An InterState Analysis," IJAE 32:107 (1977).

13. H.P. Binswanger, The Economics of Tractors in South Asia, An Analytical Review, Agricultural Development Council, New York and ICRISAT, Hyderabad, India (1978).

14. G. Blyn, "The Green Revolution and Social Structure in India," in M.D. Chaudry, ed., Rural Development: Contribution to Asian Studies, Vol. 13 (E.J. Brill, Leiden, The Netherlands, 1979).

15. S. Mehra, "Some Aspects of Labour Use in Indian Agriculture," IJAE 31:95 (1976).

16. A.S. Kahlon, "Impact of Mechanization in Punjab Agriculture with Special Reference to Tractorization, IJAE 31:54 (1976).

17. S. Tyagi, "Growth of Agricultural Output and Labour Absorption in India," J. Devel. Stud. 18:104 (1981).

18. K. Somel, "Technological Change in Dryland Wheat Production in Turkey," Food Res. Institute Stud. 17:51 (1979).

19. H. Gencaga, I. Kapil, S. Duman, and C.K. Mann, "Introducing New Agricultural Technology on the Anatolian Plateau: Some Preliminary Findings," Discussion Paper No. 11, Economic Staff Papers, United States Agency for International Development, Ankara, Turkey (1973).

20. V.W. Ruttan, "The Green Revolution" Seven Generalizations," Int. Devel. Rev. 13:18 (1977).

21. K. Kalirajan, "Benefits from the High Yielding Varieties Programme and Their Distribution in Irrigated Paddy Areas," IJAE 35:70 (1980).

22. R.M. Pastores and J.P. Powelson, "Green Revolution in the Philippines," Cultures et Developpement 11:671 (1978).

23. J. Goody, "Rice-Burning and the Green Revolution in Northern Ghana," J. Devel. Stud. 16:136 (1980).

24. H.P. Binswanger and J.G. Ryan, "Efficiency and Equity Issues in ex ante Allocation of Research Resources," IJAE 32:224 (1977).

25. P.M. Shingi, F.C. Fliegel, and J.E. Kivlin "Agricultural Technology and the Issue of Unequal Distribution of Rewards: An Indian Case Study," Rural Sociology 46:430 (1981).

26. K.B. Griffin, The Political Economy of Agrarian Change (Macmillan, London, 1979).

27. C.G. Swenson, "The Distribution of Benefits from Increased Rice Production in Thanjavur District, South India," IJAE 31:1 (1976).

28. D. Singh, "Imbalance in Agricultural Growth," IJAE 36:1 (1981).

29. M.L. Dantwala, "Agricultural Policy Since Independence," IJAE 31:50 (1976).

30. B. Bowonder, "The Myth and Reality of High Yielding Varieties in Indian Agriculture," Development and Change 12:300 (1981).

31. N.V. Namboodiri and S.N. Choksi, "Green Revolution-Change in the Supply Sources and Per Capita Availability of Protein Calories," IJAE 32:27 (1977).

32. J.G. Ryan and M. Asokan, "Effect of Green Revolution in Wheat on Production of Pulses and Nutrients in India" IJAE 32:8 (1977).

33. J.G. Ryan, "Human Nutritional Needs and Crop Breeding Objectives in the Semi-Arid Tropics," IJAE 32:85 (1977).

34. S. George (Rapporteur), "An Issues Paper Contributed by the Food Study Group of the GPID Project," in M.B. Wallerstein, ed., Interdisciplinary Dialogue on World Hunger (United Nations University, IPDHW-1/UNDP-229, Tokyo, Japan, 1981.

35. V.W. Ruttan, "The International Agricultural Research Institute as a Source of Agricultural Development," Agricultural Administration 5:293 (1978).

36. B.M. Koppel, "Food Policy Options for Secondary Regions: A Framework for Applied Research," Food Policy 6:33 (1981).

37. C.K. Mann, "Packages of Practices: A Step at a Time with Clusters," METU Studies in Development, Fall 1977.

38. R.W. Herdt and R. Barker, "Sources of Growth in Asian Food Production and an Approach to Identification of Constraining Factors," in Interfaces between Agriculture, Nutrition, and Food Science, Proceedings of a 1977 Workshop, Jointly Sponsored and Published by The United Nations University and the International Rice Research Institute, Los Banos, Philippines (1979).

39. Food and Agriculture Organization of the United Nations, Agricluture: Toward 2000 (FAO, Rome, 1981).

40. Sir C. Pereira, "The Changing Patterns of Constraints on Food Production in the Third World," in T.W. Schultz, ed., Distortions of Agriculture Incentives (Indiana University Press, Bloomington, Indiana (1978).

41. B.M. Koppel, "The Changing Functions of Research Management: Technology Assessment and the Challenges to Contemporary Agricultural Research Organization," Agricultural Administration 6:123 (1979).

42. J.H. Sanders and J.K. Lynam, "New Agricultural Technology and Small Farmers in Latin America," Food Policy 6:16 (1981).

43. V.W. Ruttan, "Reviewing Agricultural Research Programmes," Agricultural Administration 5:1 (1978).

44. W. Ladejinksy, "The Green Revolution in Bihar, the Kosi Area: A Field Trip," Economic and Political Weekly 4:39 (1969).

REGIONAL RESEARCH ON CEREALS AND NUTRITION

PHILIP C. WILLIAMS

INTRODUCTION

ICARDA is not only concerned with developing new varieties of cereals and legumes, but also in research on farming systems for the benefit of the countries in the region of its mandate and their estimated 400 million people. Many of these countries have their own programmes for the improvement of crop production, and ICARDA is already making available germ plasm for these national and regional programmes. Of the 22 countries of the ICARDA mandate (Table 1), 19 produce cereals in significant quantities, while 10 are also producers of food legumes.

In the ICARDA region cereal production has increased by 33 percent in the past 10 years. Food legume production has, however, declined by three percent, partly because of deficiencies in the system of marketing and lower incentives to farmers to produce legumes rather than cereals or other cash crops. Certain trends in population and cereal and legume consumption and legume production and importation in Middle East countries are apparent for the ten-year period from 1971-1981 (1). Based on the formula (net production + imports - exports) that is presumed to represent consumption, use of cereals as food is increasing at a rate of 5.5 percent per annum, a rate that is outstripping the population growth. During the ten years from 1970 to 1980, total per capita cereal consumption averaged 279 kg per year. Wheat represents about 54 percent (152 kg/person) of this amount. The present trends in cereal utilization and per capita consumption project an increase from the present 113 million tonnes to over 200 million tonnes by the year 2000. This volume of grain will have to be stored, marketed, distributed, processed, and administered. Data for pulse production and consumption indicate that per capita consumption of food legumes in the ICARDA countries is, in most areas, substantially lower than that of cereals; these food legumes are consumed mainly in urban areas where population density is high and meat is expensive.

The great diversity of peoples and local foods throughout the region makes screening and evaluation for quality rather complicated, and even bread is consumed in many different varieties. Improvement of yield and production is of little value unless two main prerequisites are met. First, the higher-yielding genotypes and improved farming practices should provide grains that conform to the recognized and preferred quality characteristics in the regions for which they are intended. Second, systems must be developed for efficient storage, marketing, and transportation of the production in excess of local consumption. The first prerequisite calls for research into the types of foods preferred in individual locations and the methods of processing the new material and preparation of these foods. Once this fundamental resarch has been completed, the next step is to establish the inherent quality characteristics that make certain varieties and types of grain or seed suitable for the preparation of individual foods. The third step is to develop testing methods to screen and evaluate large numbers of early generation material and smaller numbers of advanced and parental material on the basis of their physical and chemical characteristics to identify lines that are satisfactory or superior. The fourth step is to develop methods for the preparation of some of the major foods used, and their evaluation. Finally, it is necessary to introduce new genetic material to consumers and to test whether it is acceptable.

The second prerequisite deals with postharvest technology (see also Parpia, page __), an area that most governments and many agencies tend to neglect. The main reasons for this are expense and the degree of organization required. To increase productivity is a relatively simple process: it involves purchasing or acquiring some land on which to grow crops employing scientists and ancillary personnel and providing offices for them. This can be achieved for an outlay of 10 to 20 million dollars together with an ongoing annual outlay of from 5 to 40 million, depending upon the magnitude of the operation.

On the other hand, the postharvest care and technology of the crops produced is far more complicated. This involves studying the processing methods and foods used throughout the region, the provision of incentives for the farmers to grow the extra crops, and the establishment of marketing and distribution systems. In most cases, whether large volumes (millions of tonnes) of grain are expected to be imported or exported, silos and other forms of bulk storage must be built and railroads and roads developed to service them. Wharves and shipping facilities may be needed. These types of facilities require large numbers of ongoing and even more seasonal staff. Costs of establishing an efficient postharvest system to service a region as big as the Middle East are astronomical compared to the costs of simply increasing production of agricultural crops. In addition to the generation and administration of billions of dollars in establishing and maintaining such a system, there are difficult local, national, and international political obstacles to overcome and major international economic agreements to establish. These difficulties can be overcome, as is shown by Turkey's success in increasing grain production and distribution since 1971. It must be borne in mind, however, that when countries in the ICARDA region increase food production to a level where they can export it to other countries, the balance of economic power may swing in their direction and competition for markets will likely become more intense.

Quality Evaluation Objectives

ICARDA's objectives are to improve quantity and quality of four cereals (bread wheat, durum wheat, triticale, and barley), three food legumes (broad beans (*V. faba*), chickpeas, and lentils), and forage plants for animal feed together with improvement in the farming systems involved in the cultivation of these crops.

The major uses of cereals in the countries of the ICARDA region are for the production of single and two-layered flat breads, raised breads, couscous, burgul, and pasta products. The most important legume-based foods include purees such as *homos biteheneh*, stewed bean dishes such as *ful*, and *ful medames*, and soups (Table 2). When new varieties are introduced, in addition to fully acceptable processing quality, it is essential that the nutritional quality is at least maintained and preferably improved. Determination of the nutritional quality of a food measures the potential of that food to provide, either alone of in combination with other components of the diet, the energy, protein (nitrogen and essential amino acids), fibre, minerals, and vitamins necessary for growth and maintenance. In many cases, low levels of some nutrients in certain dietary components may be complemented by adequate amounts of these nutrients in other components. The quality laboratories at ICARDA began operating in June 1980, and methods are in use for the screening and evaluation of cereals, legumes, and forages found in the region served. Pioneer work carried out at the Grain Research Laboratory in Winnipeg, Manitoba, Canada, revealed the chief physical and physiochemical characteristics required for the preparation of the traditional Arabic-type 2-layered breads and for single-layered breads (2). Research is under way for the local investigation of the forms or types of foods in which the various grains are eaten. The laboratory evaluation of advanced lines and potential new parental material includes the preparation from these lines of the more common foods.

Quality evaluation programmes involved both the screening of large numbers of early generation lines by using simple test procedures and the more comprehensive evaluation of more advanced material. It is essential that both processing and nutritional quality be evaluated in crop breeding and improvement programmes in developing countries, because increasing the quantities produced is of little value if the people do not accept these foods, or if they are nutritionally deficient or carry excessive amounts of anti-nutritional factors. Often the screening of single plants and F4 lines is handicapped by only small amounts of material being available for testing (Table 3). For example, single lentil plants may yield only 2 or 3 grams of mature seed, most of which is required for re-planting. On the other hand, a single bean plant may produce fairly large weights of seed, but the validity of test results is subject to excessive inherent variability among the individual seeds. As far as possible, early generation screening tests are limited to nondestructive methods, and chemical analysis is performed on small amounts of material. At ICARDA the new technique of near-infrared reflectance (NIR) spectroscopy for the measurement of protein and fibre components is used, and shortly a programme for screening lentils for methionine using the NIR technique will begin. Tables 4 and 5 summarize the tests performed in the laboratories at ICARDA on cereals and food legumes; 32 different tests are carried out, most of which are described in the appendix. Standard procedures for some tests are used and references for these are provided. Full details of all ICARDA tests are embodied in a comprehensive operations manual (3). Many of the chemical and physiochemical tests are routinely carried out in other quality evaluation laboratories throughout the world, but the baking and cooking tests are specifically aimed at the evaluation of the advanced line of germ plasm from crops used in the ICARDA region.

It is difficult to document all, or even a significant proportion, of the foods eaten in all of the countries served by ICARDA, but a start has been made. Baking formulas and recipes have been assembled from about fifty bakeries in seven of the countries, which represents over 30 percent of the population of the region. An Arabic-style baking oven has been built at ICARDA, and Arabic two-layered flat breads are baked using a formula representative of the bakeries in Syrian cities. By controlling the temperature, it is also possible to prepare Baladi bread and North African baguettes in this same oven. <u>Tannour</u> is baked in the village near the ICARDA Experiment Station by local women who have much experience in the baking of this type of bread. Flour for <u>tannour</u> is milled to 100 percent extraction in the village stone mill. Within the next two years, it is anticipated that more comprehensive information will be gathered from most of the countries within the ICARDA region concerning the principal forms of cereal breads and other cereal uses, and legume foods, together with the recipes used. Typical formulas for two-layered Arabic and Baladi breads and for raised baguettes (pain francais) are given in Table 6. A wide range of formulae have been found for baking Arabic bread. Baladi breads are fermented using a yeasted sour dough and are characterized by very high water content and use of high (87%) extraction flour.

<u>Tannour</u> and other types of single-layered breads are made in villages, usually in private homes, but occasionally on a commercial basis; for example, the "mountain" breads of Lebanon. The formulae are very simple and consist usually of wholemeal flour, sour dough, a little salt, and water. The water is added

until the dough reaches a consistency at which the bakers (usually women) judge that the dough has good handling properties that will enable them to manipulate it into round, flat sheets of up to 80 cms diameter for baking in a kiln or on a saaj. For ICARDA's evaluation of triticale and occasionally durum wheat lines, the village formula is considered satisfactory, especially because it is at the village level where the acceptability of the triticale and durum lines has to be judged; about 60 percent of all of the people in the ICARDA region live in villages. The evaluation of triticale in this manner is different in approach from the conventional methods, which are usually centred around milling white flours and making raised breads, crackers, or biscuits. Introduction of triticale via the medium of village foods eliminates the two most important processing deficiencies found with triticales, namely the very low milling extraction and poor bread-baking quality.

Triticales tend to accumulate the poorer quality characteristics of their parents, wheat and rye, particularly those of the rye. Both durum and rye proteins are weak and will not form strong enough gluten for satisfactory baking. In addition, the mature starch granules often have radial fissures that make them highly susceptible to alpha-amylase. Consequently, loaves made from triticale flour are dark in crumb and crust colour, have low volume, and a dense, waxy texture. If common wheat genes are introduced the quality improves, but there is usually a significant reduction in yield, and consequently triticale offers no advantage over common wheat or barley. There is growing consensus that, by the time breeders have improved its acceptability for normal bread-making, its quality will closely approximate that of wheat and it will have lost the yield advantages of triticale. Triticale research at ICARDA has, however, already produced lines that are acceptable for the baking of village single-layered flat breads. The only complaint is that the colour of the bread is too dark. Breeders are trying to correct this deficiency by using white rye parents in their crossing strategy. The use of triticales for making these types of breads could spearhead the acceptability of high-yielding triticales on a scale that has not been achieved before. This could be of significant assistance in realizing the potential of triticales to meet the demands for increased production and improved nutritive value of the diet in the dry land areas of the Middle East. However, the production of tannour and saaj in villages in Syria is declining. Farmers receive up to 135 piastres per kilo for bread and durum wheats, whereas government-subsidized two-layered Arabic bread is available at 55 piastres per kilo. It is easier and more economical for the village dwellers to travel to the nearest town by tractor or other vehicle once or twice per week to fetch a bulk supply of bread than it is to use their own grain to make tannour. Such a government subsidy may be necessary in some areas, but it encourages the importation of bread wheat or flour. It also tends to inhibit the potential use of a high-yielding and nutritionally beneficial type of grain.

Advanced lines of chickpeas are evaluated through the medium of the familiar homos biteheneh. Homos is made using a standard formula including 20 percent pureed sesame, 2 percent citric acid, and 2 percent salt. The chickpeas are soaked overnight and then blended for three minutes. Flavour, appearance, texture, and odour are evaluated by means of taste panels consisting of up to twenty-five individuals. Sample numbers are rearranged, and one person enters the laboratory at a time to prevent collusion. A maximum of four lines are evaluated at a time, and the Syrian local commercial chickpea variety is included as a randomized control. The organization of ICARDA's quality taste panels is described in a separate report (4). Similar taste panel techniques are employed for the evaluation of khobz, tannour, and homos, except that a higher proportion of people from villages are "conscripted" for tannour taste panels.

Determining nutritional quality of all cereals and food legumes is an inherent part of ICARDA's research programmes. Routine tests are carried out at all stages for protein content, and facilities are available for the determination of all types of fibre components such as crude fibre, acid and neutral detergent fibres, cellulose and lignin. All of these constituents can be determined in forages and straws by NIR spectroscopy. Recent work at the Grain Research Laboratory has enabled the determination of lysine, threonine, and methionine with very good accuracy in barley and peas. This technology was developed using the Neotec Feed Quality Analyzer, Model 51A, interfaced with a Research Composition Analyzer, Model 6350. The calibration data are transferable to the Model FQA51A in the ICARDA laboratory, which now allows screening for these amino acids in even early generation material at the rate of 200 to 300 samples per day. In developing countries it is advisable to study this possibility for improving nutritive value, particularly for the inhabitants of rural areas. In cities it is economically and practically feasible to supplement bulk foods such as breads with amino acids rather than attempt to develop cereal lines rich in these constituents. Lysine and methionine are readily available in the world market, and an additional advantage of supplementing is that normal raw materials can be used to prepare the foods. For example, because many city-dwellers in developing countries acquire 60 to 80 percent of their calorie intake from various forms of breads, these represent a convenient medium for supplementation of diets. Dr. A. Khorshid of the Agricultural Research Centre in Giza, Egypt has established that spraying of lysine onto shami-type, two-layered breads fresh from the oven results in far less destruction of the lysine than when it is added to the flour (personal communication).

The same principle is likely to apply to a number of other commercially prepared foods. Breeding for higher concentrations of amino acids in grains and seeds would be of more benefit to rural dwellers, who do not have access to commercially prepared foods. This is a lengthy process, involving screening of a very large amount of potential parental material and early generation lines. Furthermore, historically the propagation and development of genotypes high in lysine have resulted in higher proportions of lysine-rich protein components relative to the total protein, and the concomitant decrease in the storage proteins present in normal genotypes has resulted in decreases in processing quality. Yields of these lysine-rich lines are usually lower than those of normal lines. If a lysine-rich or methionine-rich genotype could be produced combining the higher amino acid concentration with enhanced yield, such as is the case with some triticales, this could be beneficial to rural populations, as their methods of baking and cooking are less demanding than those defined commercially as good processing quality. The introduction of NIR spectroscopy for determining amino acid content will simplify the search for, and development of, amino acid-rich lines of cereals and legumes.

In summary, both the processing and nutritional quality evaluation practised at the ICARDA laboratories encompass a comprehensive series of tests aimed at the screening and evaluation of both early generation and advanced genetic cereals, food legumes, and forages. The laboratory work is complemented by continuing regional investigations into the types of foods eaten in urban and rural regions of the countries of the Middle East and also by taste panels for products made from new cereal cultivars but based on common recipes. The expansion of NIR spectroscopy into the testing of constituent substances that are normally laborious to determine, such as fibre components and amino acids, will simplify and extend the development of genetic material with more desirable concentrations of these constituents. At the same time, laboratory baking and taste panel-testing will ensure that processing quality is maintained.

Appendix

Methods Used in ICARDA Quality Laboratories.

A. Cereals

1. Thousand kernel weight (TKW) manual. For all cereals count duplicate sets of 200 whole kernels, weigh.
TKW = weight of 200 kernels X 5.

2. Vitreous kernel count (VKC) - durum wheat only. From the 200 kernels for TKW separate and count all kernels with opaque patches.
VKC = (200 - M) : 2.
Note: Damage by wheat (suni) bug, *Eurygaster* ssp. leaves opaque patches. The opaque patches must be studied carefully to determine whether they are "true" opaque patches, which are caused partly by low fertility and partly by genetics, or whether they represent suni bug damage.

3. Protein - Near Infrared (NIR). All grains, cereals, and food legumes. Grind 20-25 g of grain in a Udy Cyclone grinder. Be sure that the sample is completely ground. Large seeds, such as beans or kabuli chickpeas, may need pre-reduction with a pestle and mortar. Mix well, fill the sample cell of a calibrated NIR instrument, place in the instrument and read the protein content.
Calibration. Assemble 40 to 50 samples with uniform distribution of protein across the range expected in future analyses. Grind as above; read optical data. Perform Kjeldahl protein evaluation on all samples. Use multiple linear regression to compute calibration constants, which are regression coefficients of optical data on Kjeldahl protein. Set constants into instrument. Verify accuracy by reading 10 to 12 further samples of known Kjeldahl protein. Adjust intercept as necessary.

4. Protein Kjeldahl. Reference 5. Acid normality adjusted so that 1 ml of titration = 1% protein (Normality = 0.1142 for N X 6.25, and 0.1253 for N X 5.7).

5. Wheat meal fermentation time, WMFT bread, durum wheats, triticale. Prepare a 5% suspension of fresh baker's yeast, or a 3% suspension of dried yeast. Weigh 3 g of cyclone-ground wholemeal, add 1.8 ml yeast suspension and mould into a tight doughball. Place into 125 ml water in a 200 ml Berzelius beaker in a 30° C water bath. Note time. Doughball will rise to surface, and after a while will disintegrate and/or sink to the bottom of the beaker. Note the time. Difference in minutes between doughball immersion and sinking is WMFT. Strongest wheats take longest time. Wheats with times of 120 to 160 minutes are suitable for Khobz and Baladi baking. Stronger wheats are better for baking raised breads.

6. Kernel hardness by particle size index, PSI. Bread, durum wheats, triticale. Weigh exactly 10 g of cyclone-ground wheat onto a 200 mesh (75 micrometer) sieve. Add about 20 g whole wheat kernels. Sieve 10 minutes on mechanical shaker. Sieved particles X 100 = PSI. Range in PSI is approximately from 25 (very hard) to 80 (very soft).

7. Appearance. Triticale. Visually grade 50 to 100 g of triticale kernels for degree of shrivelling. Assign grade of 1 (very smooth surface) to 5 (very shrivelled).

8. Size distribution. (Barley only). Sieve exactly 50 or 100 g of well-blended barley sample for 5 minutes on normal sorting sieve apparatus with

oblong apertures of 2.8, 2.5, and 2.2 mms. Weigh what is retained on each sieve, and what has passed through a 2.2 mm sieve. Samples with more than 5% through 2.2 mm unacceptable for malting potential. Samples are subgraded on basis of percentages of largest kernels. Full details of grading system are contained in reference 3.

9. Husk percentage. (Barley only). Accurately weigh 20 g barley kernels. Pearl 15 seconds in Strong-Scott Barley Pearler. Weigh pearled kernels (loss in weight X 5) = Husk %.

10. Pigment. Reference 5.

11. Mill Flour. Bread wheat and triticale. Buhler mill procedure. Measure moisture content of wheat using Motomco or similar electronic moisture meter. Temper wheat (500 to 5000 g accurately weighed) according to hardness (PSI) of wheat (see below), leave overnight.

Wheat PSI	Temper To
70+	13.5
60-70	14
50-60	14.5
40-50	15.5
Up to 40	16

Next day blend well, start mill, add wheat to hopper. After 5 minutes brush down break side entry, tap both sieve units with rubber hammer. After 10 more minutes repeat, and also clean reduction entry. Tap with rubber hammer. After 5 more minutes repeat cleaning reduction side, tap with rubber hammer. Repeat after 5 more minutes. Stop mill, weigh all streams, bran, and shorts. Use bran finisher if available. Weigh bran/shorts flour and add to total. Blend thoroughly. Record all weights and calculate extraction.

$$\text{Extraction} = \frac{\text{Total weight of flour X 100}}{\text{weight of wheat + tempering water}}$$

12. Mill semolina. (Durum wheat only). Reference 3.

13. Farinograph. Reference 3. Farinograph stability of 4 to 7 minutes in association with fall in resistance after 15 minutes (delta R) of 50 to 80 indicates flours suitable for Khobz baking. Stronger flours with stability of 6 to 15 minutes are suitable for baking raised breads and blending with ("carrying") weaker flours.

14. Khobz baking. ICARDA procedure. Weight 500 to 1000 g well-blended flour. Add 1% salt. Weigh 0.75% (3.75 to 7.5 g) of dried baker's yeast, and 1% sugar, mix, transfer to 400 ml beaker, add 200 ml warm (34° to 40° C) water, mix, and let stand 10 minutes. The yeast will start to work. Transfer flour to mixer and add yeast suspension. Start the mixer and add warm water to 50 to 55%. Flours from stronger and harder wheats (farinograph and PSI data) need more water. Mix for 15 minutes, and during the first two minutes use a plastic spatula to scrape down flour and dough adhering to the sides of the mixing bowl. After mixing, mould into a ball and place in a fermentation cabinet (plastic sheet may be substituted). Record dough-handling properties. Leave 45 minutes, then divide into pieces of 225 g, form into balls. Record dough handling properties. Return to fermentation cabinet or plastic sheet, leave 10 minutes. Set

sheeting rolls at 1.0, 1.5 or 2.0 mm, depending on dough-handling at dividing. Strongest doughs need thinnest setting. Pass through sheeting rolls twice, to produce round flat dough pieces about 30 cms in diameter. Record dough-handling properties. Cover with plastic and leave 25 minutes. Bake at 450° C for 45-60 seconds. Cool 20-30 minutes. Judge from aspects of texture, appearance, odour, taste, evenness of layers and internal crumb structure according to Reference 3. Next day fold at least two Khobz to assess keeping quality.

15. Pasta quality. (Spaghetti). Weigh 50 g semolina and transfer to mixer. Add 16 ml water (32% absorption). Mix 1.5 minutes, scrape pieces of dough down into bowl. Close bowl with plastic lid and apply vacuum to 600 mm mercury. Continue mixing for another two mintues at 69 rpm. Mixing bowl and extrusion cell should be water-jacketed at 50° C. After mixing, transfer to extrusion cell, cap cell, and compress dough to 200 psi for 9 minutes. Replace blank cell cap with teflonized extrusion cap, and extrude spaghetti. Place strands (about 40 cms) of spaghetti over peices of 1.5 to 2 cm dowel, and dry in special temperature/humidity-controlled drying cabinet overnight. Alternatively, dry four hours at 40° C in presence of high humidity, then overnight at 80° C. Cook pieces (5 cm) of spaghetti in boiling water for 12 to 13 minutes. Test for "bitability", stickiness, and colour. Taste panels may be used.

16. Baked tannour. This is carried out for ICARDA by experienced women bakers in Tel Hadya village, and the procedure is described in reference 6.

17. Damaged starch. See reference 7.

18. Flour ash. Reference 8.

19. Diastatic power (barley only). Reference 3.

B. Food Legumes

1. Seed size.

a. Chick peas and lentils. Count duplicate sub-samples of 100 seeds. Weigh. Seed size = weight of 100 seeds : 100.

b. Faba beans. Count 100 seeds for small beans, or as many seeds as are available for large beans. Weight : no. of seeds = weight per seed.

2. Seed size distribution. (Chickpeas and lentils only). Accurately weigh 50 or 100 g of cleaned grains. Place on uppermost of a nest of four round-hole sieves. Sieve 3 minutes on automatic sieve shaker. Weigh seeds remaining on all four sieves, and all seeds passing through the smallest sieve. Calculate percent size distribution. Separate sets of sieve sizes are selected for chickpeas, large lentils, or small lentils as follows:

Chickpeas	Large Lentils	Small Lentils
8 mm	7 mm	4.5 mm
7	6	4
6	5	3.5
5	4	3

Seeds are graded according to Reference 3.

DRA-S

3. Protein NIR. As for cereals.

4. Protein, Kjeldahl. Reference 5. Sample weight is 0.5 g for all food legumes.

5. Hydration capacity. Count 100 seeds and weigh. Transfer to a 250 ml Erlenmeyer flask (500 ml for beans) and add 100 ml tap water (250 ml for beans). Cover lightly and let stand overnight. Drain, remove superfluous water with absorbent tissues, and reweigh all swollen seeds.
Hydration capacity = weight per seed (wet) - weight per seed (dry).

6. Hard seed coat. From hydration capacity test, record percentage of seeds that did not swell. This is the percentage of hard-coated seeds.

7. Swelling capacity. (Mg/seed) Weigh 100 seeds, transfer to 100 ml graduate cylinder (250 ml for beans). Pipette in 50 ml water. Record volume. Volume per seed = (volume - 50) : 100. These seeds can be used to test hydration capacity. After drying stage of hydration capacity test, return seeds to graduate cylinder. Pipette in 50 or 75 ml water. Record volume. Swelling capacity (ml/seed) = volume/seed (wet) - volume seed (dry).

8. Cooking time.

a) Chickpeas. Boil 30 to 40 chickpeas under reflux (Labconco crude fibre equipment is suitable), using 200 ml tap water in 600 ml Berzelius beakers. After 45 minutes remove one pea, press with fingers until cotyledons separate. If pea is uncooked, centre of cotyledon will be white. Cooked area will be yellow. Continue testing every 10 minutes until peas are completely cooked. When cooking is thought to be complete, test at least 5 peas to verify. Times range from 55 to over 200 minutes.

b) Lentils and beans. As for chickpeas, but test for cooking with fingers for hardness only. Commence testing lentils after 20 minutes, beans after 60 minutes. Verify that cooking is complete by testing at least 5 seeds as for chickpeas.

9. Husk %. (Lentils and chickpeas). Soak 20 seeds overnight in water. Drain, remove testa manually. Dry testa/pericarps and cotyledons. Weigh, and calculate % testa/pericarp.

10. Loss in weight on decortication. Lentils only. This is tested by means of a laboratory decorticater developed by H. Nakoul at ICARDA. Decorticate 50 g lentils for 1 minute. Pass mixture of husk and decorticated lentils through Carter Dockage tester using wheat screens. Weigh husks and lentils. Record degree of decortication of lentil seeds and husk percentage.

11. Methionine. Lentils only. NIR method. Reference 9.

12. Vicine/convicine. (Beans only). NIR. Reference 3.

13. Protein digestibility. Reference 3.

14. Homos biteheni quality. Chickpeas only. Soak 100 g of chickpeas overnight in about 70 ml tap water. Drain if necessary, add 2 g citric acid, 2 g salt, 30 g tiheni (pureed sesame seed) and blend for 3 minutes in Waring blendor (high speed). Transfer to a plate or large petri dish.

Test for taste, appearance, texture, and appearance. Taste panels may be employed.

15. Taste panel technique. Reference 3.

REFERENCES

1. Food and Agriculture Organization, Bulletin of Statistics, issues from 1975-1981 (FAO, Rome).

2. P.C. Williams and W. Blaschuk, "Comparison of Seven Different Methods for Screening Wheat for Khobz-Type Flat Bread Making," Cereal Foods World, 25:527 (Abstr. No. 155), 1980.

3. ICARDA Quality Laboratory Operations Manual, Revised Version, P.C. Williams, October 1982.

4. Cereal Laboratory Methods, Method 46-12, The American Association of Cereal Chemists, St. Paul, Minnesota, 1969.

5. Cereal Laboratory Methods, Method 14-50, The American Association of Cereal Chemists, St. Paul, Minnesota, 1969.

6. P.C. Williams and F. Jaby El-Haramein, "Quality Evaluation of Triticale for Single layer Flat Bread Baking," J. Sci. Food Agric., 1984.

7. E.A. Farrand, "Flour Properties in Relation to the Modern Bread Process in the United Kingdom, with Special Reference to Alpha-Amylase and Starch Damage," Cereal Chem. 41:98, 1964.

8. Cereal Laboratory Methods, Method 8-01, The American Association of Cereal Chemists, St. Paul, Minnesota, 1969.

9. P.C. Williams, S.L. MacKenzie, and P.M. Starkey, "Determination of Methionine in Peas by Near-Infrared Reflectance Spectroscopy," J. Agric. Food Chem., 1984.

TABLE 1. Population Changes of Countries of ICARDA Region (1970-1980)

	Thousands			% Increase		
	1970	1975	1980	1970 to 1975	1975 to 1980	1970 to 1980
Afghanistan	16978	19280	22038	13.6	14.3	29.8
Algeria	13307	15686	18594	12.9	18.5	39.7
Bahrain	214	256	302	19.9	18.0	40.5
Cyprus	615	639	651	3.9	1.9	5.9
Egypt	33329	36916	41995	10.8	13.8	26.0
Ethiopia	25450	28776	32601	13.1	13.3	28.1
Iran	28359	32743	38082	15.5	16.3	34.3
Iraq	9355	11020	13084	17.8	18.7	39.9
Jordan	2299	2702	3190	17.5	18.1	38.8
Kuwait	744	1002	1372	45.4	36.9	84.4
Lebanon	2469	2799	3161	13.4	12.9	28.0
Libya	1982	2436	2977	22.9	22.2	50.2
Morocco	15126	17305	20296	14.4	17.3	34.2
Pakistan	60449	70207	82441	16.2	17.3	36.4
Saudi Arabia	6198	7180	8367	15.8	16.5	35.0
Sudan	14090	16015	19371	13.7	14.7	37.5
Syria	6258	7354	8644	17.5	17.5	38.1
Tunisia	5127	5608	6363	9.4	13.5	24.1
Turkey	35321	40063	45346	13.4	13.2	28.4
United Arab Emirate	227	558	796	144.9	42.7	250.7
Yemen	4836	5282	5926	9.2	12.2	22.5
Yemen DR	1497	1654	1896	10.5	14.6	26.6
Total	284231	325541	377493	14.5	16.0	32.8

Source: Food and Agricultural Organization, FAO Rome.

TABLE 2. Principal Types of Foods Eaten in Countries of ICARDA Region

A. Cereals

Wheat	Triticale	Durum	Barley
2-layer breads (Khobz, Baladi)	Unknown, but generally as for wheat.	Pasta	Feed
Single layer breads (Tannour, Saaj, Mountain Bread, Merahrah)	Feed	Cous Cous	Soups
Raised breads Baguettes, Sponge Bread)		Feed	Breads
Patisserie			Beer
Cous Cous			
Feed			

B. Food Legumes

Beans	Chickpeas	Lentils
Ful Medames	Homos Biteheneh	Soup
Ful	Felafel	Splits
Canning	Others	Others
Others		

TABLE 3. Seed Weights

Lentils	Beans	Cereals Chickpeas
2mg	2g	Intermediate
Sample Limited	Sampling error high	
3-10 g/plant	10-70 g/plant	8-40 g/plant

TABLE 4. Quality Screening and Evaluation Tests Used for Cereals

Test	F2 - F4				F5 - Advanced and Parental[1]			
	Bread Wheat	Triticale	Durum	Barley	Bread Wheat	Triticale	Durum	Barley
Kernel	X	X	X	X	X	X	X	X
Appearance		X		X		X		X
Size distrib.				X	X			X
Vitreous, %			X				X	
Hardness	X	X			X	X		
Protein	X	X	X	X	X	X	X	X
Pigment	X	X	X		X	X	X	
Wheatmeal ferm.	X	X			X	X	X	
Pearling index				X				X
Mill flour				X	X	X		
Mill semolina							X	
Farinograph					X	X	X	
Bake Khobz					X	X	X[3]	
Bake Tannour						X[2]		
Diastatic power				X				X
Damaged starch					X	X		
Colour (flour)					X	X		
Colour (semolina)					X	X		
Make pasta							X	
Malt								X[4]

1 Advanced series of tests are applied to selected earlier generation material as requested by breeders.
2 Baked from 100% wholemeal in 50% blends with Stork durum wholemeal.
3 Khobz baked in blends with 60% commerical 82% extraction flour.
4 Contracted to Grain Research Laboratory, Winnipeg, Canada.

TABLE 5. Quality Screening and Evaluation Tests Used for Food Legumes

	F2 - F5			F5 - Advanced and Parental		
Test	Bean	Chickpea	Lentil	Bean	Chickpea	Lentil
Seed size	X	X	X	X	X	X
Size distribution	X	X	X	X	X	X
Hardness		X	X		X	X
Protein	X	X	X[1]	X	X	X
Hydration capacity	X	X		X	X	
Appearance (Colour)	X		X	X		X
Cooking time				X	X	
Husk, %			X[2]			X
Loss on decortication			X[2]			
Cook homos					X	X[2]
Cook ful				X		
Methionine			X[1]			
Vicine/convicine				X		
Fibre			X[2]			X
Protein digestibility				X	X	X

Notes: 1 Simultaneous NIR determination.
2 One of these tests will be eliminated after one full season of study. Fibre can be tested by NIR.

TABLE 6. Typical Baking Formulate for Khobz, Baladi, and Pain Francais Breads

	Khobz	Baladi	Pain Francais (baguettes)
Flour	100[1]	100[2]	100[3]
Water	54 +/- 10%	80 + 15%	55 + 5%
Yeast	2.25 + 00.8%	10 - 15%[4,5]	1 - 2.5
Salt	0.75 + 0.5%	1	1.5 - 2
Sugar	0[3]	-	-
Dusting flour	-	2 - 2.5%	-
Mix	25 + 10 min.	20 + 10 min.	20 + 5 min.
Stand (ferment)	35 + 20 min.	60 + 30 min.	10 - 35 min.
Divide	X	X (195 g)	370-400 g
Ferment	10 + 10 min.	50 + 17 min.	0-20 min.
Sheet	X	Flatten by hand	X
Final Proof	20 + 17 min.	-	20-30 min.
Bake	57 + 24 sec.	1-2 min.	20-30 min.
Temperature	420°C + 30°C	400°C + 30°C	200-270°C

Notes: 1 82% extraction.
2 87% extraction.
3 75% extraction.
4 Usually zero, but up to 1.5% in cool weather.
5 Sourdough.

DISCUSSION

SESSION V - FOOD PRODUCTION VERSUS NUTRITION

NEVIN S. SCRIMSHAW

Somel has quoted eloquently from Ladejinsky of the factors impeding the use of green revolution techniques, including lack of distributive justice, of extension services, of stable farm markets and prices, of access to water, and poor land-tenure practices, exorbitant rentals, high cost of inputs, poor legislation and government policies. All of these problems exist and cannot fairly be blamed on agronomists and plant breeders. At the same time, however, we can all cite examples where the early policies of the green revolution seem to have played into the hands of the privileged and against the small farmer. The most charitable view of many of the problems is to say that it is easy to apply hindsight without appreciating the considerable foresight and the initiative that was exercised in the early years. Nevertheless, I think we must acknowledge that there was also some tunnel vision and some plain stubbornness that may or may not have been fully justified by the need to concentrate efforts on cereal yields in order to produce quick results.

In this sense ICARDA is fortunate in that it was developed as a later generation International Centre. Certainly, ICARDA's emphasis on farming systems, on-farm trials, food legumes, local grain uses, on cooking quality, and on taste panels is totally different from the programme of an international agricultural centre in the early 1960s. With its current programme ICARDA is not likely to encounter problems comparable to the lack of acceptability of IR8 rice because of poor cooking quality and taste or the rejection of Opaque A-2 maize after large-scale introduction in Colombia because of its poor storage characteristics.

It is worth noting that as soon as the effects of the green revolution began to emerge there were a number of very perceptive articles, mainly by agricultural economists, indicating the difficulties. One that I like, in part because of the title, "The Green Revolution: Cornucopia or Pandora's Box", written by Clifton Wharton in 1969,[1/] indicated at that time some of the reasons for believing that the new technology would not spread as widely or as rapidly as some thought. Among limits to the spread of new high-yielding varities he pointed out were the problems of water availability and distribution, the cost of large irrigation projects, adequate markets to handle the increased production, the effects of price structures, and the adoption of new technology by farmers growing primarily for family consumption. Such farmers were understandably reluctant to experiment with the very survival of their families. He also described the difficulties of learning new farming skills and the expertise of a higher order than that needed for traditional farming methods. Also, changing the cropping patterns and being able to practice multiple cropping means changes in the customary agricultural cycles and even in the religious and traditional habits that are part of their culture. Most significantly, he emphasised very

1/ Foreign Affirs Quarterly, 47 (3):464-476, 1969.

strongly that the failure of countries to make major institutional reforms would be a likely handicap. He then detailed some of the institutional and structural problems of introducing the green revolution into Latin America and India, and pointed out the need to expand the entire complex of services of industries to achieve higher production.

The goals of increased food production are frequently couched in terms of some desirable minimal standards of nutrition. Such goals are commendable but can only be obtained by individuals who have the income available to purchase a better diet. The demand for food depends on both the income of the consumers and the price of the food, and Wharton goes on to speak of the food problem as both a problem of food production and supply and of demand and income. He also questions the effect of the green revolution on the displacement of rural peoples that has heightened the pace of migration to the cities, and like so many others, he was concerned that emphasis on the potential of the green revolution would decrease attention on the urgent need to reduce population growth. He was a prophet who has since been recognized even in his own country.

There is now widespread agreement that there have been certain other undesirable characteristics of the early green revolution, such as the neglect of legumes. It is also clear that there was a neglect of farmer and consumer preferences and of the applicability of the new technologies to small farms. There has also been a consistent failure to take into consideration nutritional factors and the role of women in agricultural production. Meeting the nutritional needs of each member of the community means changing the structure of production and division of labour between the sexes. This new orientation must take into account the role of women in both reproduction and production and the influence of changes in agricultural practices on the course and outcome of pregnancy or breast-feeding and on women's energy requirements during these periods of physical stress. Seasonal variation in the demands on women's time is also important. In traditional agricultural societies where women are recognized as food producers, the need is to lighten both the productive and reproductive tasks of women through appropriate technologies, among which those in the green revolution package should be influential. There are many other labour-saving technologies that need to be made available to women. Examination of the specific food requirements of women means admitting that the multiple stresses make them nutritionally vulnerable and that their excessive physical, physiological, and to some extent psychological burdens in most agricultural societies should not be seen as just a natural part of the society but rather a matter of concern.

I would like to close by reference to the green revolution in Mexico. In a fascinating article in the Scientific American in 1976[2/] entitled "The Agriculture of Mexico", Wellhausen portrayed the green revolution as having plateaued, and the task ahead for Mexico for food production seemed to be not just formidable but almost impossible. As one of the pioneers of the green revolution techniques in Mexico, as director of both the original Rockefeller Foundation Research Programme there and the director of CIMMYT, he noted that increases in corn and wheat production had been spectacular in the 1950s and the early 1960s. Corn production, for example, increased from 1,000,800 tons in 1940 to 1,000,900 tons in 1945, i.e., only a 100,000 ton increase in five years! By 1960 production due to green revolution technology was up to 5,500,000 tons, and reached 9,000,000 tons between 1965 and 1970.

Then this growth stopped and even fell to 8,400,000 in 1975. The wheat yields continued to increase a while longer and then plateaued as well.

2/ Vol. 235 (3):128-150 (1976).

The production of basic food crops in Mexico in 1941-45 was 150 kg per capita, by 1961-65, this increased to 250 kg and in 1966-70 to nearly 300 kg. Then in 1971-75 it dropped to 275 kg. During this time, population kept increasing at nearly three percent and the irrigated land that was suitable for green revolution techniques in Mexico had largely been used up. The corollary to this was that Mexico exported food in the early 1960s, by 1967-69 it had no more food to export, and by 1971 it was spending 50 million dollars on cereal imports alone. In 1972 this jumped to 190 million dollars; by 1974, the last year for which the information was available, Mexico was spending 500 million dollars for food imports. Furthermore, this curve looked as though it were heading upward ever more steeply, and with the population increase, there was no end in sight to the amount of additional food imports that would be needed.

In January 1982, at a North-South Round Table meeting in Washington, D.C., Cassio Luiselli, who was in charge of the Mexican Agricultural Systems, reported that policy was changed under the Government of Lopez Portillo to make credit and inputs available to the small farmer, to direct the extension services toward the small farmer, and to assure favourable prices for the producer. These have begun to show results to the extent that real imports in 1980 were 9 million tons, much smaller than the 18 million tons predicted in 1977. In 1981 these imports were down to two million tons, and it was predicted that in 1982 Mexico would not need food imports. This is attributed mainly to this policy shift, designed to help the small holder.*

Another point is that this increase has been achieved largely without the varieties developed at CIMMYT. If you visit the Puebla Project, which is now quite a successful effort to increase the ouput and well-being of small-holding farmers, you find varieties of corn that are tall because the farmers have an urgent need for fodder as well as grain. If you visit CIMMYT, a few kilometers away, you will find a concentration of dwarf high-yielding varieties. You will also find farmers interplanting legumes, which was against earlier advice, but is now being shown in the Puebla Project to work very well. The lessons to be drawn from this are obvious.

<u>Alderman:</u> I would mention what I think is a medium-term problem. According to FAO estimates, in the medium-term, agricultural production will grow at a rate of 3.1 percent and possibly at a rate of five percent. In the long-term, however, in a number of countries five percent is rather optimistic. The average growth rate in the USA is about two percent. Growth in Japan even during the Meiji Era, which was an expansive time period, agricultural production rose about two percent per year. However, population growth rates are two to three percent in the Middle East and per capita income is growing at a rate of five percent or more. This means another two or three percent increase in the demand for food.

In addition, there is a growing demand for meat, and feed for animals is a major component of the grain market. This requires a five to six percent annual growth in agriculture, a very large task for agricultural researchers. For that reason we would expect food imports to be substantial for many years to come and to adopt a policy goal to stop imports could be very dangerous. For example, while India has not imported grain for the last two to three years, no one would say that this policy has been a real nutritional success. The same is true in the Philippines.

---

* More recently the economic crisis in Mexico and altered policies of the new government have reversed this favourable trend.

The second point I would like to make is that this great demand for grain is putting significant pressure on prices. Without government intervention such as subsidies, this upward pressure on prices will continue, and imports will decrease or even stay at the same level. The result is, of course that the poor will be hurt the most. We need to target policies and programmes towards the poor, because the market is not likely to offer a short-term or medium-term solution for them.

Williams: With all due respect, I doubt if many people are aware of the necessity for increasing food availability in this region. As I mentioned earlier, the region will need 100 million tons of food imports by the end of the century and there is no place capable of supplying that amount. That is the problem. When Russia was recently denied 17 million tons of grain by the U.S. there was no other place to get that 17 million tons and a lot of their cows were slaughtered. It is true that U.S. and Canada control 91 percent of all the grain exported in the world, and they will presumably continue to do so, but there is a limit to how much we can continue to increase our own production. Eventually there will be no place to get it from. Meanwhile, the population is increasing at an annual rate of about three percent.

Somel: One thing that compounds the situation is that, unless production shifts to the areas of deficit, imports will not be adequate to solve nutrition problems unless there are direct food transfers. Without this modestic increase in production, there may be no effective demand with which to pay for imports.

Srivastava: The examples of green revolution application in Mexico and in the Puebla Project are those of high-input, high-resource technology that were developed to get the maximum benefit from a favourable situation. In this part of the world where ICARDA is concentrating its efforts, conditions are less favourable. High input technology requires better moisture conditions, and therefore the green revolution touched irrigated areas of high fertility in the Middle East but did not really reach the vast areas of rainfed agriculture. ICARDA's major thrust is to develop technology for moderate to lower rainfall areas using less sophisticated resources.

In the last four years in Syria we have conducted barley, durum wheat, and bread wheat trials, about 200 in all, in different rainfall areas. We have found that, using simple inputs, even in rainfall zones with only 250 mm annual rainfall we could double the production of barley. Therefore, there is ample scope to increase the productivity of the region provided that the policy is right.

Somel mentioned that we need more policy adjustments to increase production. Let me give you an example from Syria. I understand that subsidized fertilizer is available on irrigated land at a rate of 20 kilograms per hectare. Yet, for nonirrigated lands, the drier zones, fertilizer is not subsidized. The majority of the area where the crops are grown in Syria is rainfed, but there is a policy that discourages fertilizer on these lands. In general, these are the poorer farmers who would benefit greatly by production increases. Therefore, policy makers have to be informed that 20 kg per hectare of nitrogen in areas with 250 mm of rainfall is very effective. The final example is from Algeria. Six months ago, about 48 to 50 kg of wheat were required to buy 1 kg of meat. If I were a farmer in Algeria, I would certainly not grow wheat. I would grow grass and bring in some sheep and let them graze it. The production of cereals in Algeria is going down again even though there is sufficient technology. What Algeria lacks is a firm policy.

In conclusion, there is plenty of production potential in the Middle East, but this potential has not been exploited because proper technology and proper policy have both been lacking. Given the two, there is enormous scope for production increases. I am optimistic that we can produce the 100 million tons that Williams says will be required.

Nygaard: To carry on one more step with what Srivastava has just said, generally, we treat agro-climatic conditions, rainfall for example, as fixed things that we cannot control. At the same time we treat socioeconomic characteristics, land tenure for example, as something we can control. If we draw a rainfall distribution pattern for North Africa, we may find that parts of Tunisia and parts of Algeria have similar agro-climatic conditions for wheat production. However, we know that there are socioeconomic differences (that encompass political differences) between the two countries, and thus there are different incentives that affect farmer behaviour. The point is, we develop new technologies to fit the agro-climatic environment, but we try to change the socio-economic environment to fit the technologies that have been developed. This would not necessarily be a problem if we could change conditions as we pleased, but we have absolutely failed to convince policy makers to change socio-economic conditions. No one has the ability to change prices in Algeria or land tenure in Tunisia, so we blame low production levels on slow adoption rates or poor agricultural incentives and not on inappropriate technology.

Thus I believe we have two choices. We have to increase our efforts greatly in the area of agricultural policy so that we can change economic conditions, which I believe Dr. Srivastava is suggesting. This is sound and could be successful. However, if we decide that we cannot change socioeconomic conditions, we have to accept them as given just as we do rainfall and try to develop new technologies consistent with the socioeconomic and agro-climatic environments.

Gerhart: One point I would like to mention is the question of inter-regional disparities in income. This is one problem that I think is particularly unfair to blame on plant breeders. The obvious potential for any plant depends largely on the available moisture, the quality of the soils, and the physical resources. Not all areas have the same potential. In East Africa, where I was a planning officer, we were told that we had to develop maize varieties for the non-rainfed areas as well as for the low-rainfall areas. This was extremely difficult to do. One of the breeders said that the best crop for this area was grass, which I thought was an honest response.

The reason this is such a problem is that in most areas of the world, particularly the developing world, for example sub-Saharan Africa, ethnic boundaries are very closely correlated with ecological boundaries. The origins of tribal boundaries in Africa are different ecological systems. Therefore, when you introduce a new technology that greatly increases the value of land and the value of production in one area, you are most likely also to be affecting the income of particular ethnic groups. This engenders either increased resentment and jealousy in the less developed area or increased capacity to exercise power on the part of those in the wealthy areas. One effect of more wealth is improved education. In Africa the best educated people are all in the highlands because this is where the high-value cash crops can be grown. Also, the missionaries preferred to locate in these highlands because they were outside the malarial zones.

Nevertheless, many of the problems are ethnic conflicts as a result of differences in income. In many parts of the developing world with low levels of income, including India and virtually all of sub-Saharan Africa, I do not think anyone in good conscience could argue that one should withhold improved crop varieties because it is going to increase income from 100 dollars to 200 dollars per capita in one district but not in another. However, if governments want to avoid ethnic conflict within their borders they must look for ways to spread the benefits of these technologies more widely, spread social services more broadly, and if possible, develop improved technologies for the poor resource areas. I think it is in this last category where Srivastava said that there is room for action. There is if you put a premium, not on output, but on political stability, which could be obtained by increasing research efforts in the resource-poor areas.

It is very hard for the market to do this because these areas are generally sparsely populated and thus the demand is not as great, nor is production potential. Nevertheless, it is a case where the research institutes, national governments, and donor agencies have to take this larger national good into account and direct, or if you like, misdirect, resources into these impoverished or less productive areas.

Khattab: With respect to Somel's paper, I would not like to think that we would leave this conference frightened by what happened in the green revolution, and therefore sit idly by and accept agricultural production as it is now. I think there is a great potential to increase food production in this region. To do this we have to use modern technologies and adapt them to suit local conditions. This includes mechanization because there is going to be a shortage of labour for agriculture. Of course, one has to learn from what has happened elsewhere by making sure that, while focussing on production, socio-economic effects are considered, including equitable distribution of income. I am really impressed by the work that is being introduced on the quality of cereals and legumes, as discussed in Williams' paper. This is a very important aspect for ICARDA because we need to increase not only the quantity but the quality of our food crops. The only thing missing, in my view, is that we need to have food technologists as part of the research team to look into the preparation of these food crops. This includes improving the food quality and curbing the losses that can occur in the preparation process.

Pinstrup-Andersen: I would like to add to Nygaard's comment regarding socio-economic conditons and the extent to which we should focus technology on fixed socioeconomic conditions.

First of all, I think he raised a very important issue as far as the International Agricultural Research Centres are concerned. Until fairly recently, many of these centres would not even think about policy analysis or policy advice. The argument was that these centres were neutral technical centres that should not in any way get involved in politics. Now this of course was at a time when a number of the many leading scientists from these institutes, including Norman Borlaug, were giving large amounts of direct policy advice to governments on such things as fertilizer imports, fertilizer prices, etc. In fact, such advice was very successful in turning governments toward much more effective public policies. Nevertheless, in general, the centres then and some of them now would argue that we must stay away from analysis and advice on national policy matters. I think this is wrong and this will probably not surprise you, since I come from IFPRI where everything we do is related to national food policies. The fact is that we need to look at the adaptation of both technology and policies as an integral set of activities. We must keep in mind that changing priorities in agricultural research usually takes a long time and we cannot give the plant breeders objectives one day, change them on the next, and expect them to have a new variety in two weeks time. This research has a long-term horizon, whereas changes in public policy can be very abrupt and frequently happen in a matter of weeks or months. It seems to me that as scientists from International Agricultural Research Centres interested in this general area, we need to sort out the things that we are unlikely to change in the socioeconomic environment over fairly long periods of time.

To give you an example from Latin America with which I am more familiar: to wait for appropriate land reforms to take place would be quite ridiculous. Therefore we must take into account that this is probably one of the socio-economic factors we are not going to change. Any adaptation will have to come from technology. On the other hand, I think pricing policies can be fairly easily manipulated, if we can provide solid analytical evidence to back up advice, and particularly if the advice is given by highly respected and prominent people in the field of agricultural research. I am of course referring to the Borlaugs of this world because governments tend to listen to people who have been successful.

The International Centres have a responsibility to include policy analysis in their work, because they are upsetting the system, it is hoped for the good, but in doing so guidance in issues such as public policy must also be provided. I do not think the International Centres can hide behind a technical and neutral facade. We are beyond that kind of situation.

To comment on Somel's paper, I have done my utmost to come up with something upon which we could disagree. There is a lot more evidence available now concerning some of the points on which Somel has not really taken a firm stand. For example, we can say that the biological-chemical technology that provided the basis for the green revolution was labour-using. I do not think there is any question that the demand for labour went up as a result of the new technology. Because the demand for labour rose in areas where there was a seasonal or permanent labour scarcity, or where there was inelastic labour supply, wages went up and that was why labour-saving mechanization was introduced. It was not the biological-chemical technology that in and by itself introduced labour-saving technology. It was because in certain areas there were not enough labourers to go around and labour-saving mechanization was required. This was a logical and obviously a correct response to increasing labour demand. This is a point where we can be much more concise. There is much misunderstanding on this point in the literature, and people with vested interests argue that the green revolution caused labour-saving technology that pushed many workers out of employment. This is just not true.

Second, as Somel pointed out, the pie has definitely increased. What he fails to point out is that the absolute size of the piece of pie available to the very poor has also increased. There is not any doubt about that. The share of this new pie may be smaller or larger, but the absolute net benefit to the poor is higher now, in my opinion, than it was before the green revolution.

Third, I agree that we need to focus our attention on *ex ante* assessment of new technologies. It is always nice to know what happened in the past and it helps us to design the future, but we now need to focus much more clearly on prior assessment. I think the International Agricultural Centres are very much aware of this need -- there is work of this kind going on I believe in almost all, if not all of them, but there is a real problem at the national level. The national agricultural research institutes in many countries do not yet realize that following the traditional approach of merely doing research without paying any attention to what the effects will be is not useful. What we need to concentrate on, relating to Nygaard's point, is the interaction between policy and technology.

Somel: My response would be to ask for references because I did a computerized literature search and did not come across any strong evidence on the second point that you mentioned. A larger pie may be available, but whether this becomes accessible to the poor is a different matter. There is no evidence of that. I note in my paper that only one reference said something in this respect, but it was not a micro-study. In this study there was a methodological problem of inconsistency between the premises and the results, but I really do not know of any studies that say specifically, based on concrete evidence, that the poor now have more to eat.

Scrimshaw: Pinstrup-Andersen indicated that the Centres are only now beginning to be concerned with policy, and I mentioned a number of other things that were missing in the early programmes at the Centres. One we have not discussed is the lack of research on postharvest food conservation. FAO also neglected this problem area, and this was one of the reasons why the UNU made this one of the three priorities of its Hunger Programme in 1975. Actually, the workshop at IRRI was the first explicit recognition that I know of by an Institute Director that this would be an appropriate part of the activities of the International Centres.

Parpia, who was the architect of the UNU postharvest food conservation programme, has asked for the floor next and I will give it to him.

Parpia: I would like to raise a question with Williams. He mentioned that it is much cheaper to increase agricultural production than it is to build a network for the postharvest system. If this is the case, we will never build a balanced multisectoral economy that can support agricultural development in the long-run and generate employment as a means of earning income to provide more food for people. Today one reason that the United States is able to produce so much is that only four percent of its population is directly involved in agriculture. Thus, it is possible to support, directly and indirectly, the development of agriculture. I think this is one lesson the developing countries can learn. However, the types of technologies to be used in developing countries would be different. Agriculture should be used as a means of developing other sectors that will support it. We should not advise people to forget this and emphasize only agriculture.

Williams: The U.S. and Canada are net exporters of grain, and we built our systems of railroads, canals and elevators years ago. Today the biggest problem Canada has is moving grain -- not growing grain -- but moving it. We have two railroads that go across the country, but we may have to build a new one. No one knows where the money is going to come from as it will cost about a half billion dollars to build. We still have to build it because we will have to export about twice as much grain by the end of the century as we do now.

Growing grain is not a serious problem in Canada; our breeders and agronomists are convinced that we can double yields if we need to. At this stage, there is no incentive for farmers in Canada to increase yields because they have to store it. We once did a survey in the Canadian prairies on the age of grain in storage on farms and we found some 13-year-old wheat. It was still all right; bread could be made from it because Canada has the biggest "refrigerator" in the world with the exception of Siberia. Apart form the cost of building a transportation and grain-handling system, billions of dollars are involved. It is a colossal undertaking. The grain commission runs the grain industry in Canada, sets all the specifications, and monitors it. As the chemist in charge of protein work, I advise the commission and thus the government, what should be done because only governments can get anything done. I think it is definitely the prerogative of International Centres to advise governments as long as they know they are right before they give the advice.

Somel: I have a comment to make about the investment requirements for agricultural development. As Williams said, this is an expensive proposition, and I noted in the paper that the projections call for a 60 to 80 billion dollar investment per year between now and the year 2000. Is this possible? A news commentary I heard recently indicated that the expenditures on armaments in the developing countries purchased from the developed countries in 1981 totaled 44 billion dollars.

Pellett: I am very impressed with the activities and successes of the International Agricultural Research Centres and I am wondering whether Scrimshaw and others can suggest why we have not been so successful with this type of international activity in the field of nutrition? It seems we are always saying we do not have enough information, we do not know what really happens to the poorest of the poor in terms of their intake, or their purchasing power, and widespread malnutrition persists. We have the example of INCAP and one or two other institutions, but we certainly do not have anything that is as functional as groups of international scientists working together to deal with the nutrition problems of the world or to deal with the policies that are needed as well.

Scrimshaw: Possibly it is because health is even lower on the list of priorities than food. There has been some recent effort towards a health consortium comparable to the CGIAR system, and UNDP has been supportive, but there are some formidable obstacles.

Nygaard: To play the role of devil's advocate and ask my favorite question: If we had $5 for research we would probably give one dollar to the nutritionist, one to the social scientist, one to the breeder, one to the agronomist, and....

Somel: One to administration!

Nygaard: Yes, at least one to administration. My question is, if we only had one dollar and we could not split it up, what would we do with it? I assume that we follow the advice of Somel and spend it on socioeconomic research.

Scrimshaw: Who wishes to respond?

Williams: I think we ought to spend it on postharvest technology.

Gerhart: I would not dare respond to that. I would like to question the figure Somel quoted from the FAO survey about the enormous cost to achieve a high level of nutrition. To reduce the incidence of undernutrition to very low levels, say 1 percent of the population, it would take an economic growth rate of over 10 percent annually to the year 2000. I wonder if the FAO figure is not based on an estimate of reducing malnutrition by increasing income alone, and whether or not that cost could be substantially reduced with targeting projects to special groups. It is totally unrealistic to achieve a 10 percent growth rate in the developing countries for the remainder of this century, but I do not think it is unrealistic to think about virtually eliminating malnutrition in developing countries.

Scrimshaw: I think we have to remember that China has largely eliminated clinical malnutrition and hunger with a per capita availability of food less than that in India.

Somel: There is a paper I have not been allowed to quote because it is still in draft form that addresses this issue. It does say that unless other measures --not only in the field of nutrition such as targeting, but also other technical and socioeconomic policies -- are taken this is the growth rate that will be required. You are right in saying that, by itself, growth will not reduce problems that are based on inequitable income distribution, but will only increase it.

Ali: We always throw the ball back to the policymakers, who are human beings like us. The only way to convince the policymaker it to show him something of a practical nature. In this workshop all of us are saying that research findings are quite different from the findings of the farmers. There is a big difference between the research level and practical level. If we can bridge that gap, not only in the field of production, but also in the fields of technology and nutrition, then we can change the minds of these policymakers.

Nahal: I totally agree with Somel that the term "green evolution" is the term that we should use because it is well adapted to the situation. What we really need is to maintain the stability and the productivity of the ecosystem that we are managing and exploiting. In fact, the green revolution in arid and semi-arid zones, particularly in the developing countries, has not always been successful with respect to its effect on the environment and on the productivity of these lands in the long term. This is because of the special characteristics of these ecosystems, which are fragile and should be approached carefully. For this reason, adapted technology should be used. Take as an example the irrigated areas in the Third World. We find that there have been adverse consequences of the green revolution. The reason is that these ecosystems have evolved very slowly and they have reached their stability and equilibrium in arid conditions. When we add water we are disturbing all these interrelationships between the different components -- physical components or biological components and micro or macro components. To manage these very costly irrigated projects, research should be of an interdisciplinary nature and should be oriented to adapted technology. This technology should be in harmony with the characteristics of these special ecosystems. I think that we have the possibility in the region to cooperate with the national, regional, and international research centres and find the right technology for this kind of ecosystem.

Scrimshaw: I would like to ask Bressani why the green revolution appears to have had so much less impact on Central America than on Mexico, and whether there may be some parallels with its applicability to this region?

Bressani: To me the green revolution means that by using the appropriate kind of technology we are really able to increase yield. This should not be surprising because in countries like Canada, the U.S., and some others, they have had a green revolution for the last 40 to 50 years. The problem that arises in our countries in Latin America is that we do not seem to have an integrated system of using the outputs of the things produced. We do not try to diversify the uses of what we are producing. We produce a lot of some things but we have ignored others, and we have not been able to integrate the system to achieve equilibrium.

In some of the Latin American countries, for example, the production of food legumes during the last 10 years has been decreasing and we have had to import high amounts. One of the reasons we have not been able to produce more is that we have not been able to develop the infrastructure that is needed. In Nicaragua large amounts of land are being used for bean production with the latest technology, fertilizer, irrigation, harvesting by mechanization, etc., but they do not know what they are going to do with the grain and they do not build the facilities to store it. To summarize, I think we need to integrate the whole system if we want to be more successful.

Singh: I am very glad that the social scientists are making a strong attempt to analyze the green revolution. I am also glad they encourage it rather than discourage it. I would like to point out that the green revolution has not been brought to all the crops nor to all areas. In general, it has been confined, particularly in the developing world, to wheat and rice and to areas that are irrigated. I can quote an example from India. In Punjab State where irrigation facilities are available, the average productivity of wheat and rice almost doubled, whereas in some parts of Bihar and Orissa where irrigation facilities are completely lacking or in short supply, few effects of the green revolution can be observed. Thus the effects have been very much localized. Wherever the facilities were available and the government encouraged loans for the purchase of fertilizer and other things, productivity went up.

Somel mentioned that poor people have not benefited from the green revolution. I do not agree with him. I do not have any facts, or a paper to quote from, but I would like to mention that the average life expectancy in India in 1950/51 was 21 years and now it is 60 years. How has this been achieved? Although there have been some improvements in medical facilities, in the last thirty years the total grain production in India increased from 34 million tons to 135 million, by three times. Meanwhile the population increased by only 75 percent. In 1950/51 we were importing food grains on the order of 10 to 12 million tons, and in 1981 India imported only two and a half million tons of food grain. I would say again that the benefits of the green revolution have not been equally distributed, but it would be wrong to say that poorer people have not benefited.

Wages are another example. In Punjab State the wages are almost two and a half times greater than in Orissa State. Most probably this is the effect of the green revolution. Farmers are able to produce more, and they are willing to pay more because they are in need of labour. Where is the imbalance? The imbalance in the green revolution is that certain crops were improved and the farmers grew more because they saw a clear benefit from doing so. For other crops where a breakthrough was not achieved, for example, food legumes, productivity has not risen up. In Session IV, I mentioned that productivity or yield in chickpeas has increased by 24 percent, but the overall production in the last 30 years in the world has not changed, whereas the effect of the green revolution on wheat and rice caused both total production and productivity to increase. Therefore an attempt should be made to achieve that breakthrough in food legumes and other crops that are not part of the green revolution.

In Nygaard's question of where the one dollar should be spent, I would like to suggest that is should be spent for increased productivity on those crops that up to now have been ignored.

Scrimshaw: I would like to suggest that we are in the process of moving from a concern for the inequalities in distribution of food and a variety of other resources between the nations of the North and the nations of the South, to a concern about the inequality of distribution among developing nations, and further, to concern with the inequalities of distribution among regions within nations. Eventually we will move into a phase where the unit of our concern will be the inequality of food availability among households. A nutritionist's concern then becomes the distribution of that food within the household and particularly for the vulnerable groups.

Salameh: I have a question on the origin of the term green revolution. If it came from a developed country, and I think it did, there are many revolutions rather than only one and we have to have many terms. We do not need the term green revolution if it developed in a developed country. But if it came from a developing country, we need this term and we need to find out who gained and who lost by these changes.

Amir: I am confused by the terminology we are using; terms like green revolution and evolution. To me, the green revolution is turning the desert green rather than changing or increasing the yield on a particular piece of land. We are trying to expand our irrigated areas into the desert and there is much more effort going into this. For the latter category, I would use acclimatization, so evolution is probably a better term than revolution.

It was mentioned that in Egypt we mix fenugreek and lentils with wheat to make bread. We used to grow enough lentils in Egypt, and to export them. Now however, we are importing them and I do not think that they are used in the rural areas anymore. So where is the evolution in producing more lentils?

Somel started his speech with some optimism but ended on a note of pessimism. He stated that the increases in production have not only satisfied the minumum requirements but also the affluent requirements. What region is he talking about? Is this at the level of the developed countries or at the level of the whole world? One could use average figures for the world and speak of enough food, even though one cannot really say that we have satisfied the requirements of everyone. Therefore, I think one has to look particularly at the places where help is needed.

Next comes the question of imports. We have talked of importing "junk food" although the word junk also has different interpretations. When I was in Saudi Arabia I found something that looks like rice and tastes like rice when you cook it, but it states on the package that it is artificial rice. It is imported from the U.S. and I would like to know whether this is agricultural production or not. Did the plant breeders ever play a role? In the case of wheat, Egyptians do not like to eat dark bread and that is why we accept a lower level of extraction, about 70 to 75 percent. If we had wheat with a whiter colour we could have 90 to 95 percent extraction and then have the benefit of micro nutrients that are now lost in milling. I would be grateful to have a loaf of that kind.

Parpia: To address the point raised by Amir, it is possible to develop composite flours using those raw materials that provide higher nutrition and are easier to grow. The technology developed at Mysore that was later used in Brazil and Indonesia, to make the "rice" Amir referred to, used tapioca flour, ground nut flour, and wheat which were then shaped. Proper vitamins and minerals can be added to it in order to make a very nutritious product. Therefore, technology can contribute to increasing the availability of food from various resources.

Alderman: What is the price of that mixture? Is it cheaper than rice itself?

Parpia: No, it was about the same price.

Somel: I doubt that these would be available to the rural poor, but rather would be directed to the urban poor.

Parpia: If it adds to the food supply and urban people need less of other grains, there is more available for the rural poor, too.

Pinstrup-Andersen: I was fascinated by Williams' point that one of the ICARDA chickpea lines does not taste good. The mere fact that he did not mention the name leads me to believe that it is one of the more promising ones, maybe even the most promising one. Therefore, you have a clear trade-off here between taste and yield. This is pure speculation. The point I want to make here is that, since one of the objectives of this workshop is to identify research priorities, here is an area that has priorities for multiple breeding objectives. We know virtually nothing about how decisions are made under such circumstances. Is there a screening system such that a high-yielding chickpea variety would never be released unless it tasted good? How does this whole system work? When we add nutrition we add three or four other breeding goals. How does decision-making operate in this area? I propose that this would be a very fruitful area for research if it is done in such a way that social scientists do not evaluate biological sciences but let it remain a multidisciplinary effort.

Williams: First I would like to respond to Amir's comments. It is possible in the villages of Egypt that they reach nearly 100 percent milling extraction rates. They mill in stone mills in which wheat goes in at the top and comes out the bottom, and that is what they eat. Of course, if you use white wheat, the bread is whiter. ICARDA is trying to produce a lighter coloured triticale and lighter coloured bread wheat because it is more acceptable. Of course, if people get hungry enough the colour is not too important. The flavour is important and the texture is, the colour less so. In Egypt they also eat barley bread in the cities, and that is quite dark. It is made from 87 percent extraction flour. The reason why it is not available all over Cairo is that they simply cannot make enough of it. They do not have the technolgoy to automate the processing of barley. For example, barley bakers in Cairo divide the dough by hand, which is a lot of work. On the other hand, they have automated the processing of two-layered shami-type breads that are very much like Syrian bread. The technology of baking is to produce food for large populations, and automation is essential.

Pinstrup-Andersen asked about decisions and breeding goals. Usually the breeder discusses what to do with the food technologist who does the work. In the case of this particular chickpea it was not the taste, it was the texture. The taste was fine. However, if you have two types of bread, one is like leather and the other one soft, you are not going to eat the one like leather. In the case of this chickpea my advice to the breeder is to go ahead because the increase in yield was so far above the normal material that the small difference in texture certainly was not significant. In another example, we found that changing the agronomic practices resulted in a considerable decrease in protein but dramatic increase in yield. My advice would be exactly the same, because the production of protein per hectare increased by about 40 percent.

Nygaard: Williams, you still have not told us the name of that chickpea variety!

SECTION VI

POSTHARVEST PROCESSING AND PROBLEMS

REDUCTION OF POSTHARVEST FOOD LOSSES

HUSAIN A.B. PARPIA AND S.K. MAJUMDER

INTRODUCTION

It has been increasingly recognized that most problems, especially those concerned with food and nutrition, are interdisciplinary, but what needs to be stressed even more is that a multidisciplinary approach is needed to find meaningful solutions. The causes of hunger, poverty, and malnutrition are very complex and need to be understood not only in relation to the natural sciences involved, but also the socioeconomic problems of each country and each region. Study of these issues should involve the decision maker at government and planning levels, the scientists and the implementers. Once the problem is made halfway clear to all those concerned with finding the solution, a meaningful attempt can be made to mobilize the available resources in men, materials, institutions, and finances to find lasting solutions that would make a real impact. This approach will help to strengthen the capabilities to increase self-reliance in research, training, and transfer of technologies.

Recognizing the limitations, especially of human and institutional resources in developing countries, the effort of the United Nations University is to build them with attention to the creation of inter-institutional networks where the required disciplines can be mobilized in a cooperative effort, at the same time involving scientists, policymakers, and those who will use the results. Such an effort avoids unnecessary duplication and maximizes use of competence and resources. In the context of this approach, the subject of postharvest-technology needs to be examined in relation to agriculture, nutrition, and other related disciplines.

The present world population of 4,300 million is expected to exceed 6,000 million by the year 2000. The challenges for the twenty-first century to feed mankind and improve the quality of life will be of a much larger magnitude and will require a qualitatively different approach. The current forecast of 1,400 million tons of cereal production will have to be doubled by 1990 and doubled again by the turn of the century (1). This amount of food will be very difficult to achieve through increased production alone. Other means, in which prevention of postharvest losses is very important, deserve a great deal more attention than they have received.

Although nearly two-thirds of the human population live in the developing countries, they share barely 15 percent of the world's income; income disparities within these countries are also large. In 40 developing countries for which data were available, the upper 20 percent of the population received 55 percent of the benefit from the rise in national income, while the lowest 20 percent received only 5 percent (2). As these income groups became larger, starvation increased. Without reducing poverty, hunger and malnutrition cannot be eliminated. Increasing agricultural production alone does not seem possible in many developing countries and obviously presents many problems. These countries use barely 15 to 20 percent of the world supply of chemical fertilizers (1). In many of them fewer than 20 percent of the farmers are able to buy fertilizers, and an even smaller number can afford pesticides. These countries will not be able to purchase large amounts of fertilizers, not only because of the shortage of foreign exchange, but because of the high costs. If the Western pattern of fertilizer use were introduced, such as that in the USA where 300 litres of crude petroleum are used to produce one acre of corn (3), the cost of food in developing countries would become so high (4) that it would be out of reach for a large portion of the population. Therefore, a totally different approach will be needed, scientifically, socially, and economically.

It is paradoxical that densely populated parts of the world, such as Japan, West Germany, and the United Kingdom, do not suffer from very severe deficiencies, whereas several countries in Africa, Latin America, and the Near East with a low population density-to-land ratio are short of food (5). The factors that have prevented increased land cultivation and greater production to the extent desired are many and need careful analysis if the Near East region is to become self-reliant.

The estimates of postharvest losses vary greatly (6), and very few systematic assessments have been made. The criteria and the methods of assessment used differ and should be standardized in order to obtain comparable figures. In many cases, for political and other reasons, governments are hesitant to provide data even when they are available. However, the obvious need not be proved in order to take action. Present information concerning postharvest losses using limited data and intelligent estimates more than adequately justifies action to prevent these losses. The results of prevention would be substantial. It may, however, be emphasized that even intelligent estimates for the Middle East are lacking, except perhaps for Sudan.

Instead of discussing losses in all different types of food an effort has been made in this paper to give greater attention to cereals and legumes as they provide the largest portion of calories, proteins and other nutrients to most of the human beings on earth. If the current food grain production is to be doubled by 1990 it will yield a total of about 280,000 million tons. Even if the preventable loss figure at this level of production is assumed to be as low as 10 percent, this would mean adding 28,000 million tons to world food supplies. Although prices of different creals vary and legume prices are quite high, based on the assumption that the average price would be $300 per metric ton, the cost of losses would be nearly $8,400,000 million. This justifies an annual investment of at least 1 percent of this amount for research, development, training, technology assessment and transfer over the next ten years.

World production is nearly three times above the requirement for primary foods in terms of calories, but consumption patterns vary, as illustrated by two examples from Borgstron (7) shown in Tables 1 and 2. In the developing countries the consumption of cereals in 1970 averaged 170 kg per capita, almost all of which was consumed directly. In countries like Canada and the US, the annual per capita cereal consumption was about 1,000 kg per capita, of which barely 70 kg was consumed directly. The 374 million tons of grain used by these countries to feed livestock in 1969-71 was greater than the total requirement for food grain to feed the population of India and China combined. If the food losses occurring at various stages (Table 3) can be prevented through the development and/or use of improved technologies, it should be possible to increase the food supplies by 10 percent at least. The shortage of food in many deficit countries is only about 4 to 6 percent. Some estimates of losses in different countries are given in Table 4 and further estimates have been made by FAO (8).

Insects and rodents not only physically consume materials from the crops and reduce the weight of the edible and commercially useful components, but also inflict qualitative losses through degradation, which encourages further biodeterioration by moulds and mites. All this reduces the hygienic quality of the food grain and lowers the nutritive value. A list of common pests in rural and urban areas in tropical countries is given in Table 5 (9,10).

The adoption of plant protection measures, in addition to providing immediate economic benefit, ensures optimum returns on other inputs like seeds, fertilizers, and efforts at improved cultivation. These measures also ensure protection of the crop against the risks of irretrievable damage from any unpredictable pest out-breaks. Optimum benefits can be obtained when the three essential inputs, improved seeds, adequate irrigation, and optimum quantity of fertilizers, are employed in proper sequence. If plant protection measures are inadequate, the yield potential created by these inputs cannot be fully realized, resulting in high production costs. Pest control measure have become absolutely essential, especially because the high-yielding varieties are more susceptible to pests.

Food losses occur in the field, as well as during the total postharvest system. The sequence of organisms inflicting injury to the growing crop and in the postharvest period of handling, processing, storage, and distribution causes aggregate losses that vary between 20 to 60 percent in many countries of the world. The losses are mainly caused by weeds, insects, moulds, rodents, and other pests. These estimates of losses have already been discussed in great detail in several publications. Some examples are cited (11) in Table 6. In the case of insect infestation, the loss in quality is much greater when the food standards for the assessment of edible quality are applied.

Insects produce uric acid, innoculate fungi and bacteria, and leave fecal matter, cast skin and foul odour in the commodities. Quinones and other harmful substances are produced in the infested products. Many fungi produce harmful metabolites such as mycotoxins (12), of which aflatoxin, islandotoxin, and citrinin are quite common. The toxic effects of fungal and bacterial metabolites, some of which are carcinogens, deserve much greater recognition in order to prevent harm to the consumers (10-12).

As a result of insect infestation (M. Swaminathan, C.F.T.R.I., Mysore, India, personal communication), the protein efficiency ratio of wheat drops from 1.86 to 1.36 in a period of four weeks, and that of grain legumes that serve as protein supplements to cereal diets, from 2.21 to 1.85. The nature of other qualitative damage inflicted upon food grain by various infesting agents as a result of production of different harmful and undesirable metaboltes is given in Table 7.

Infested food grain results in higher losses during subsequent milling and processing. Chickpeas with a kernel damage of 15 percent gave a milling yield during their splitting and dehusking as low as 65 percent compared to 82 percent, when the insect damage to the grain was 2 percent (Table 8) (13). Similarly in the case of groundnuts, insect infestation results in reduction of viability, increase in fatty acids, and lower oil extraction yields.

It is thus clear that the approach of postharvest food and agricultural technology to food losses in the Third World has to be very different from that in the advanced countries. It also becomes obvious that research priorities and personnel traning needs will have to be considerably different in developing countries (14).

At this point, it is worth examining the interrelationship between pre-and post-harvest technologies and some selected areas of postharvest technology that deserve priority and that would make the maximum possible impact on improving food supplies as well as contribute to socioeconomic transformation of predominantly subsistence agricultural economices into mixed agro-industrial economies. Such an approach, besides providing more food, would ensure more balanced and faster economic growth. The technologies to be used must be based on modern science, but they must be socioeconomically viable and appropriate if they are to succeed in achieving the objective of a better quality of life.

INFESTATION CONTROL

Rodent Control. Among the agents responsible for loss of food in the field and during storage, rodents appear to take the largest toll. There has been a considerable amount of discussion on rodent control over the last few years, but the actions taken, especially in the developing countries, have left much to be desired. Their potential for reproduction is enormous. They breed at the age of three to four months and probably continue to breed up to the age of 18 months. The gestation period is 21 to 25 days. The females come into heat about every five days and can breed within a day after giving birth. The young are weaned when three weeks old, very often just prior to the arrival of another litter. A female averages between five to seven litters per year, each containing eight to ten young. However, litters may contain as many as 20 young, and 14 litters per female have been recorded. Many of them die, but in one year, a pair of rodents often produce 60 to 70 offspring that survive to maturity. While breeding "seasons" are evident during some periods of the year, usually 20 to 30 percent of the female rats in a colony are pregnant.

The gestation period of the house mouse is approximately 21 days. An average of five young are born in each of five to eight litters per year. Juveniles are dependent upon the mother for about three weeks and reach maturity in two to three months. Sometimes, two or more females may produce young in the same nest at the same time. It is probable that few wild mice survive more than a year.

It is fortunate that ecological conditions are not wholly suitable for the survival of the entire rodent progeny; otherwise man would have had to fight a major battle against rodents for his survival on earth. With increases in food production, the conditions for the survival of rodents are beginning to be more favourable, but the measures for their control are not improving in the same proportion. On the contrary, natural enemies of rats, such as snakes, have been systematically exterminated by man. Thus, the full benefits of high-yielding crops cannot be realized under present conditions without a sound multinational programme of rodent control.

There are very few scientific surveys on rodent population, but some intelligent estimates based on field studies indicate that between 46 and 78 percent of a crop can be destroyed by rats. This damage can be done at different stages of growth, i.e., freshly sown seed, seedling, half-blade, and during various storage stages. Even in a conservative estimate, India is said to have a rodent population of 2,400 million, and six rats can eat the food supply of one person. Tropical climate conditions are particularly favourable for rodent multiplication, and most of the developing countries are located in the tropics.

An emergency had to be declared on the Island of Mindanao in the Philippines in 1953 when close to 70 percent of the rice crop was destroyed by rodents. Press reports in March 1976 from the Philippines also indicated that heavy losses in the rice crop had been caused by rats. An emergency was declared on the island of Madagascar in 1965, when 80 percent of the crop was destroyed by rodents in that year. In 1975 rodents caused havoc in Senegal. It is quite obvious that there are many places where such damage may have occurred and gone unreported.

Control of rodents in the field can be achieved by the well-known technique of gas fumigation of burrows, combined with the newer method of liquid fumigation. The latter is especially suited for varieties of rats that erect barriers in their burrows. Baiting should also be used simultaneously with rodenticides, such as norbormide, zinc phosphide, or barium carbontate incorporated in a low protein bait. Safe methods for baiting that would avoid harm to children and farm animals under rural conditions in developing countries have been worked out. Physical methods of rodent control such as trapping are also quite successful when applied with skill and knowledge of rodent behaviour. In some rural areas traditional techniques of control are quite ingenious. For effective control, a combination of such methods should be worked out under different circumstances based on a sound knowledge of rodent behaviour and propagation, combined with training of personnel to prevent rodent destruction of food.

With urbanization of rural areas as a result of the growth of cities and towns, the rodent population has migrated to them and is causing greater losses at postharvest stages.

At the postharvest level some measures for control of rodents have proved quite effective. With certain structural improvements, a warehouse can be made rodent-proof. A 10 centimeter-long rat guard skirting the warehouse above ground level successfully prevents rodent entry. This technique has been adopted in the construction of a number of new warehouses and has proved successful. Old warehouses can also be made rat-proof by putting a 15-centimeter polished band of cement on the surface of the wall at a height of about 1.5 to 2 metres around the whole building, and by separating the steps from the main strucutre by 50 centimeters.

In addition to the use of well-accepted techniques of baiting, poisoning, fumigation of burrows, etc., it is possible to make jute bags rodent-repellent by treating them with a composition of chemicals containing malathion in heavy oil. This also makes baiting more effective.

Insect infestation control. Crops are protected against diseases and pest infestations during growth. This involves application of foreign chemicals, the xenobiotics, synthesized by man. During the last three decades, an enormous amount of literature has appeared on the repercussions of chlorinated, phosphatic, carbamate and organo-metal compounds because of their potential effect on the environment and ultimately on human populations. Rachel Carsons' Silent Spring and the interdisciplinary reports of the international and national committees have amply pointed out the possible consequences of overuse and misuse of such chemicals, particularly the residue type, and also of compounds that undergo potentiation and form terminal residues of higher persistence and toxicity than the parent substances. These terminal residues find access to both fresh and processed foods. The "pesticide cycle" is indicative of the distribution of the substances in our environment even when they are not directly applied to food crops. Thus, there is a possibility of migration of such pollutants to areas where they are not used.

Similarly, the products elaborated by insects and microorganisms in the preharvest period may subsequently find access to the harvested product. Mycotoxins such as the aflatoxins, islandotoxins, citrinin, ochratoxin, gibberalin, etc, are some examples of the saprophytic or semi-saprophytic and parasitic organisms that cause the problem of contamination of produce harvested for fresh consumption or for use as raw materials for the food processing industry.

Low-quality infected or infested materials are often fed to animals without consideration of the possibilities for ingestion by man via these animal food products.

Pre-harvest infestation by insects and fungis is common in the tropical and subtropical belts, and their problems differ from those in the developed, temperate areas of the world. In tropical developing countries, the small size of landholdings and the various socioeconomic systems do not allow mechanization, such as the use of combine harvesters and mechanical driers. Therefore, before harvest, grain crops are left on the panicles and allowed to be conditioned for hand-harvesting with sickles. In manually operated agricultural systems, the problem of pre-harvest field infestation is quite common. Groundnuts present a peculiar problem even where the climate is dry because the population of soil arthropods is abundant. Under high irrigation, many of the dry-soil arthropods cannot survive, but the loose, dry soils of the sub-Saharan areas, the millipedes, centipedes, termites, and many other soil insects survive very well and attack the crops during growth. These examples are directly related to the pre-harvest agricultural practices affecting the postharvest quality of food.

The drying method used has a critical influence on the postharvest storage characteristics of harvested grain. Every grain attains equilibrium with the humidity of the atmosphere. The equilibrium moisture content may give rise to free moisture content within the kernel, especially with diurnal fluctuation of temperatures. This moisture can support the growth of both fungi and insects. The technology available for moisture control, the drying system, and related processes differ from area to area, depending on the traditional agricultural practices and the system for handling harvested grain. A mechanized, large farm with combine harvesting facilities uses mechanical handling and bulk transport systems. Each step is dovetailed to the next and geared to large-scale operation methods. The intake of bulk-harvested grain from the field and the reduction of moisture to a safe level before filling silos fits into the system of unit operations and their capacities.

In contrast with this silo-cum-elevator storage system, the small holdings in many developing countries require the development of drying methods and storage structures compatible with the harvesting equipment and the speed of operations. Individual farm-oriented storage stuctures have to be designed according to the size of the harvest, the marketing and distribution system, and the local purchasing capacity. Usually, subsistence-level farm structures are built with local agricultural materials -- straw, bamboo, timber, mud (clay), bricks, or tiles. The holding capacity of such strucutres does not normally exceed two tons. With an agricultural holding of about 2.5 hectares, an individual farm would not need a storage structure of more than 5-ton capacity. It should be built to have the stability and strength for holding such quantities. Apart from the size of the structure, the availability of energy input of animal and human power will determine the handling system. The technologies for aeration of grain, loading and unloading, and disinfestation operations have to be compatible with the available tools and resources.

It is estimated that the cost of these structures, if kept within 10 percent of the value of the produce, can provide a favorable cost-benefit ratio. Since the sturcture in itself cannot prevent internal infestation, appropriate prophylactic measures suitable for use by a small farmer, have to be developed and used to ensure good-quality produce for the market and wholesome raw materials for food industries. Here linkage with the pre-harvest condition will determine the design of the structure as well as the size of milling and processing equipment for postharvest use.

In developing countries, the agricultural systems should include hygienic practices for preventing field oviposition by stored-product insects and infection by fungi. For this purpose a suitable measure for pre-harvest prophylaxis has been proposed. Such prophylactic treatment by malathion and fungicidal sprays like captan or similar products can produce clean grains, free from internal infestation, and safe for storage in farm containers. Pre-harvest prophylaxis in conjunction with insect and rodent-proofing of containers such as burlap bags, high density polyethylene bags, hessian and laminates, including straw bags, can be employed for preventing cross-infestation during subsequent handling and storage.

Another prophylactic method that has proved effective is use of liquid fumigants possessing ovicidal properties. However, not many are available. The best known are chloropicrin, ethylene dibromide, methyl iodide, ethyl formate, and methyl bromide. Inorganic fumigants such as sulphur dioxide, chlorine, ammonia, and phosphine are not ovicidal. Under temperate storage conditions these non-ovicidal fumigants are satisfactory, as the climate itself is effective in inhibiting insect life cycle and delaying damage.

In order to cope with fluctuations in food grain production, the state and central (federal) food departments have to plan for procurement, storage, processing, and distribution. These agencies cannot use small unit structures for storage of food grains, but need larger ones for holding the stock for distribution and also as buffer stock for food security purposes. Operational requirement and the economical limits of these large-scale storage structures have been described by Majumder (15).

CONSERVATION PROCESS COMPATIBLE WITH SIZE AND TYPE OF PROCESSING INDUSTRY

Low temperature itself in the temperate climate acts as a preservative for harvested produce, while in tropical belts, the life cycle and survival of insects and moulds with higher reproductive potentials throughout the year confront the producer with a greater challenge to protect food commodities. In the vast Asian region the losses might be lower than in other regions because the climate is dry in most of these countries.

In European countries and North America, raw grains and their primary milled products find little place in day-to-day cooking in average households. The system of postharvest processing and handling is mostly linked in these countires with centralized, large-scale milling and processing and super-market distribution systems. The flour mills and bakeries are part and parcel of the integral system of producing bread or confectionaries. Storage and sanitation measures under these production systems are based on elevator, hopper, pneumatic conveyors, cleaning, conditioning, packaging, fumigation, aeration systems, and related unit operations as an organized industry.

The utilization of wheat, particularly whole wheat flour, for traditional breads such as chapaties, kisara, or other preparations such as couscous are more oriented towards obtaining raw, clean wheat and subjecting it to custom milling as and when required. In the rural areas, custom milling is a cottage scale or an individual family-oriented operation. Similarly, rice mills, oil mills, legume mills follow the same pattern. In rural areas of some developing countries and in growing urban centres there is a possibility of developing cooperative milling for 100 to 500 households in a centre. Appropriate technologies to suit the scale of operations for using the raw materials from a group of villages for rural industrial processing need to be developed more systematically. The success of such efforts has already been demonstrated where appropriate technologies have been devleoped along with the required entrepreneurship.

The major food processing industries (dairy, fruit, vegetable, meat and fish) manufacturing such products as baby foods, breakfast foods, weaning foods, and enriched foods that operate primarily in developed countries in temperate zones have few of the problems encountered in the tropics. Many of the typical problems under tropical conditions occassioned by infestations of *Tribolium castaneum* in milk powder, *Ephestia cautella* in corn flakes, *Calossobruchus chinensis* in dehydrated peas, and *Tribolium castaneum* and *Oryzaephilus surinamensis* in special food supplements are some examples. Corn flakes, noodles, and the many pasta goods are not free from attack by insects. In the dairy industry, particularly in milk-processing plants, flies, roaches, termites, woodborers and bandicoots invade the installations. Unless the plants are specially designed, pest activities expose the products to unhygienic conditions and losses. Similarly, fruit and vegetable processing plants are invaded by *Drosophila*, common flies, roaches and rats. The standard of sanitaion required and the design of the building, waste disposal, and disposal of effluents are problems in tropical countries that pose difficulties of a different order.

The choice of pre- and post-harvest equipment and machinery for handling and processing systems, the unit operations involved, and the size and speed of operations have to be adjusted to an appropriate balance in terms of input and output of materials and energies. Modernization in the developing countries in the tropics has, therefore, to be based on pre-harvest technologies using efficient energy inputs together with optimum postharvest low-energy handling, conservation, and processing.

Nutritional problems, particularly protein-calorie malnutrition, vitamin-A and iodine deficiencies, nutritional anemia, and related diseases are widespread in most developing countries. In this context, the role of food protection combined with productivity of agricultural crops should not be underestimated. It is known that malnutrition is the result of a combination of different factors, foremost of which are inadequate production, inadequate availability of food, and low income levels. Therefore, any applied nutrition program must be backed by optimum productivity of the soil and postharvest conservation and alternative income generation. The combined effects of these developments will provide sufficient calories, protein, and food supplements for maintenance of health and to ensure socioeconomic growth for the benefit of all sections of the population. In the world today, several organizations have recognized the potential for prevention of food losses as a measure towards achieving adequate food supplies and minimizing nutrient losses in foods. FAO in particular initiated an effective program for prevention of food losses in 1978.

A more appropriate system that includes technical cooperation among developing countries in the tropics in particular will have to be developed on the basis of appropriate technologies for pre-harvest production and protection, with equal attention to postharvest and conservation processes. Modernization in the developing countries in the tropics will, therefore, have to be based on developing traditional technology into modern scientific technology, adaptation of other available technolgies, and development of entirely new, adaptable, and economical technologies through sound programs of national research. In this effort, attention must be given to overall energy balance.

APPROPRIATE TECHNOLOGIES FOR TROPICAL REGIONS

In the tropics and subtropics, where most of the developing countries are, the present state-of-the-art techniques of postharvest food production systems that are capital- and energy-intensive cannot be adopted. They are culturally incompatible and do not generate employment. The scale and types of most Western postharvest technologies for conservation, processing, packaging, distribution, and utilization of cereals, pulses, oilseeds, bakery and dairy products, fruit and vegetable raw materials, and processed food products are such that they cannot be absorbed without adaptation and modification. This will also require creation of human capabilities, institutional capacities, and a suitable research and development infrastructure appropriate to the needs. Many of the processes, products, techniques, and systems for adoption in tropical and subtropical areas have been described by Hall (16).

IMPROVEMENTS IN PROCESSING TECHNOLOGY OF FOOD GRAINS

Processing rice. Most developing countries use obsolete and ill-maintained rice milling equipment. A large number of mills are so small that they cannot produce sufficient quantities of bran and husk to be utilized efficiently to manufacture byproducts. Table 9, based on studies in India, shows that it should be possible to raise the milling yield by 1.5 to 5 percent. If the rice-milling industry can be modernized, even at the present level of rice production, rice-consuming countries should be able to overcome almost half of their rice shortage.

Developing countries are often very short of fats and oils as well as cattle feed, for which rice bran is an excellent potential source. It is important that rice bran be utilized soon after milling in order to prevent the development of hydrolytic rancidity. If the rice mills are large enough, or if several of them could be grouped together in an industrial estate, it should be possible to obtain at least 10 tons of bran per day and utilize it rapidly and economically for solvent extraction of the oil. Wherever a number of small mills are located at longer distances from the solvent extraction plants, it would be necessary to inactivate the lipase by suitable treatments that are now available. This would help to increase the supply of high-quality fat for human consumption. At present, populations in developing countries of Asia consume barely 15 to 18 grams of fat per capita, which is probably less than half the desirable levels. Furthermore, the extracted rice bran containing about 15 percent protein could be used for the manufacture of composite animal feed and ultimately result in the supply of additional food for human consumption. With the heavy pressure of population on land, agricultural byproducts are of great value for production of animal foods for people in developing countries. A well organized rice milling industry could also result in development of other allied industries, such as manufacture of activated carbon from the husk and also of hard board, both of which are required today in sufficiently large quantities to justify development of such industries.

Over 50 percent of nearly 50 million tons of rice produced in India and almost the entire rice production of Bangladesh is consumed in parboiled form. The traditional process consists of soaking paddy for two to three days followed by steaming, drying, and milling. This has the advantage of fixing the vitamins present in the peripheral bran layers into the kernel. The traditional practice, however, has several disadvantages in that the product develops off-odour due to microbial fermentation, and fungal contamination results in production of mycotoxins. While there are several sophisticated processes for parboiling in existence, a simpler process has been developed that consists of soaking paddy at 70°C for four to five hours, steaming, and mechanical drying. This not only speeds the entire process, but yields a product of high quality. If larger quantities of rice were to be parboiled in the world, it would not only improve the nutritional quality of the diet through making more vitamin B available in the rice, but also reduce considerably the breakage during milling.

The modern simplified technique of parboiling eliminates the need for sun-drying, wherein dehydration is not uniform, and losses to birds are quite heavy.

In fact, improved parboiling gives a somewhat higher yield that covers the additional cost involved.

Processing of grain legumes. Grain legumes are the second largest source of protein in many developing countries of the world. Rich in lysine, they provide a valuable supplement to the cereal diet. The traditional milling (dehusking and splitting) techniques frequently result in losses due to breakage and powdering. An improved process has now been developed that involves conditioning the skin for its easy removal and employs the pearling technique to prevent breakage. Table 10 shows the improvement in milling yields of various legumes. By adopting this procedure, about a million tons of good quality food could be added to the food supplies of India alone.

Milling of wheat. Wheat production, although the largest among world cereal crops, is mainly confined to more temperate climates. Production and consumption of wheat in the developing countries is, however, increasing. Because of urbanization, the use of bread is becoming quite widespread. For the most economical use of wheat, it is desirable that the milling of flour be restricted to about 85 percent extraction, as was done in the United Kingdom during World War II. This flour is also more nutritious. In fact, in many developing countries such flour is more suitable for making traditional products.

FISH CONSERVATION

A large proportion of fish caught in the world is used in animal feed production. Every effort needs to be made to use a larger proportion of this protein-rich resource for direct human consumption. Considering the limitations under which developing countries have to work, appropriate technologies that can make small-scale operations economically feasible have been developed. An insulated reusable basket made of traditional materials proved successful in packaging and distributing fish along the western coast of India. In this basket iced fish can be distributed on bicycles over a radius of 40 kilometers. This has nearly tripled the distribution radius. The basket can also be transported as far as 400 kilometers on top of buses that travel to internal markets.

Improvements have been made in traditional techniques for sun-drying. After proper cleaning and treatment with sorbic acid, the shelf-life of dried fish has increased from three to nine months. Such products also have good markets in several countries of Southeast Asia and offer export potential.

TECHNOLOGY TRANSFER

Developing countries urgently need to make proper use of appropriate technologies to build food and agricultural product processing industries. For this they must develop their capabilities to build a national institutional infrastructure for the purpose. Such efforts must be combined with the development of sound management and competence in plant operation, marketing, and finance utilization. Without proper use of all these skills in balanced form, it is very difficult to build a successful enterprise. An important prerequisite for this is the formulation of an enlightened policy that would stimulate agro-economic development. This is a joint responsibility of the government, entrepreneurs, and technologists. It calls for laying down priorities in terms of the social and economic benefit to be derived through the use of limited resources to produce results of maximum value.

An institutional framework needs to be built that can identify problems and help overcome constraints to the developmnt of agro-industries. Programmes of action should be formulated and implemented within time targets according to priorities. This would help to optimize use of national resources and international and bilateral assistance. A system of technology selection to meet the requirements of agro-industrial development is a vital component of this effort. Transplanting inappropriate technologies obtained on unfavourable terms can have a negative effect on development and impede future progress. A number of costly mistakes of this type have been made that could have been avoided by many developing countries had a proper policy been formulated to build necessary infrastructure and achieve competence for assessment and transfer of technology. The experience of the less developed among the advanced countries and of the more developed among the developing countries who have made the transformation, or are in the process of doing so, could be of particular value. For example, countires like Ireland, Yugoslavia, Mexico, India, Egypt and Nigeria may be in a special position to assist the Third World.

RESEARCH AND DEVELOPMENT

Nearly 95 percent of research and development expenditure in the world takes place in advanced countries and is essentially geared to developing know-how suitable for their own needs. The small- and medium-scale technologies that were used by the industrialized countries during the last century or in the early part of the present century have become obsolete. A large proportion of the modern, capital-intensive and high-energy technologies available are not appropriate for the developing countries in many areas of food conservation and processing because their needs are different. Thus, modern appropriate technologies have to be developed that will help to build economically sound, employment-generating, capital-saving conservation and processing industries.

One of the largest energy resources available to the developing countries, especially in rural areas, is human energy. Therefore, other sources of physical energy to be employed in industrial development should be reduced to the minimum, keeping in view product quality and economy. it is essential to set up research and development organizations in the area of food science, technology and nutrition in the developing countries and to strengthen the existing ones. Their main objectives should be to:

1. Select and identify the most appropriate technologies from advanced and developing countries that would meet, to the largest possible extent, the social requirements for the development of food and agricultural product conservation and processing industries. These could be purchased or obtained on suitable terms for setting up industries and also used as the starting point for further technological development. Terms of technology transfer that would keep the know-how secret or "captive" should be avoided as far as possible.

2. Build adequate competence so as to test, modify, and adapt the selected technologies to the needs of conservation and processing industries and to the raw materials available in the country.

3. Undertake technological research based on available scientific knowledge that would help to build new, appropriate technologies.

4. Undertake basic research oriented to improving and upgrading existing technologies.

5. Undertake fundamental research that would provide new technologies within 5 to 10 years after making certain that the available resources can sustain them.

6. Train personnel in the areas of food science, technology and nutrition, plant operation, management and marketing skills required for industry, government departments, and research institutions.

If the above programme is to be successful, scientists and technologists cannot be allowed to remain in isolation from the policymaking machinery of government and industry in either the private or public sector. They must form a part of the top-level national policymaking bodies where the decisions are made. Their involvement would improve the quality of the decisions from the scientific, technological, and other relevant points of view, and would also place responsibility on them for providing the required know-how and advice on its effective utilization.

In advanced countries, research and development institutions came into existnece because industry required them to sustain progress. In developing countries these institutions have another important role, that is, to develop industries. This requires a special effort to establish pilot and prototype plants so as to minimize the risk involved for small and medium entrepreneurs whose resources for covering risks are very limited.

If the postharvest technologies for the Third World have to be different scientifically, socially, and economically from those in the Western world, the training required to identify, develop, and utilize them must also be different. Food technology training in the North has, perhaps, created problems because the education provided is related to the types of packaging, preservation, flavouring, colouring, texture, and mouth-feel problems associated with processing of convenience foods for advanced countries. This results in the creation of the indigenously born "foreigner" who has to undergo a process of reeducation to be useful to developing countries. Brain drain occurs in this process unless utmost care is taken to provide the right kind of training. A major example of an effort in training food scientists and technologists under the right conditions that has made a significant contribution is the FAO International Food Technology Training Centre at the Central Food Technological Research Institute in Mysore. Also, the success achieved at the Institute in applying modern food science and technology to conditions in Asia has been notable. The recent contributions of the United Nations University under its World Hunger Programme have also been valuable.

Training in entrepreneurship should constitute a part of the package of technology transfer. Without sound entrepreneurship, agro-industrial development cannot proceed on firm foundations. In fact, this is the area of major weakness in many developing countries at present. It is not possible for a shopkeeper or a merchant to become an industrial entrepreneur overnight without training and providing him with the appropriate atmosphere and conditions for this purpose. In general, progress in this direction is quite slow, but it could be speeded up through an enlightened policy and action programme to bring about much needed transformation.

Because of limited resources available in the developing countries, establishment of inter-country cooperation among them for technology transfer, research, development, and training at regional or sub-regional levels could be of great value. This type of organization should have close links with national institutions and provide them with every possible assistance to build their own competence. Creation of "banks of technology" at the regional level needs priority consideration. They could collect the required "know-how" that could be supplied on comparatively short notice on request. It must be recognized that scientific and technological self-reliance is a prerequisite for economic self-reliance. The UN agencies, particularly the Food and Agriculture Organization, can play a vital role in developing mechanisms for cooperation among developing countries, building networks of research and development institutions, ensuring greater cooperation of advanced countries, and raising the competence of human resources to stimulate development towards self-reliance. The initiative and responsibility of the developing countries themselves in this effort is the key factor.

SUMMARY AND CONCLUSION

The benefits of developing a postharvest system for handling food on a sound techno-economic foundation in the developing countries would be:

1. Increase and improve food supplies without additional demand on land.
2. Raise nutritional quality of food with consequent improvement in nutritional levels, especially of the low-income population.
3. Increase employment in the conservation and processing industries especially in rural areas, and reduce employment pressure on agriculture.
4. Raise the income level of the producer by ensuring a more stable market, making it possible for him to use greater inputs for increasing production.
5. Stabilize prices and provide food to the consumer at a reasonable price.
6. Ensure better utilization of the storage, milling, processing, and distribution capacities for optimal use of the machinery and the system.
7. Ensure more efficient use of agricultural residue for manufacture of by-products for use as food and feed.
8. Increase foreign exchange earnings and improve balance of trade.
9. Protect the environment by eliminating pollution.
10. Speed up socioeconomic transformation to create more balance between agriculture, industry, and other sectors.
11. Ensure more efficient uses of energy resources in production, conservation, and distribution and harness nonconventional energy resources to increase and improve food supplies.
12. Encourage greater multidisciplinary information exchange and documentation, research and development, education and training, technology assessment and transfer.

REFERENCES

1. Food and Agriculture Organization, Agriculture: Toward 2000, Twentieth Session of the FAO Conference, Rome, 10-29 November, 1979 (FAO, Rome, 1980).

2. R.S. McNamara, Address to the Board of Governors of the World Bank, Nairobi (1973).

3. D. Pimentel, L.E. Hurd, A.C. Bellotti, M.J. Forster, I.N. Oka, O.D. Sholes, and R.J. Whitman, "Food Production and the Energy Crisis," Science 182: 443 (1973).

4. J.S. Steinhart and C.E. Steinhart, "Energy Use in the U.S. Food System," Science 184: 307 (1974).

5. E.P. Eckholm, Losing Ground: Environmental Stress and World Food Prospects (Northern, New York, 1976).

6. H.A.B. Parpia, "Post-Harvest Losses and the Impact of Their Prevention," Biblio. Nutr. Diet. 28: 58 (1979).

7. G. Borgstrom, "The Price of a Tractor," Ceres 7(6): 16 (1974).

8. Food and Agriculture Organization, "An Analysis of an FAO Survey of Post-Harvest Losses in Developing Countries" (AGPP:M1SC27) (FAO, Rome, 1977).

9. C.M. Christensen, ed., Storage of Cereal Grains and Their Products, (Amer. Assoc. Cereal Chem., St. Paul, 1974).

10. S.K. Majumder, "Control of Microflora in Moist Grain," Central Food Technological Research Institute, Mysore (1974).

11. S.K. Majumder and H.A.B. Parpia, "Prevention of Food Losses and Potential," in Symposium on Science and India's Food Problems (NIS, India, 1967).

12. S.K. Majumder, K.S. Narasimhan, and H.A.B. Parpia, "Microecological Factors in the Microbial Spoilage in the Occurrence of Mycotoxins on Stored Grains," in G.N. Wogan, ed., Mycotoxins in Foodstuffs (MIT Press, Cambridge, Massachusetts, 1965).

13. M. Milner, ed., Nutritional Improvement of Food Legumes by Breeding (The Protein Advisory Group of the United Nations, New York, 1973).

14. H.A.B. Parpia, "Food Technology Problems in India and Other Developing Countries," Food Technol. 22: 62 (1968).

15. S.K. Majumder, "Storage in Relation to Tropical Developing Countries," Pesticides Annual 56: 78 (1978).

16. D.W. Hall, "Handling and Storage of Food Grains in Tropical and Sub-Tropical Areas," FAO Agriculture Development Paper No. 90 (FAO, Rome, 1970).

TABLE 1. Primary Calories in Energy Balance Per Caput 1971-72*

	Food Primary Calories per day (PP)	Food Kg CE p.a.	Energy Account Kg CE p.a.	Primary Food Calories as Energy Account
India	2,643	140.6	186	75.6
Mexico	4,372	232.2	1270	18.3
Italy	7,729	411.9	2,682	15.4
U.S.A.	11,886	623.3	11,244	5.5

*Source: Reference 7

TABLE 2. Calories in Food Intake Per Person Per Day (1970)*

	I Total Calories (I+III)	II Plant Calories	III Animal Calories (-fish)	IV Feed Calories	V Total Primary (II+IV)
U.S.A.	3,300	1,869	1,431	10,017	11,886
India	1,990	1,871	109	763	2,634
Difference	1,310				9,252
Mexico	2,614	2,321	293	2,051	4,372
Italy	2,995	2,206	789	5,523	7,729
Difference	381				3,357

*Source: Reference 7

TABLE 3. Estimates of Quantitative Losses During the Handling and Processing of Rice in Southern Asia*

Operation	Range of Losses
Harvesting	1 - 3
Handling	2 - 7
Threshing	2 - 6
Drying	1 - 5
Storing	2 - 6
Milling	2 - 10
	10 - 37

*Source: D.B. DePadua. University of the Philippines at Los Banos, College, Laguna, Philippines, personal communication, 1975, to IDRC, Canada.

TABLE 4. Some Estimates of Losses in Different Countries

Country	Material	LOSS Percentage*	Value
Nigeria	Sorghum	46	-
	Cowpea	41	-
U.S.A.	Stored Grain	-	$500 million
	Packed food	-	$150 million
	All crops	-	$3500 million
India	All crops		
	Field Loss	25	-
	Storage loss	15	-
	Handling and processing loss	7	
	Other losses	3	-
Germany	Harvested grain	-	DM 77.4 million
Sierra Leone	Rice	41	-
	Maize	14	-
Tropical Africa	All crops, Storage and Handling	30	-

* These percentages refer to postharvest losses unless otherwise stated. Although the figures refer to specific crops, they indicate the scale of the problem.

TABLE 5. List of Common Pests in Rural and Urban Stores of the Tropics*

Storage Insects and Mites	Common Storage Fungi	Rodents
Sitophilus oryzae	*Mucor* ssp	*Rattus rattus*
Oryzaephilus surinamensis	*Rhizopus* ssp	*R. norvegicus*
Sitotroga cerealella	*Fusarium* ssp	*Mus musculus*
Rhizopertha dominica	*Alternaria* ssp	*M. booduga*
Trogoderma granarium	*Botrytis* ssp	*Bandicota indica*
Laemophleus minutus	*Ambylosporum* ssp	*B. bangalensis*
Laetheticus oryzae	*Chladosporum* ssp	*Nesokia indica*
Stegobium paniceum	*Scopulariopsis* ssp	
Araecerens fasciculatus	*Aspergillus* ssp	*Milardia meltada*
Lasioderma serricorne	*Penicillum* ssp	*M. gleadowi*
		Tatera indica
Pachymerus chinensis	*Trichothecium* ssp	
Alphitobius rufipes	*Nigrospora* ssp	
Necrobia ssp	*Syncephalastrum* ssp	
Tenebrio molitor	*Curvularia* ssp	
Carpophilus dimidiatus	*Verticillium* ssp	
Tenebroides mauritanicus	*Absidia* ssp	
Tinea granella	*Sporendonema* ssp	
	Stachybotrys ssp	
Ptinus tectus	*Candida* ssp	
Attagenus piceus	*Paeculomyces* ssp	
Typhea stecorea	*Trichoderma* ssp	
Corcyra cephalonica	*Thamnidium* ssp	
Ephestia cautella	*Syncephalastrum* ssp	
	Citromyces ssp	
Plodia interpunctella	*Gibberella* ssp	
	Minilia ssp	
	Cephalosporium ssp	
	Sporotrichum ssp	
Mites:		
Acarus siro		
Tyroglylphus ssp		
Tyrophagus putrescentiae		
Caloglyphusberlesei		
Glycyphagus destructor		
Acaropsis ssp		
Typhlodromus ssp		

*Source: References 9 and 10

TABLE 6. Some Examples of Kernel Damage and Losses in Food Grains*

Commodity	% Kernel Damage	% Weight Loss
Beans	39.5	6
Jowar (sorghum)	34	14
Maize	0	-
	10	2.7
	30	8.2
	70	19.1

*Source: Reference 11

TABLE 7. Qualitative Damage Produced on Food Grains by Infesting Agents

Insect	Mould	Mites
Uric acid	Apparent uric acid	Guanine
Moisture	Moisture	Foul Odour
Exuvae	Discolouration	Allergens
Chitin	Mycotoxins	
Dead Insects	Thermogenesis	Pathogen Vector
Frass	Musty odour	Debris
Killed Germ	Loss of viability	
Microflora		

TABLE 8. Effect of Insect Infestation on the Yield of Dehusking and Splitting Chickpeas*

	% Kernel Damage	% Dhal Yield
Chickpea (uninfested)	2	82
Chickpea (infested by insects)	15	65

*Source: Reference 13

TABLE 9. Average Milling Yields of Rice from Paddy in Conventional and Modern Mills

Types of Mills	Raw		Parboiled	
	Total %	Head %	Total %	Head %
Modern rubber roller	72.5	55	73.5	70
Conventional disc sheller type	71.0	50	73.0	68
Engelberg type "huller"	69.0	45	72.0	66

TABLE 10. Milling Losses of Grain Legumes in India

Legumes	Yield by	
	Traditional Method %	Improved * Method %
Chickpea (*Cicer arietinum*)	75	85
Pigeon Pea (*Cajanus cajan*)	72	87
Green Gram (*Phaseolus radiatus*)	65	85
Black gram (*Phaseolus mungo*)	71	85

* Bench scale results

REGIONAL RESEARCH ON LEGUME PROCESSING AND NUTRITION

RAJA I. TANNOUS*

*Dr. Tannous was not present at the meeting, but the paper was read for him by a member of the ICARDA staff

INTRODUCTION

Food legumes have been recognized as an important contribution to human diets since the beginning of agriculture. However, their importance and use as food has been limited to certain regions of the world. Many countries today use legume species as animal feed only, but the Middle East is an area where grain legumes constitute a very important part of the daily diet, perhaps more so than in any other region of the world. In some countries grain legumes have been referred to as the "Poor Man's Diet". There were some good reasons for that. However, today grain legumes are no longer inexpensive but they constitute one of the most important sources of food nutrients to people in many countries of the world, particularly in this area. Their main nutritional importance is that they are a main source of dietary proteins. Grain legumes are also good sources of the vitamins, thiamin and niacin, and of calcium and iron; but contain little fat, carotene, or ascorbic acid. However, what limits their utilization in human diets are objectionable endogenous factors present in the seeds, namely, antinutritional components, flatulence, poor cooking qualities as well as poor digestibility of some legumes.

The importance of grain legumes in the Middle Eastern diets has thus prompted intensive research in several institutions in the region, notably in Lebanon and Egypt, to evaluate and improve the role of legumes in local diets.

The food legumes that are most important to the Middle Eastern region are faba beans, chickpeas, and lentils. To a lesser extent some varieties of peas and common beans are also consumed, and occasionally lupine and fenugreek are utilized. Legumes are also widely consumed as immature green seeds or as green pods with the immature seeds enclosed. More often the green pods or seeds are cooked to make a stew.

A list of the food legumes that are commonly consumed in the Middle East is given in Table 1. One or another of these food legumes may be consumed daily by many families in the Middle East. During the harvest season, the green seeds of faba beans and chickpea are consumed raw, as a snack. Similarly, lupine seeds are consumed as a condiment, particularly in a very popular Armenian food (Basterma). Peas and common beans are used in a stew with meat and usually consumed with rice.

The most common dishes consumed containing faba beans, chickpeas and lentils are given in Table 2, namely, faba bean dip (foul moudemas), chickpea dip (hommos bitehineh), rice and lentils (mujaddarah) and lentil soup, falafel and common bean stew. Other ingredients and amounts used in each dish are also shown in Table 2. These dishes are very popular. In many countries in the Middle East foul moudemas is frequently consumed for breakfast. In Lebanon, hommos bitehineh is consumed with almost any kind of meal. A falafel sandwich is often eaten in the evening as a supper. At homes, schools and other institutions, mujaddarah and bean stew are common.

STUDIES ON THE NUTRITIONAL QUALITY OF FOOD LEGUMES

Most of the studies reviewed in this section are concerned with dry legume seeds and dishes made from them, but a few studies have been done on the green seeds that are consumed occasionally.

Nutritional Composition of Grain Legumes. Nutritional analysis of food legumes consumed in the region have been reported (2). They are important as a protein source because they contain 20 to 40 percent protein, which is two- to four-fold the average protein content of cereals. The fat content is, however, low except in chickpeas and lupine.

Studies have also been conducted on the developing green chickpea seed (3), and show that the fat content increased until 21 days after flowering, after which time it remained the same. Protein remained unchanged, but changes did occur in important amino acids such as lysine and the sulfur amino acids. Lysine was much higher 14 days after flowering, while sulfur amino acids were higher after 42 days.

Although the protein content of legumes is high, the amino acid composition of their proteins is also of importance, especially in their high content of lysine (2,4) because this amino acid is normally low in cereal based diets. Most dry grain legumes are good sources of thiamine but are poor in carotene and vitamin C. However, green chickpea is relatively high in both vitamins and is also high in iron and other minerals (2).

Nutritional Evaluation of Legume Dishes. Since grain legumes are consumed with other foods, the nutritional value of the composite dishes is of importance and analyses have been reported (2). The nutritional significance of these dishes also lies in the frequency with which they are consumed. For example, foul moudamas or falafel are consumed daily by very large numbers in Egypt and elsewhere. For overall nutritional evaluation, factors such as digestibility, physiological availability of certain nutrients, presence of antinutritional factors, the problem of flatulence, and the effects of processing, all become important. In addition, where legumes provide the major source of protein in the diet, the nutritional quality of the legume protein may become a limiting factor; the protein quality of chickpea is however much higher than that in faba beans or lentils (4,5), so the frequent consumption of chickpea dip may be nutritionally significant.

The supplementation of other protein foods with legumes is of major importance, for example, the consumption of legumes with bread is superior to either one alone. Fortunately, most of these dishes are consumed with bread; and in the case of mujaddarah, lentils are cooked with rice. Following the same reasoning, certain deficiencies in legumes become important and they should be remedied by the inclusion of other food items in the diet that are rich in these nutrients, namely carotene and vitamin C.

The availability of dietary iron in some legume dishes is shown in Table 3 (6,7). Again, not all the iron found in legumes is available to humans. However, in comparison to some other vegetable foods, the availability of iron in these foods seems to be adequate.

Effects of processing on nutritional quality. Uncooked legume seeds contain antinutritional factors that can be toxic if large amounts are consumed, (5,8). Table 4 shows only hemaglutinating and antitrypsin activities, although there are other factors that may as well be responsible for the mortality of animals fed uncooked beans. However, proper cooking of the seeds renders them safe for consumption. In a recent study (9) on the effects of fermentation on toxic factors in legumes, it was observed that this process could reduce the hemaglutinating factor in faba beans and the antitrypsin factor in chickpeas.

It was demonstrated in some of our studies many years ago that the cooking of legume seeds also has an effect on their protein quality. The data indicated that chickpea was superior in protein quality to faba bean and lentils and that cooking improved the protein quality, but severe cooking did not improve their quality further. It was also observed that autoclaving legume seeds had no effect on amino acid content of lentils or chickpeas (5,8).

Utilization of grain legume flours as supplements. Because grain legumes are a good source of dietary proteins, flour prepared from legumes is a useful protein supplement to other local foods to improve their protein quantity and quality.

Several investigations were carried out at the American University of Beirut (10,15), where grain legumes were utilized as protein supplements in weaning food mixtures, Arabic bread, biscuits, and other foods. In these investigations, protein isolates and concentrates were also prepared from these legumes for use as supplements (16,17).

The general conclusion drawn from these investigations is that legume flours can be used in limited amounts to improve the protein quality of local foods without seriously affecting their taste, acceptability, or other quality factors.

PROCESSING AND COOKING QUALITY OF FOOD LEGUMES

Regional research in this area has been limited to the cooking quality of faba beans (University of Alexandria, Egypt) and lentils (American University of Beirut).

Normally, dry legume seeds require a long time to cook. Seeds of faba beans, chickpeas, common beans, and, to a lesser extent, lentils are soaked in water overnight before they are cooked. Sometimes small amounts of sodium bicarbonate ($NaHCO_3$) are added to chickpea and faba beans to reduce their cooking time.

The cooking process softens the hard seed by improving the plasticity of the cell wall, thus facilitating cell expansion and reduction of intercellular adhesion. Legume seeds that are difficult to cook are thought to be influenced by the presence of insoluble pectins in the middle lamella of the cell wall. Large amounts of insoluble calcium and magnesium pectates are formed in the middle lamella of the cell walls when the seed is high in Ca and Mg, or when the cooking water is high in these elements.

Mattson (18) and Mattson et al. (19) reported that cooking quality may be associated with the ratio of monovalent to divalent cations, and with the contents of phytin and phosphorus in the seed. They reported that high available phosphorus in the soil contributes to high phytin content in the seed and consequently to good cooking. Fowler (20) suggested that phytin has a softening action on peas during cooking by acting as a Ca absorbent, consequently preventing the formation of insoluble calcium pectate. It was suggested that the softening of peas during cooking takes place through a reaction between Na/K phytate (present in cotyledons) and insoluble Ca/Mg pectate (present in the cell wall) that converts the latter into the soluble Na/K pectate (3,18). Besides the relative contents of phytin, Ca, Mg, and free pectin, Muller (21) reported that the thickness of the palisade layer and the contents of lignin and alpha-cellulose in the seed coats are probably important factors in the cooking quality of pulses. Burr et al. (22) found that the cooking quality of dry beans was not influenced significantly by storage time and temperature when the beans' moisture content was maintained at 10% or less. However, moisture contents above 10% eventually caused deterioration in the cooking quality.

Cooking quality of lentils. The influences of mineral nutrition on growth regulators and the stage of maturity, dehulling, canning, and freezing on the cooking quality of lentils were investigated at the American University of Beirut. The effect on cooking quality of various combinations of major and trace elements at different concentrations was investigated in a plant growth experiment utilizing an acid-washed sand/perlite mixture as a plant medium. The studies on the effects of growth regulators and stage of seed maturity were done in the field.

Cooking quality was determined by adding 20 ml distilled water to a 2 g seed sample in a 250 ml Erlenmyer flask, submerging the flasks in a boiling water bath and maintaining a boil for 43 minutes. The seeds were then removed, dried with blotting paper, and their tenderness and texture assessed by feel after pressing the individual seeds with the back of a spoon. Well-cooked seeds did not form a paste. Results of this test were expressed as cooking index with scores of 1 to 15; good cooking quality was indicated by lower scores.

The cooking quality, expressed in quality index scores, as influenced by various nutrient solutions is summarized in Table 5. The data show that cooking quality was significantly influenced by mineral nutrition. Adequate levels of major and trace elements contributed to good cooking. Plants watered with adequate levels of N, P, K, Ca, Mg, S, B, Cu, Fe, Mn, Mo, Zn, and a high level of K (210 ppm) produced the fastest cooking lentil seed. A combination of high levels of K and Na in the seed was associated with good cooking. However, levels of the divalent elements, Ca and Mg, had no correlation with cooking quality. Thus, cooking quality was related to levels of monovalent elements, and to some extent to the ratio of monovalent to divalent elements. No direct relationship was found between phytic acid content in the seed and the cooking quality (23).

The effects of various growth regulators and the chelating agent EDTA on cooking quality are reported in Table 6. The data show no significant effect of these chemicals (applied as foliar sprays at two intervals during early development) on the cooking quality.

A preliminary field experiment was undertaken to study the effect of stage of seed maturity on the cooking quality of a hard-cooking variety of lentils. Seeds were harvested at soft, mid-soft, mid-hard, and very hard stages and their cooking quality tested. The results shown in Table 7 demonstrate that cooking time decreased with the increase in seed maturity. The very hard mature seed cooked twice as fast as the very soft immature seed.

Cooking quality of broad beans. Cooking quality of broad beans has been extensively investigated by the Faculty of Agriculture, University of Alexandria, Egypt, mainly by Dr. Shehata. In their studies the cooking quality of broad beans as measured by penetrometer readings has been correlated significantly with percentage hulls, relative densities, and hydration coefficients (Shehata personal communication).

Processing quality. Lentils are mainly available as unprocessed dry seeds, but dehulled lentils are often found on the market and are used in lentil soup. There are limited studies on the processing of lentil seeds (10,11). Dehulling is known to increase the digestibility and to reduce cooking time. If the germ is removed during dehulling, loss of thiamine may occur.

In a study to develop a process for the preparation of precooked lentil seeds (24), the seeds were steam-blanched and then soaked at 50°C. This resulted in a higher water uptake than soaking at a room temperature of about 20°C. (Table 8). Sodium meta-bisulphite was found to be effective in maintaining colour of lentils; other seeds acquired a darker colour during processing.

The best processing conditions observed by Karkanawi (24) were, successively, steam blanching for 25 minutes; soaking for eight hours at 50°C in a solution containing 1% NaCl, 0.5% Na_3PO_4, 0.75% $NaHCO_3$, 0.25% Na_2CO_3 and 0.5% Na_2SO_5, then steam-cooking for 15 minutes. The lentils were then dried at 45°C for four hours or at 75°C for six hours to a final moisture content below 10 percent. The cooking time for precooked lentil seeds was reduced to eight minutes from the 60 minutes required for unprocessed seeds in an open cooker.

In another study, the soaked seeds were cooked for 15 minutes then dried to a moisture content of 7 to 10 percent. Precooked seeds were either refrigerated or frozen. Refrigerated seeds proved to be unsatisfactory, while those that were frozen had a long shelf life. Cooking time for the precooked lentil seed was reduced to four minutes in an open steam cooker. The level of hemagglutinins was significantly reduced by precooking and freezing. The level of protein in the precooked frozen lentils was reduced by about 1 percent. The texture and taste of the precessed products were satisfactory.

In a study by Pao (11), four canned legume dishes were studied (hommos, foul, mujaddarah and fassoulia). The addition of a thickener to the brine had the most significant effect on thermal processing characteristics.

Research Outlook

Although lentils are a commonly used grain legume in the diets of millions of people, very limited research has been done on their quality in relation to human nutrition. Priorities in research should be given to screening numerous lentil lines for amino acid content, antinutritional factors, flatulence factors, and also for speed of cooking. In addition, genetic and environmental factors, as they influence seed decortication, should also be investigated together with seed-processing and supplementation studies.

REFERENCES

1. M.V. Kuzayli, J.W. Cowan, and Z.I. Sabry, "Nutritive Value of Middle Eastern Foodstuffs. Composition of Pulses, Seeds, Nuts, and Cereal Products of Lebanon," J. Sci. Food Agric. 17:82 (1966).

2. P.L. Pellett and S. Shadarevian, Food Composition Tables for Use in the Middle East, American University of Beirut (Heidelberg Press, Beirut, Lebanon, 1970).

3. S. Abu-Shakra, S. Mirza, and R. Tannous, "Chemical Composition and Amino Acid Content of Chickpea Seeds at Different Stages of Development," J. Sci. Food Agric. 21:91 (1970).

4. J. Jamalian and P.L. Pellett, "Nutritional Value of Middle Eastern Foodstuffs. Amino Acid Composition," J. Sci. Food Agric. 19:378 (1968).

5. R.I. Tannous and M. Ullah, "Effects of Autoclaving on Nutritional Factors in Legume Seeds," Trop. Agric. 46:123 (1969).

6. J.W. Cowan, M. Esfahani, J. Salji, and A. Nahapetian, "Nutritive Value of Middle Eastern Foodstuffs. III. Physiological Availability of Iron in Selected Foods Common to the Middle East," J. Sci. Food Agric. 18:227 (1967).

7. M.S. Mameesh, S. Aprahamian, J. Salji, and J.W. Cowan, "Availability of Iron from Labelled Wheat, Chickpea, Broadbean, and Okra in Anemic Blood Donors," Amer. J. Clin. Nutr. 23:1027 (1970).

8. M. Ullah, Effect of Autoclaving on the Protein Quality of Legume Seeds. M.Sc. Thesis, Faculty of Agricultural Sciences, American University of Beirut, Beirut, Lebanon (1960).

9. A.B.M. Moslehuddin, Effect of Fermentation on Toxic Factors in Legumes. M.Sci. Thesis, Faculty of Agricultural Sciences, American University of Beirut, Beirut, Lebanon (1978).

10. H.A. Hussein, Effect of Thermal Processing on the Cooking Quality of Lentils. M.Sci. Thesis, Faculty of Agricultural Sciences, American University of Beirut, Beirut, Lebanon (1976).

11. S.K. Pao, Variables Affecting the Thermal Processing of Selected Lebanese Foods. M.Sci. Thesis, Faculty of Agricultural Sciences, American University of Beirut, Beirut, Lebanon (1972).

12. U.M. Shibaklu, Utilization of Legumes in Weaning Food Mixtures. M.Sci. Thesis, Faculty of Agricultural Sciences, American University of Beirut, Beirut, Lebanon (1972).

13. R.I. Tannous, S. Shadarevian, and J.W. Cowan, "Rat Studies on Quality of Protein and Growth-Inhibiting Action of Alkaloids of Lupine Lupinus termis, J. Nutr. 94(2):361 (1968).

14. R.I. Tannous, J.W. Cowan, F.R.Y. Asfour, and Z.I. Sabry, "Protein-Rich Food Mixtures for Feeding Infants and Preschool Children in the Middle East. I. Development and Evaluation of Laubina Mixtures," Amer. J. Clin. Nutr. 17:143 (1965).

15. S. Tukan, Infant Food Mixtures Based on Burghol and Lentil. M.Sci. Thesis, Faculty of Agricultural Sciences, American University of Beirut, Beirut, Lebanon (1969).

16. R.F. Daqqaq, Chemical and Biological Studies on the Protein Isolates of Broadbean, Chickpea, and Lupine. M.Sci. Thesis, Faculty of Agricultural Sciences, American University of Beirut, Beirut, Lebanon (1977).

17. H.Y. Nuwayhid, Nutritional Evalution of Biscuits Prepared from Chickpea and Broadbean Protein Isolates. M.Sci. Thesis, Faculty of Agricultural Sciences, American University of Beirut, Beirut, Lebanon (1975).

18. S. Mattson, "The Cookability of Yellow Peas. A Colloid-Chemical and Biochemical Study," Acta Agric. Scand. 2:185 (1946).

19. S. Mattson, E. Akeberg, E. Eriksson, E. Koutler-Anderson, and K. Vahtas, "Factors Determining the Composition and Cookability of Peas," Acta Agric. Scand. 1:40 (1950).

20. H.D. Fowler, "The Characterization of Phytin in Peas," J. Sci. Food Agric. 7:381 (1956).

21. F.M. Muller, "Cooking Quality of Pulses," J. Sci. Food Agric. 18:292 (1967).

22. H.K. Burr, S. Kon, and H.J. Morries, "Cooking Rates of Dry Beans as Influenced by Moisture Content and Temperature and Time of Storage," Food Technol. 22:88 (1968).

23. N. Wassimi, S. Abu -Shakra, R. Tannous, and A.H. Hallab, "Effect of Mineral Nutrition on Cooking Quality of Lentils," Canad. J. Plant Sci. 58(1):165 (1978).

24. M.N. Karkanawi, Studies on Improving Cooking and Nutritional Qualities of Some Legume Seeds. M.Sci. Thesis, Faculty of Agricultural Sciences, American University of Beirut, Beirut, Lebanon (1974).

TABLE 1. Food Legumes Commonly Used in Middle Eastern Diets.

Common Name	Scientific Name	Arabic Name
Broad Bean	*Vicia faba*	Foul
Chickpea	*Cicer arietinum*	Hommos
Lentils	*Lens esculenta*	Adas
Fenugreek	*Trigonella foenumbraecum*	Hilbeh
Lupine	*Lipunus* ssp (termis, albus)	Tummos
Peas	*Pisum sativum*	Bazella
Common Bean	*Phaseolus vulgaris*	Fasulya nashef

TABLE 2. Common Recipes of Some Popular Legume Dishes (in grams)*

Faba bean dip (Foul Moudamas)	
Broadbeans	360
Sodium Bicarbonate	1
Water	350
Salt	35
Garlic	5
Lemon juice	250
Olive oil	25

Chickpea dip (hommos bitehineh)	
Chickpea	750
Water	775
Tahineh	400
Salt	25
Lemon juice	300
Garlic	12
Olive oil	200

Rice and Lentils (mujaddarah)	
Rice	200
Lentils	150
Water	500
Olive oil	33
Onions	100
Salt	5

Common Bean Stew	
Common beans	350
Water	450
Butter	30
Meat	450
Onions	200
Tomato paste	60
Salt	6
Pepper	1

Falafel	
Faba beans (dry)	700
Chickpeas	300
Dry Red Onion and Green Onion	500
Garlic	50
Salt	40
Black & White pepper	5
Wheat flour	75
Oil	50

Lentil Soup	
Lentils	385
Water	1500
Salt	5
Pepper	1
Butter	15

TABLE 3. Physiological Availability of Iron in Some Legume Food*

Legume food	Relative availability**
Chickpea dip (<u>hommos bitehineh</u>)	58%
Lentils and Rice (<u>mujaddarah</u>)	68%
Fried bean patties (<u>falafel</u>)	46%
Ferrous Sulfate	100% (assumed value)

* Source: References 6, 7.
** Determined by hemoglobin regeneration in anemic rats

TABLE 4. Effect of Cooking (Autoclaving at 121°C) on Antinutritional Factors in Legume Seeds*

Legume	Hemagglutinating activity		Antitrypsin activity		Mortality**	
	None	20 min.	None	20 min.	None	20 min.
Broadbeans	80	0	0	0	1	0
Chickpea	0	0	8.4	0.6	0	0
Lentils	640	0	0	0	4	0
Pea	80	0	8.4	0.8	3	0
Common bean	8200	20	9.6	0.8	10	1

* Source: References 5, 8.
** Number of rats dead, from a group of 10, after 4 weeks.

TABLE 5. The Cooking Index, Sodium and Potassium Content of Lentil Seeds Grown in Sand/Perlite Culture as Influenced by Various Nutrient Solutions

No.	Treatment*	Average** Cooking Index	ppm Na	K	Na+K
1	AME+ATE	1.9	32	218	250
2	LME+ATE	3.3	11	180	191
3	AME+LTE	2.1	42	206	248
4	AME+ATE+H Na	1.9	37	197	234
5	AME+ATE+H K	1.9	28	212	240
6	AME+ATE+H Na+H K	1.6	28	200	228
7	AME+ATE+L Na	2.4	10	197	207
8	AME+ATE+L K	2.2	29	201	230
9	AME+ATE+L Na+L K	2.4	14	194	208
10	AME+ATE+L Ca+L Mg	1.5	23	195	218
11	AME+ATE+L Ca+L Mg+H K	3.5	15	188	203
12	AME+ATE+L Ca+L Mg+H K+H Na	1.9	23	219	242
13	AME+ATE+L Ca+L Mg+H Na	1.5	33	220	253

* ATE = Adequate trace elements, B, Cu, Fe, Mn, Mo, Zn.
LTE = Low trace elements
AME = Adequate major elements, N,P, K, Ca, Mg, S.
L = Low
H = High

** Measured on a 1-5 scale; the lower the score the better the cooking quality.

TABLE 6. Effect on Cooking Quality of Growth Regulators Applied on Lentil Plants Grown in the Field, Beqa'a, Lebanon

Growth Regulators (kind and concentration)		Cooking Index	Growth Regulators (kind and concentration)		Cooking Index
I AA			MH		
	100 ppm	6.45		.04%	6.62
	500 ppm	5.97		-	-
G A_3			EDTA		
	50 ppm	6.61		0.002M	6.43
	250 ppm	5.88		0.1M	6.27
N AA			CCC		
	100 ppm	6.08		200 ppm	6.38
	500 ppm	5.87		1000 ppm	6.00
2,4-D			Ethyl		
	10 ppm	5.50		200 ppm	5.88
	100 ppm	7.10		1000 ppm	6.03

TABLE 7. Cooking Quality Index Scores of Lentils Harvested at Four Stages of Seed Maturity

Maturity stage	Mean
Soft	10.50
Mid-soft	8.00
Mid-hard	6.13
Very hard	5.87

TABLE 8. Effect of Temperature of Soak Water on Water Uptake by Seeds at Different Soaking Periods

Soaking Period (Mins.)	Water Uptake (%)	
	20°C (approx.)	50°C
5	17.5	13.9
10	22.4	21.5
15	25.4	35.1
20	28.1	40.6
25	28.4	54.6
30	28.8	57.1
60	45.5	81.7
120	53.2	93.3

Source: Reference 24.

DISCUSSION

SESSION VI - POSTHARVEST PROCESSING AND PROBLEMS

MOHAN SAXENA

We have had two very interesting presentations -- one on postharvest losses and the other on the regional perspective on the utilization of food legumes and its effect on nutrition. From the presentations made so far, it has become clear that there is a need for increased availability of food to meet the demands of an ever-increasing population. However, the scope for achieving this primarily by increasing production is limited, as this would require expensive inputs that are more or less out of reach of the majority of farmers in the developing countries. An alternative is to reduce or altogether eliminate the losses to which food is exposed from the stage when it is produced to the moment at which it is finally consumed. This point is very clearly brought out by Parpia in his presentation.

The total quantity of nutrients available from a specific quantity of food depends upon the magnitude of a number of factors that negatively affect the quantity and quality of the food as it passes through the food chain. At the same time there are ample opportunities for regulating these losses by following an interdisciplinary research approach that includes agricultural scientists and nutritionists. Let me elaborate this point by using a diagram that shows the relationship between the food produced and the food available for nutrition.

If we assume that a certain amount of food is produced, as shown in the Figure by a solid horizontal line, we can see that differential amounts of the total nutrients are available for consumption (shown by broken line). This depends upon the magnitude of the negative factors listed above the solid horizontal line. Parpia's paper lists the postharvest steps at which losses could occur. For our discussion we start from the harvest stage. During the process of harvesting, losses in food legumes could occur by pod shedding and pod dehiscence. After harvesting, the produce has to be moved to the threshing floor for threshing and winnowing. The losses here would depend upon the transport facilities, the threshing technique, and the methods of winnowing.

The above losses can be reduced or eliminated by research by several different disciplines. The plant breeders can provide genotypes that may permit minimal harvesting and postharvest handling losses of pods and seeds. In lentils, for example, we have seen that it is possible to develop genotypes that show a low level of pod shedding and dehiscence. The agro-technologists can provide inputs in devising methods of harvesting, threshing, and winnowing that could reduce these losses. Simple technologies and small changes, such as timely harvesting, transporting the crop quickly to the threshing floor, developing inexpensive harvest methods such as use of a blade cutter for harvesting lentils, or threshing the produce with stationary threshers rather than by hand or by animals could result in considerable savings.

Once the produce is threshed, some of it is kept by the farmers for home consumption and the surplus is sold in the market. In both cases, the produce is stored for varying lengths of time, and and losses during storage and handling at this stage can seriously affect the net availability. Parpia clearly indicated the magnitude of losses caused by rodents, insects, secondary infections from fungi because of changes in moisture content, and/or secretions and excretions of pests infesting these storage areas. These losses can be reduced in two ways. One is through the pre-harvest technology itself as indicated in the chart. The other is by use of prophylactic measures at the preharvest stage in the field which can prevent infestation of the produce in storage.

For this to occur, input is needed from agro-technologists to devise cheap and safe prophylactic measures and also from plant breeders to develop genotypes with a reasonable level of resistance to infestation by storage pests. We have some examples of the potential from genotypes that are tolerant to storage pests. It is possible that such types may not be as acceptable for human consumption, and thus the pay-off may not be high. Nevertheless, interfaces should exist between the breeders and those involved in the postharvest technology. Postharvest storage technology has had several innovations leading to the development of simple, cheap, and effective storage structures from locally available material. Parpia has highlighted these and they would definitely contribute to pushing the broken line of food availability in the figure much closer to the potential level.

The next step at which losses could occur is during the processing of legumes. For some legumes such as *Vicia faba*, there is generally not much processing of dry seed in West Asia and North Africa. However, there are other pulses where processing becomes important. A certain loss in total available food occurs during processing, such as decortication and splitting. The magnitude of loss may depend on the procedures adopted and the nature and quality of the produce used. That insect-infested chickpeas gave a poor yield of dhal and reduced nutritional quality was clearly shown by Parpia. Processing losses could also be reduced by developing genotypes that have a higher meat-to-hull ratio and where the seed coat does not stick tightly to the cotyledons. The breeders will, however, need a contribution from processing technologists to identify desirable traits and to develop simple mass-screening techniques for processing quality. At the same time, the development of a simple, inexpensive, and efficient method of processing pulses using indigenous resources needs high priority. The increased popularity of lentil cultivation in Sudan has suffered an initial setback because no facility was available for decorticating the lentils.

Finally, the overall nutritional contribution of the available food depends on the amount of utilizable nutrients present in the produce. This aspect has been covered in the paper by Tannous. In the presentations in other sessions of this workshop, we heard about the significance of such methods as precooking and blanching to enhance the nutritional availability of food legumes. Parpia mentioned possible improvement by flaking. Food technological inputs are needed to increase the nutritional value, decrease nutritional losses, and simplify the preparation of local dishes. Cooking time and digestibility of the proteins in pulses are two important considerations in addition to the content of antinutritional factors. A contribution from breeders in developing genotypes with improved quality with respect to these attributes would improve availability of nutrients.

The two presentations in this session, whose major emphasis is diagrammatically represented in Figure 1, pinpoint the opportunities for interaction among biological scientists, postharvest technologists, nutritionists, and food technologists. Since interactions among these disciplines have been the major theme of this workshop, this last session should provide an appropriate occasion for that kind of interaction. It is my belief that the two papers presented in this session will generate good discussion.

In order to start discussion, may I exercise the prerogative of the discussion leader and put the first question to Parpia? Many aspects of postharvest technology leading to increased utilization of food, and thus increased availability of nutrients for human consumption in the Indian context, were discussed. The development of small-scale technology for making dhal from food legumes is an interesting example. Realising that many simple postharvest technology innovations in India may not be easily transferable to conditions in the Middle East, could he give some specific examples from this region where changes in the existing technology may improve nutritional yields?

Parpia: I think you have really picked the most important example, because grain legumes occupy a very important place in the diet of people in this region. Technology has been developed to increase milling yield by 50 percent. Before, it was only possible to obtain a 10 to 15 percent higher return. Since a good portion of the legume that is consumed here is dehusked, this technology is entirely transferable. Someone made the suggestion in one of the earlier sessions that it is not desirable to split the legume because a portion may be lost. The technology developed at CFTRI allows one to dehusk whole grain and there is no problem with this process, but consumer acceptance in most of India is for the split grain. In Maharashtra whole grain fetches a higher price and they have been successfully using this technology.

The most important factor in milling is not only the milling equipment, but moisture conditioning. Reducing and raising moisture content loosens the glutamin layer (the sticking layer between the kernel and the husk). This was the biggest contribution of this technology to allow the use of pearling rather than the traditional village procedures. This technology has already been transferred. At a previous UNU workshop, participants from Ghana brought some wing beans they wanted milled. With a slight modification of the moisture conditioning technique and a slight readjustment of the equipment, it was possible to mill the wing bean very efficiently. The UNU thought that this technology should be demonstrated so it financed the manufacture of a small pilot mill for Ghana at CFTRI. Also, although I do not know whether rice milling presents any problem in the Middle East, but the technology from India was easily transferred to Indonesia.

In order to implement a programme to use the improved technology, a rice milling policy resolution had to be passed in India. The resolution was drafted by the Institute for the Ministry of Agriculture, discussed in the Ministry and passed into law. Since then it has been efficiently implemented.

I would like to mention another example on parboiling technology. One of the CFTRI staff members spent six months at the International Rice Research Institute (IRRI), and made certain modifications to suit the Philippine varieties of rice: the technology is now in use. In addition, most of South Asia is short of fat. Rice bran, which is obtained by this new method, is much better for oil extraction. However, many village mills were not obtaining the rice bran because they were using hull-milling. The solution to this was to introduce a shallow mill and use the normal procedure only for polishing. The result was the recovery of good bran. Since bran has a very active lipase it easily goes rancid. A small piece of equipment was developed that switches on simulaneously and generates enough heat to inactivate the lipase so that all the rice bran, which may contain 18 to 20 percent fat, was utilized. The remaining bran has about 18 percent protein and can be used in animal feed; this generated a chicken-feed industry. You can see the chain reaction from preventing postharvest losses to the benefits that can be derived.

With regard to appropriate technologies, the first objective is to identify those technologies, such as the grain legume technology, that have already been modernized and transformed to see whether they can be transferred elsewhere. The second objective is to identify traditional technologies on which research work has begun and the impact this would have on nutrition and utilization. The third objective is to undertake a systematic campaign in each region, including the Middle East, to survey these technologies properly. The fourth is to create an information system to exchange the information available. The fifth and final objective is to train people in the utilization of these technologies.

Myntii: I would appreciate it if our colleagues from ICARDA could comment on the extent to which postharvest technologies come into their work; particularly the improvement of postharvest technology. Are you involved in storage methods and facilities, e.g., buildings, as well as harvesting?

Nygaard: I can answer part of that. Since I was going to ask if we could get some help on this issue anyway, let me tell you what I was going to say. Messrs. Abdul Bari Salkini* and Ahmad Mazid* and I did some survey work on lentil production. Information that we had from the Food Legume Programme at that time suggested that harvesting was a real constraint because there was a lack of harvesting equipment. In the survey, we tried to get data on harvest costs, the loss of grain or straw from the time it is pulled out of the ground until it is put into storage. This involves a series of steps, all done by hand. We wanted to compare losses if these steps were done by a machine. We were surprised that the estimates of losses that we got from farmers were very low. Some estimates were only two to three percent and I think the average was five to six percent, while we expected the estimate to be closer to 20 percent. Either the farmers are underestimating their losses (they have been using the process for so many hundreds of years that they really do not realize the magnitude of the losses) or, in fact, there are very few losses in that traditional, very labor-intensive method, and we were overestimating the problem.

Let me briefly describe this harvest process. The farmers pull the lentils when they are still green and pliable. They pull them out, roots and all, by hand. They make piles in the fields and they leave them there for three days to two weeks. Then they are loaded onto either a donkey's back or on a cart and carried to the threshing floor and stacked in large piles. When time permits, usually after harvesting the barley and wheat, they thresh it, using one of several methods. They then winnow it by throwing it up into the air and letting the wind blow away the chaff, and then sift it to get rid of the dirt. Finally, they put Central Food Technological Research Institute for the Ministry of Agriculture, discussed in the Ministry and passed into law. Since then it has been efficiently implemented.

I would like to mention another example on parboiling technology. One of the CFTRI staff members spent six months at the International Rice Research Institute (IRRI), and made certain modifications to suit the Philippine varieties of rice: the technology is now in use. In addition, most of South Asia is short of fat. Rice bran, which is obtained by this new method, is much better for oil extraction. However, many village mills were not obtaining the rice bran because they were using hull-milling. The solution to this was to introduce a shallow mill and use the normal procedure only for polishing. The result was the recovery of good bran. Since bran has a very active lipase it easily goes rancid. A small piece of equipment was developed that switches on simulaneously and generates enough heat to inactivate the lipase so that all the rice bran, which may contain 18 to 20 percent fat, was utilized. The remaining bran has about 18 percent protein and can be used in animal feed; this generated a chicken-feed industry. You can see the chain reaction from preventing post-harvest losses to the benefits that can be derived.

With regard to appropriate technologies, the first objective is to identify those technologies, such as the grain legume technology, that have already been modernized and transformed to see whether they can be transferred elsewhere. The second objective is to identify traditional technologies on which research work has begun and the impact this would have on nutrition and utilization. The third objective is to undertake a systematic campaign in each region, including the Middle East, to survey these technologies properly. The fourth is to create an information system to exchange the information available. The fifth and final objective is to train people in the utilization of these technologies.

Myntii: I would appreciate it if our colleagues from ICARDA could comment on the extent to which postharvest technologies come into their work; particularly the improvement of postharvest technology. Are you involved in storage methods and facilities, e.g., buildings, as well as harvesting?

Nygaard: I can answer part of that. Since I was going to ask if we could get some help on this issue anyway, let me tell you what I was going to say. Messrs. Abdul Bari Salkini* and Ahmad Mazid* and I did some survey work on lentil production. Information that we had from the Food Legume Programme at that time suggested that harvesting was a real constraint because there was a lack of harvesting equipment. In the survey, we tried to get data on harvest costs, the loss of grain or straw from the time it is pulled out of the ground until it is put into storage. This involves a series of steps, all done by hand. We wanted to compare losses if these steps were done by a machine. We were surprised that the estimates of losses that we got from farmers were very low. Some estimates were only two to three percent and I think the average was five to six percent, while we expected the estimate to be closer to 20 percent. Either the farmers are underestimating their losses (they have been using the process for so many hundreds of years that they really do not realize the magnitude of the losses) or, in fact, there are very few losses in that traditional, very labor-intensive method, and we were overestimating the problem.

Let me briefly describe this harvest process. The farmers pull the lentils when they are still green and pliable. They pull them out, roots and all, by hand. They make piles in the fields and they leave them there for three days to two weeks. Then they are loaded onto either a donkey's back or on a cart and carried to the threshing floor and stacked in large piles. When time permits, usually after harvesting the barley and wheat, they thresh it, using one of several methods. They then winnow it by throwing it up into the air and letting the wind blow away the chaff, and then sift it to get rid of the dirt. Finally, they put the lentils in bags. I may be missing a step or two, but if you watch this process, it is hard to believe that losses are not more than five percent. However, we did not have the capacity to actually measure the grain lost in the process, so we are still not happy with the quality of the data we have. We would be glad to have some suggestions on how to improve this measurement process. Perhaps Parpia could tell us if there is a methodology developed that would help us better estimate post harvest losses.

Alderman: Were there any losses to rats in the piles? I have seen these piles in India and you can hear the rats in the evening eating the grain. This is a loss the farmer may not even be estimating.

---

* Research Associates Framing Systems Programme, ICARDA.

Nygaard: Since we did this survey from ten in the morning until four in the afternoon, we did not see or hear any rats. Seriously, that is a valid point --one that was not mentioned by the people to whom we spoke and about which we asked no questions.

Parpia: The best answer I can give is to exchange some practical experience. We went out to a rice field during harvest and talked to villagers in India. They also said that losses were not great. A young colleague of mine picked up a rock and threw it at a pile of harvested plants and at least 200 birds flew away. They were not just perching there without purpose. If you want some estimate of losses to birds there is a publication about this from Latin America.

When I asked the farmer why he was not cultivating millet, which gave a very good yield in that area, he said he was ready to cultivate it only if 20 other nearby farmers also grew millet. Otherwise he would lose most of his crop to parrots. If 20 farmers grew millet the parrots would share it and not hurt him so much. Clearly, this farmer was aware of the fact that these losses were occurring. On the other hand, he was not aware that the birds were eating his rice.

Rats are also a big problem and one that is difficult to measure. Once a colleague of mine, who is a specialist in rodent control, took me to a beautiful new pilot plant constructed by CFTRI. I told her I had visited the plant at least twice a day and I was sure there was no rat problem. She laid out a systematic set of traps and she said, "Tomorrow you will be the one to open the plant". I did so the next morning, and she had caught 80 rats in one night, and she said one can never catch more than 30 percent of the rat population through trapping. Rats can do a tremendous amount of damage, and as they are a nocturnal animal we normally fail to observe them.

Saxena: In the particular survey that Nygaard mentioned, where the loss was only of the magnitude of about five percent, I think the figure was true. However, there is tremendous variation in this region on the magnitude of losses occurring in a crop like lentil. At Tel Hadya we had an interesting experience in the very first year when we planted on land that had been an ordinary farmer's plot the previous year. We observed fields where the lentil stand of volunteers (seed lost in the field at harvest that germinates in the subsequent season) was as dense as if it had been planted at a rate of 200-250 kg of seed per hectare. If the average yield is about one ton/hectare, this is a loss of 20 percent. The farmer has been trying to reduce this by timing his harvest better, but this is becoming increasingly more difficult as labour is not available in sufficient numbers. Our emphasis on devising methods of harvesting lentils by alternative means that are quicker and relatively cheaper came out of this kind of experience and these surveys.

Allan: I found Parpia's paper very interesting and a good collection of examples of appropriate, intermediate, small-scale alternative technology. It is also very important because of its emphasis on energy, in which I have an interest at the moment. The more efficient use of energy and the reduction of wastes are important, and it is urgent for the developing countries to get out of technological traps such as the one mentioned by Williams in the last session. I think most of us were surprised to hear the magnitude of the costs of erecting adequate grain-handling storage and transportation facilities in the Middle East -- a cost of millions and millions of dollars.

However, with apologies to Williams, I think this is an example of Western-oriented technological transfer. If you consider the situation in North America or in Europe and assume that the Middle East has to have the same sort of facilities, you may make a great mistake. If you can convince governments to follow that policy, you may commit them to astronomical expenses that, in 30 or 40 years time, may be shown to have been very wrong.

I think the way you look at the problem is from the "bottom up" instead of from the "top down", and there are two aspects of this. One is that this grain-storage handling technology should begin at the village level, then at the district level, and then at the provincial level. All the facilities should be built up from the bottom and should be made to work properly before we install huge installations at the national level. If there is food security at the local or provincial level you will have national food security, but the converse is not necessarily true.

The second point is that Western countries have already invested huge amounts of money in their grain-handling and storage facilities. If they cannot use that to move grain all over the world, such as to export it to countries like Egypt, it is not a very good investment of their money. Thus, there is a large vested interest in continuing this movement of grain around the world quite apart from any feed aspect. When people write the history of this part of the century in 50 to 100 years time, they will be most astonished at why we spent so much money, and even worse so much energy, moving all this grain around the world when most of it could be grown right where it was needed.

Williams: Please forgive me for my excessive North American zeal in discussing the grain-handling systems. My reasons for giving these figures is that I believe that Syria, and some other countries as well, must become net exporters of grain because there are not many other areas in the Middle East that are capable of growing the necessary quantities and handling it properly. However, I would predict that the Syrians are going to find that handling grain efficiently and exporting it is totally different from importing it. For example, people who import grain buy on sample or on grade. In Canada we have a grading system and 70 years of integrity, so people trust this system and buy from us on grade. In America, most of the grain is bought on sample. A sample of, say, 5 kg is sent to the buyer who may agree to buy, hoping that the ship has the same quality grain as the sample. It usually does because we all try to be honest. The point is it takes a while to develop a good exportation system.

In this part of the world, I know that there is a lot of grain storage in the villages. Syria is a very dry country; for example, the Romans dug holes at Tel Hadya in which to store grain. It is easy to do this as long as the water table is low enough. It was very cheap, and I am sure there will be more use made of this in the future years.

In this part of the world grain storage could be done at much lower cost than in the West because labour is cheaper. But most of the facilities would have to be imported. The Russians have enough technology to send rockets to the moon but they have very poor grain-handling facilities. They are actually importing grain through Rotterdam and trucking it across Europe to Russia. They do not have port facilities and, in fact, do not have enough sea frontage. They also would have a problem of financing major development of grain-handling systems. Right now Russia needs between 30 to 50 million tons of grain a year -- a lot of which is fed to animals. To look at the world's grain industry from the outside with an objective eye, one can see the need in the future for a much larger grain distribution system.

Thomson: I would like to return to the point about losses. Livestock in this part of Syria at this time of year depend on feed supplements. They also graze fallow land and often this has a lot of volunteers growing on it. Although we may be losing a certain amount of grain out the back of a combine, this is not really lost as it is grazed by the livestock during the next spring. Farmers have estimated expected losses from combine harvesting to be 50 to 80 kg/ha. One other figure, on big plots of one to three hectares, we estimated yields at 1500 kg/ha for lentils by quadrant samples, whereas after threshing we had only about 900 kg. This is quite a big loss. I would not suggest that they are always that big, but I think they are considerable.

Parpia: To reinforce the point raised by Thomson, I would like to give an example. I happened to be on a UNU assignment in Sudan. At that time there was an FAO mission there led by a transnational corporation from Canada to construct silos. The UNDP representative whom I had met the previous day, and with whom I had discussed traditional technology, involved me in this mission. I opposed the construction of silos, partly because silos cost three to five times more than a flat warehouse, and in a country where all the food produced that year is consumed in 12 months, silos are not required. A large portion of this grain never even entered the market channels. The only silos needed were for food security.

The Sudanese government representative and the UNDP representative fully agreed with me, but the FAO and the transnational corporation representatives did not. The decision was taken not to build silos. Then we discussed several type of flat structures that the Sudanese said were similar to local ones already in use but needed to be improved. The villager in India uses inert gas storage. When the bin is nearly full of grain he places a lamp at the opening that burns an edible oil. He lights the lamp and then seals the lip of the bin with cowdung. When all the oxygen is consumed the lamp goes out and there is no problem of insect infestation during the storage period. This does not cost anything and does not need an expert from a transnational corporation; nor could such a person give this kind of advice.

Goldsworthy: I am also interested in the question Myntti raised about the extent of postharvest and storage losses. The tables Parpia gave us show that there is a dearth of information in this area, and I would invite my colleagues at ICARDA to tell us a bit more about these storage losses.

Cow peas in the Sudan and Sahel zones of West Africa are stored in the types of stores Parpia has described, very similar to the rural storage in India --earthernware silos, but they are usually not sealed. Instead they have thatched roofs. It is estimated that about one third of the total crop is lost each year. This is largely an unimproved crop, to which the International Centres only began to pay scientific attention within the last ten years. In the first 7,000 accessions of cowpeas that were screened by plant breeders, an effort was made to select for resistance to the main cause of this storage loss, a pest called the bruchid. One line was found in which the rate of increase in the population of the bruchid was only 20 percent of that in the other susceptible lines. With help from the U.K. Tropical Products Institute and the University of Durham, this resistance was found to be due to a level of about two and a half times the normal level of trypsin inhibitors in the seed. When the seed was cooked the trypsin inhibitor, being heat labile, was destroyed and did not appear to affect the value to the consumer.

Like all breeding issues, when you find something good it usually has other things wrong with it. We were dealing with a crop where we had to have resistance to viruses and other diseases. This cultivar came from an area where these diseases did not occur, and thus it was extremely susceptible. It took us nearly two years to get enough seed to work free of the virus. The breeding work has now produced a number of derivatives that combine virus resistance with agronomic types of the sort we wanted. It offers the prospect of eliminating a loss of something like $20 million worth of legume seed in storage each year, just within the West African region.

Cow peas had moved with Spanish settlements to the New World, to the Carribean, and because they can adapt to fairly harsh, dry environments, there is a relatively large production in the northeast of Brazil where IITA (International Institute of Tropical Agriculture in Ibadan, Nigeria) had one breeder based. One of the main field pests was a field weevil that was not found in Africa. A few small breeding efforts in Central America discovered two or three lines that were resistant to this weevil. The resistance was in the pods not in the seed. We found that this pod resistance also reduced the increase in the population of the bruchid to about 20 percent. Here was the prospect of combining independent sources of resistance, in the pod and in the seed, to virtually eliminate the pest. I think that is quite an exciting prospect.

I have not heard, in the short time I have been at ICARDA, of any exploration for diversity in the germ plasm. In West Africa, it was stimulated by the very severe losses that had occurred, good information on surveys of markets by university entomologists from Northern Nigeria, and work that FAO did in Ghana to quantify the extent of these losses. Thus, we had some fairly definite information to work with.

The significance of pod resistance is that the farmer stores the seed in the pod and then threshes the seed just before it goes to the market. The buildup in infestation is after threshing and on the way to the market. So pod resistance has the potential to reduce storage losses.

Srivastava: I think we should look at the losses at different stages. At planting time there are certain losses, when the crop is growing there are losses to birds, animals, and insects. At harvest there are considerable losses because of harvesting techniques of a mechanical or manual nature, and, finally, there are storage losses. There are no institutions ar the national level to seek solutions to prevent these losses -- solutions that farmers will accept. Who should accept the responsibility for this research? For example, straw that comes from food legumes and cereals is a very important component in the livestock system, and a group from FAO asked us how to improve the utilization of straw for feed. In some countries in the Middle East straw is as expensive as the grain itself, yet we have not made much progress toward improving straw use. To respond to Myntti's question we are not doing very much at ICARDA on postharvest losses and I certainly hope something more can be done.

Nordblom: I would like to congratulate Parpia on an interesting contribution, particularly for pointing out the huge losses caused by rodents and insects and for describing some ingenious methods for controlling them.

Early in the paper he made two points and then drew a conclusion that grain feeding to livestock is undesirable. The first point was that the U.S. and Canada feed animals enough grain to feed the entire populations of China and India. This is the first time I have heard this figure and it may be true; but I think it is also true that feeding livestock in North America is a very efficient operation. The second point was that high levels of meat consumption are unhealthy for humans and may lead to cardiovascular and other diseases. Thus, he concludes that if the U.S. and Canada would change their consumption habits, they would be healthier and they could export more grain. This is a common perspective, but I would like to offer a few comments on how such a conclusion is modified by economic facts.

Grain is used as feed to the extent that livestock producers find the practice profitable. Grain has been relatively cheap compared to meat and it is rational for these producers to feed grain. They will continue to feed it if the cost of animal weight gain is low enough. If people offer a higher price for that gain than the feeders are willing to pay, then the grain will move immediately from livestock feed to human food. Therefore, there is a role that prices play whereby humans can bid away the grain from the animals and the animals may bid it away from the humans.

Also, in light of the fact that meat products are highly desired by consumers, even if some people believe they are not healthy, the existence of large-scale livestock feeding is a kind of safety buffer. In time of famine when human needs cannot be met by production, feed grains or grain that would have gone to livestock are bid away for human feeding. Also, some livestock is slaughtered. Thus, the grain can be diverted quickly from livestock to humans in time of emergency. Livestock feeding means the grain industry will be maintained at an optimal stage of production. In other words the safety buffer is maintained.

From these perspectives, I personally cannot consider the profitable use of feed grains by livestock to be a postharvest loss. On the contrary, it means that a high level of grain production is maintained when effective demand for direct human consumption is not enough. Far less grain would be produced if it were not for the great demand for livestock feeding, so livestock create a huge safety buffer for us.

Parpia: Nordblom has described this from the point of view of someone from an affluent country. I would like to look at the same problem from the point of view of a developing country where the affluent few are willing to pay a high price for animal food and therefore the buying power of an animal is higher than the buying power of a poor man. Thus, you ensure his starvation by developing an animal industry. This has happened in many places and I can give you examples. The figure I quoted regarding the fact that the U.S. and Canada feed enough food grain equivalent to feed the whole population of India and China together is from the documents of the World Food Conference. It was reported also in the Development Forum.

In my view the question is that in order to create a security stock in a developing country, it is much easier to store and conserve food grains than it is to conserve and store meat. In time of surplus one stores the food grain to create security, but I can very well appreciate your point of view looking at it from an advanced country that has a huge grain surplus. It seems to me it is a question of whether it is moral for a rich country to consume meat at a time when the world is starving. I think it is a matter of human rights. At the same time, I think there is a need for more nutritional education in the developed world to see how much meat they should consume. The people in the developed world need as much nutrition education as the people in the developing countries.

Williams: In North America the technology of feeding cattle and chickens is based on feed grain and not food grain. Wheat that is fed to animals in Canada is graded as feed and it is not fit for human consumption. This is poor quality grain such as, for example, barley that has been under snow and is mouldy. The point is that this feed grain is not potential human food.

We are talking about a big bank of grain, but the bank will only last the world at most 27 days. This includes the total grain surplus for the world. This reserve can drop to about 17 days depending on the weather in North America, Russia, and China. In any case, the world reserves of grain are not very big and this is what concerns most of us who are interested in postharvest losses. Storage losses can amount to 20 to 30 percent, and if we could save that it would make a big difference to the grain surpluses in the world.

Parpia: The demand for animal feed has been rising at a rate of 5.5 percent a year as against a population increase of 2.1 percent. Because the animal has a larger buying power he gets preference, and instead of food we are producing feed grain. That is happening in the developed world, and I hope developing countries will not do this.

Williams: I would also like to make a comment about the research we are doing at ICARDA on milling. In Syria flour milling extraction is 82 percent. If you have a ton of dry grain you expect to get 820 kg of flour from it. The higher the extraction rate the better the flour from the point of view of nutrition, but the more difficult it is from the point of view of processing. In the villages, they mill 100 percent extraction. Nearly all of villages have their own stone mills. There are two stones, one is stationary and the other rotates. The miller can adjust the gap to a millimeter or even less, and these mills grind grain very finely. We are certainly going to do more research on this at ICARDA and we feel that we may mill triticale in the same way. Triticale is not acceptable at the moment because of its colour, but in every other aspect it is very good. When it comes to urban flour consumption, white types of flour are preferred in the region, and the city folk do not like more than 80-85 percent extraction flour. However, this loss is not as bad as it sounds because all the bran is used. For example, in Egypt, 87 extraction flour is dark and is only used to make bread in rural areas. About two and a half percent fine bran is used for every kilogram of fine flour, and this increases the extraction rate to 90 percent and it is very nutritious. The other brans are all used in making some form of cattle or chicken feed. I hope this information answers some of the questions about milling.

Singh: We have talked alot about grain losses. I would like to introduce another kind of loss -- an energy loss. Williams talked about the cooking time of the three grain legumes we are working on at ICARDA, and he cited an example of chickpea that takes from 55 to 240 minutes to cook, depending on the cultivar. He mentioned that soaking could reduce the time considerably, but it still takes a long time. This has been reported by him, as well as several nutritionists. Unfortunately, nobody has gone farther than this. This discovery has remained in the laboratory, the housewives are wasting energy every time they cook these grain legumes. Is there some way we could make this technology avaialble to housewives?

Parpia: India is a very large country, but I would like to point out that the technique of using bicarbonate is very common in Kashmir. A housewife knows how much to add -- the amount depends on the age of the beans. Here is a traditional technology that can be promoted and is now used in the preparation of precooked dhals, and a few factories now have been set up in Bombay. I do agree that it requires much greater publicity and a wider distribution of information.

Saxena: I thought it was a fairly common practice with housewives to use bicarbonate in cooking most of the food legumes. I am certain that the foul madames here in the Aleppo market is made using very large quantities of not only bicarbonate but other items that tenderise the beans. Maybe some other food scientists would like to make a comment on this?

Bressani: In surveys we have conducted in Latin America on how rural people process or prepare beans for consumption, we have found that they do not use bicarbonate. We even attempted to provide them with a salt mixture, very similar to the one that has been described. However, this is impossible to do in a practical way in the rural areas. We have been doing something rather new, and that is to soak the beans in a 15 percent solution of sodium chloride for 2 hours. The beans are then drained and dried. Some of the sodium ions and some of the chloride ions penetrate the beans and this gives a very good resistance to insect attack. We significantly reduce fungal contamination and the texture of the cotyledons remains very soft for a long period of time. At present we are carrying out a pilot study with the Guatemalan government at field level to see if this can be implemented. The cooking time also is significantly decreased. Instead of two to three hours it may take only 20 to 25 minutes.

Ali: In a study conducted in Khartoum we found that most people prefer the large seeded varieties of faba beans, but they indicated that these varieties have a very thick seed coat. Is it possible to breed a large variety with a thin seed coat? This would reduce the time for cooking and the water holding capacity of the beans.

Erskine: In lentils there is quite a lot of variation in seed coat thickness, but if we tried to make it thinner, I would be worried that we would increase postharvest loss to weevils and other associated problems. It is complex, but there is genetic variation, and it might be possible to use some of it in this way.

Saxena: I know there are some markets where housewives go specifically to buy lentils that are infested with weevils simply because they are easier to cook.

I would like to change the subject to an aspect that was covered by Parpia in his presentation. This is protection of the grains in storage by using different methods. He mentioned activated clay, an interesting innovation, but in this region there are other practices being followed by housewives in the villages to protect food legumes as well as other grains in storage. In Sudan, they grow a large number of Nim trees whose leaves are used in stored grain. I know in India as well, Nim leaves are used very effectively in storage. Has anyone here in the Middle East looked at this, and what are the prospects of using it? I know there are no harmful residues with this kind of protection and I think it acts more as a repellent than as a real control.

Parpia: We have looked into the Margossa or Nim leaf very carefully. It is only effective for a short time against a few moths, and it is not effective against insects infesting the grain. I would rule this out completely.

Williams: There is one thing we have not discussed and that is the paranoid attitude people have toward pesticide residues. I guess it is not quite so important at the village level. For example, I know a lot of countries still have not outlawed DDT. I have mixed views myself, as I would rather have people use DDT and kill insects than have the insects eat all the food. Canada had been exporting grain to Germany for years and suddenly Germany passed a law whereby they would not allow any trace of it in the grain. It costs us a fortune now to monitor all the ships to Germany and we may as well monitor all the rest of the shipments because we now have the equipment and the staff. Pesticide residues are building up all over and one must keep this in mind.

I like the methods mentioned by Parpia; they are safe and work well at the village level, but they are not feasible for bulk handling. In Syria I have noticed a number of grain elevators being built and I know there are two or three being built in Egypt. People are building large-scale, bulk-type grain-handling systems. There has recently been a flour mill built in the Beqa'a

Valley in Lebanon. I asked the manager there why it was built. The reason was that there are a lot of people in the valley and they are concerned that during a period of political unrest, there may not be any flour available so they have built facilities for grain storage and milling to ensure a supply.

Singh: A small comment about the use of pesticide to conserve seed from insect damage. We have observed that when grain legumes are split and the husk is removed, only the cotyledon is left (commonly called dhal in India). The damage by insects to the cotyledon is far less in comparison to that in the whole grain. This was observed at ICRISAT in both chickpeas and pigeon peas, but the entomologist could not explain why insect pests are attracted to whole grain but not split grain. If this is true, why not immediately convert the grain to dahl and then store it?

Parpia: It depends on which kind of insect it is. Certain insects are attracted to the whole grain while others are attracted to the split type, and in addition the type of infestation in pre-harvest and post-harvest stages can be different. At the same time, pre-harvest infestation can be carried on to the post-harvest stage. Frequently, oviposition that occurs in the field is one carried through. It is not quite so simple, but it is true that some varieties are much less affected than others.

Singh: In this case it concerned the bruchids, and as you said, it was not simple, which is why ICRISAT entomologists could not give a proper answer.

Karrar: I liked Parpia's intermediate technology at the village level and the preservation of seeds and food stocks. We have to be careful about chemical preservatives or chemical insecticides, particularly at the village level where people do not know safe concentrations. In the Sudan, we found an area where farmers were using insecticides, and in this area there were large amounts of residues in breast milk. DDT, for example, effects RNA and some of these chemicals are known to be carcinogenic. I think it is very dangerous to propagate potentially toxic chemicals and I think we should stay with intermediate technology.

Khattab: If one is allowed to conclude something from this very interesting discussion on post-harvest problems of cereals and legumes, it is obvious that there are a host of such problems. Since ICARDA is already interested in the quality of these grains, I think it is logical that they sould establish a post-harvest research laboratory as well.

Thomson: I would be happy to have a clarification on a few issues. One is the question of the diet in the Middle East that has evolved over many centuries. We hear that it is reasonably balanced, but in spite of this there are problems of infant malnutrition and high infant mortality. A second area concerns the possibility and the rationale for using plant breeding methods for increasing the micronutrient content of foods. Should we instead be placing emphasis more on other ways to provide nutrients required to maintain a balanced diet?

We have heard that for protein it is not so much the amino acid pattern that is important but its digestibility. Some of the work being done is looking particularly at the content of such amino acids as lysine and methionine in crops. Therefore, should we not be looking at *in vitro* methods of screening for digestibility and putting more emphasis on antinutritional factors?

My fourth point is that I, as an animal scientist, find the large increase in the demand for meat close to my own heart. This is a controversial area. We know of the probelms of saturated fats and cardiovascular diseases derived from these animal products. In this respect, I feel we should be considering leaner animals that at the same time we will increase the efficiency of utilization of our limited grain or forages.

Miladi: Diets in the Middle East are one thing and infant mortality rates are something else. In countries like the United Arab Emirates, infant mortality is high because of changing habits. Mothers are switching from breast-feeding to bottle-feeding. One hundred grams of protein baby food made from rice cost U.S. $20 on the market, whereas 100 g of milk protein costs $2.00, but these people are being influenced by advertisements so they feed the child plain rice. Without education on how to prepare bottles, problems such as the infections that Pellett spoke of are common. Therefore, the causes of infant mortality are really related to many factors.

I would like to mention what the United Nations Unversity and ICARDA are trying to do to develop manpower in the region. The University, in particular, is financing graduate work research opportunities for a number of people from several other countries in the region. These people are working on issues that are also of interest to ICARDA and some hope to do their research at ICARDA.

Saxena: The input by the United Nations University is truly commendable and I think the example of the kind of experience at CFTRI and other centres is definitely going to be of great help to the Middle East and North Africa. Now the stage is set and we expect tangible results.

I think this is the right time to conclude this discussion. When we started the session I was not really sure whether there would be that much interest generated among the participants on this topic, yet there was lively participation. This is at least partly because of the provocative papers by Parpia and Tannous.

DRY AREA AGRICULTURE AND NUTRITION

RECOMMENDATIONS

On the evening of the third day, after all the papers had been presented, the workshop participatns met in five independent groups (see below) to formulate recommendations that would give guidance to future research and development activities on these subjects for the region. The recommendations were intended to be particularly useful to ICARDA and UNU. These recommendations are reported below by each working group under the following heading:

I. Priorities in nutrition research.
II. Nutrition priorities in agricultural research.
III. Priorities in agricultural research.
IV. Nutrition priorities in plant breeding.
V. Priorities in research on postharvest technology and food processing.

I. Priorities in Nutrition Research

The main recommendation of this group is to emphasize collection of relatively simple baseline data on the "at-risk" group in the ICARDA region. This work will require manpower training and institutional support and a greater degree of interaction between specialists in nutrition, food science, and agriculture. This is required at the national level, and workshops similar to this one should be held nationally. Sophisticated physiological and metabolic studies need not be given high priority at present.

Specifically, with respect to human nutrition:

- Baseline dietary surveys should be conducted on at-risk populations, especially small farmers in the dryland farming areas. These surveys should monitor food purchases, food and nutrient availability, food habits, income distribution and the within-family food and nutrient distribution. Such baseline data are essential for monitoring changes.

- Similar baseline data should be collected on nutritional status to investigate the nutrient status of individuals, with special attention being paid to children and females of child-bearing age. If possible, birth weight data should be recorded to determine prevalence of low birth-weight infants.

- Research is needed on the relationships between food intake, nutritional status, and productivity among rural populations in selected countries of the region.

- Understanding is needed of the causes, at the local level, of the decline in breast-feeding and the associated high infant mortality rates. Development of low-cost weaning foods should be promoted, using suitable, locally available legume/cereal mixtures.

- National food policies (prices, subsidies, rationing, price-fixing, interventions, transfers, import/export, technology) should be examined in relation to their nutritional effects and their socioeconomic impact.

- As a long-term goal for the countries of the region, the establishment of nutritional surveillance units is important. This would allow the monitoring of nutrition and health in relation to the effects of changes in food production.

- In agricultural research, ICARDA and plant breeders elsewhere should continue to breed for increased yields while also contintuing to monitor quality and acceptability, to ensure that these remain at a satisfactory level. For elements like iron, it is probably easier to supplement diets by fortification rather than to embark on long-term, costly plant-breeding programs.

- There should be very strong encouragement of local processing methods for the ICARDA crops, to ensure that valuable consitutents and characteristics are retained. Local production of appropriate "convenience" foods should also be promoted to reduce women's labor.

II. Nutrition Priorities in Agricultural Research

The following recommendations are based on a recognition of the need for increased food and nutritional considerations in agricultural development. This will tend to manifest itself at different stages.

- At the agricultural project design, implementation and assessment level, all the various national agencies involved in food and nutrition should be included. Therefore, our first recommendation is to hold interdisciplinary workshops at the national level with objectives similar to those of this workshop.

- At another level is the need to modify curricula of institutions specializing in agriculture, economics, food and nutrition in order to give their students a broader educational base and thus foster interdisciplinary cooperation. Thus, steps should be taken to encourage such changes in regional institutions. As a positive step in this direction, ICARDA should include nutrition-related activities in the current training program.

- Food and nutrition problems that have been identified can be alleviated by designing relevant nutrition program, possibly using mass media methods.

- One way to proceed with the goal of including nutritional considerations in agricultural projects is to have a model agricultural project that incorporates the principles that have been discussed in the workshop. Nutritionists and economists should play a role, not only in implementation and project assessment, but more importantly in project design. Methodologies for successfully enhancing the nutrition consequences for the target areas that have already been identified as nutritinally deficient should be developed and tested.

III. Priorities in Agricultural Research

- To ensure the maintenance of balanced diets, agricultural and food research should take into account the principal commodities in the production systems and consumption patterns of target populations.

- To ensure long-term maintenance of food supplies, agricultural research should take into consideration agro-climatic and socioeconomic differences among agricultural zones.

- Research priorities should be established as a joint effort among biological and social scientists of the research institutions, using the best possible analytical approach and taking into account equity and efficiency considerations.

- To facilitate the improvement of levels of nutrition, agricultural and food research should assist and interact with governments to formulate sound policies for producer and consumer prices, input and consumption subsidies, and trade policies, including in particular the ways in which production and consumption patterns of the poorest groups differ from those of the population as a whole.

- In regions where, characteristically, the amount of rainfall is limited and varies greatly from one season to another, maintenance of food supplies requires that priority be given to the development of crop stability to ensure food supplies from year to year.

- Agricultural experiment station research should include agro-economic surveys on production practices, storage practices, on-farm trials, in order to improve food production on farms, with particular attention to small farmers.

- More research on environmental issues, soil, water and nutrient management and crop-livestock interactions is needed to imporve the stability of the resource base in semi-arid and arid zones, avoid desertification, and ensure maintenance of food supplies.

- Human nutrition would benefit from research on improved range management, with focus on livestock and livestock by-products production.

IV. Nutritional Priorities in Plant-Breeding

- The highest priority for plant breeders should be to increase the availability of food through improving productivity of staple food crops without decreasing nutrient levels. To this end, breeding objectives aimed at increasing and/or stabilizing economic yields should be emphasized.

- High- and stable-yielding cultivars will only be adopted if they have acceptable quality characteristics. Therefore, further research is needed in order to determine consumer preferences throughout the region and to develop appropriate screening procedures. As more is known, adequate quality testing as a vital component of breeding programs should be refined.

- In breeding for increased yield, advanced materials should be monitored to ensure that nutritional and processing qualitites are maintained at an acceptable level. Nutritents that should be monitored include protein (both quanity and quality) and the essential minerals and vitamins that are known to be limiting in diets of certain populations in the region.

- Further research on micronutrients is required before firm recommendations can be made to breeders. Special attention should be given to iron availability in view of the high incidence of anemia in the region.

- Protein digestibility in food legumes should be monitored and if possible improved through breeding. The role of polyphenols in reducing protein digestibility, and the role of grain legume carbohydrates in reducing cholesterol levels require further study.

- Through routine monitoring of nutritional factors in agronomic and breeding trials, much basic information will be generated on genetic and environmental effects and their interactions. This information could be of considerable value for future applied research, and it is recommended that efforts be devoted to this end.

- Greater attention should be given in research on faba beans to factors responsible for the favism disease that is endemic in the region. Toxic factors in other food crops of the region (e.g. millet) should also receive some attention.

V. Priorities in Research on Postharvest Technology and Food Processing

There is a need for a multidisciplinary approach to increasing and improving food supplies, in which postharvest technology is an inherent factor. Postharvest technology is the process that begins at harvest and ends with food consumption. The following recommendations are made in acknowledgement of the fact that this is an often-neglected area among many facets of the food system.

- It is recommended that an institutional framework be established that addresses the problems of postharvest technology at national and regional levels. This is envisaged as a network of isntitutions and individuals. It would involve the disciplines of food technology, nutrition, agricultural engineering, industrial design, socioeconomic research, and other areas, as needed. ICARDA and the UNU could be insturmental in the creation of such a network.

- The factors involved in postharvest loss must be researched and remedies sought. For major crops the losses should be studied from field to home by crop and under regional and local conditions. It is recommended that emphasis be given to development of a methodology to assess postharvest losses, and use of the methodology should be promoted throughout the region.

- There is a definite need to assess and promote the role of women in postharvest systems from the aspects of both loss and food production. The establishment of local industries with women as an important part of the labor force should be encouraged in the face of modern technological change. Such industries would be based on the promotion and improvement of traditional technologies, but should not preclude the possibilities of the creation of new income-increasing sources. Such industries would generate employment and income, and must be energy conserving, economically viable, and utilize all aspects of modern up-to-date technology.

- Methods of communication, training and education on aspects of postharvest technology, food production, and local processing at mini-industrial levels should be developed. These would be aimed at all of the facets of rural communities in particular, but certain aspects would be applicable to the reduction of losses and wastage and the improvement of food production in urban areas.

CONCLUSIONS

The interaction of thoughts and opinions during the workshop resulted in stimulating a process that should achieve a greater understanding among agriculturalists, food scientists, nutritionists, and social scientists. The recommendations made will require action to build capabilities of human resources and strengthen the interdisciplinary capacities of institutions. This, in turn, needs the development of unconventional interdisciplinary programs of advanced training involving a network of institutions and universities. There is also a need to formulate research and development projects involving institutions with different disciplines so that they can work together to find solutions that would accelerate the development process based on agriculture, food science and technology, and contribute to socioeconomic transformation for a better quality of life. It is hoped that the institutions involved will modify their rules and regulations that act now as impediments to such action and make advanced training possible for individuals where they could work at more than one institute and specialize in the areas of their work with much greater understanding of several disciplines. This will make their contribution more effective and meaningful. In building such understanding and networks, it is hoped that the United Nations University will continue to be involved and will develop further cooperation with other institutions within the ICARDA region.

GLOSSARY OF TERMS

Aflatoxins

A group of toxic compounds are produced by molds, especially *Aspergillus flavus*. They are thus mycotoxins and have been demonstrated to be *potent carcinogens*, whose major target organ is the liver. They were initially discovered as contaminants of peanut meals, but they can be classified as contaminants over a wide range of food materials.

Aggregate Demand Analysis

This type of economic analysis takes place at the level of a region or a country. It gives useful estimates of total demand for that area and the important componenets that create that demand. It can be extremely useful for studying government policies. However, it does not consider differences among different groups within a society and generally presents an incomplete picture of the welfare of the population.

Amino Acids

Amino acids are the fundamental units from which proteins are made. These are defined as *essential* (indispensable) or *nonessential* (dispensable), depending on whether they can be manufactured by the body (nonessential) or whether they must be supplied by the diet. These categories are not clear-cut, but normally isoleucine, leucine, lysine methionine, phenylalanine, threonine, tryptophan, and valine are considered essential for the human adult. Histidine should be added for the child and perhaps for the adult; however, in the adult long-term deprivation is needed before it becomes essential. Often cystine and tyrosine are included with the essential amino acids becuase of their close association with methionine and phenylalanine, respectively. The nonessential amino acids are necessary for protein to be synthesized, but they can be made from glycose and a source of nitrogen. These include alanine, arginine, aspartic acid, glutamic acid, glycine, and proline.

Amylases

Amylases are enzymes that can split starch into smaller fractions. They exist in alpha and beta forms that split different linkages in starch. Amylases exist in the digestive tract, but can also be found in molds and cereal products from which they can be used for food processing, as for example in the malting of barley.

Anemia

This is a condition in which the concentration of hemoglobin in the circulating blood is below normal. This may be caused by a large variety of factors. One of the most common causes is insufficient iron to meet the needs of hemoglobin synthesis. Regardless of the cause, all types of anemia produce many similar signs and symptoms because of the blood's reduced capacity to carry oxygen. Iron may be present in apparently adequate amounts in the diet, but for various reasons may have poor bioavailability (qv).

Anthropometry

Measurement of the human body. In the context of this book, it means the use of body measurements as an index of nutritional and health status. Amongst the most used indices are weight-for-age, height-for-age, weight-for-height, and arm circumference. All are compared with standard values from healthy, well-nourished populations.

Antinutritional Factors (Antiphysiological Factors)

These may also be called naturally occurring toxicants. Toxic is here used in the widest sense of meaning any adverse physiological response that can detract from the nutritive value of a foodstuff. Many of these adverse effects can be reversed by the appropriate cooking or processing of the foodstuff. Amongst the most well-known of these factors are trypsin inhibitors, found especially in soya bean products. Phytohemaglutinins (lectins) come from various beans, and lathyrogens fro the lathyrus pea. The effects produced range from inhibition of growth in test animals to intoxication and paralysis. A wide range of other factors also exist, including the compounds causing favism found in *Vicia faba*, gossypol in cottonseed, and cyanide from lima beans and cassava. Attention has only recently been directed to polyphenolic compounds in beans. They not only have an antophysiological role, but may also affect cooking time and insect infestation during storage.

Arteriosclerosis

Hardening of the arteries characterized by patchy, nodular thickening by fat and cholesterol deposits of the inner layers of the arteris (atherosclerosis). More common in affluent societies and in the rich of poor societies, the condition may relate to the type of diet consumed as well as to other aspects of life style. May lead to coronary thrombosis (qv).

Ascochyta Leaf Blight

A fungal leaf disease that causes small, white lesions on the leaves and can also affect other parts of the plant. Its effect is very severe; in the Middle East one can frequently find chickpea fields that have been completely destroyed by the disease.

Availability

(See Bioavailability)

Back Cross Method

A breeding method of improving plant characteristics in a stepwise fashion where previous gains are not lost. It is rapid, requires a small number of plants, and is predictable. Its major limitation is that it does not permit the achievement of unusual combinations of genes from two or more varieties.

Basal Metabolic Rate (BMR)

Defined as the energy output of an individual under standardized resting conditions: bodily and mentally at rest, 12 to 18 hours after a meal, and in a neutral thermal environment. More loosely used to imply the energy requirement of individuals under resting conditions when food has not recently been consumed. This should be more accurately called Resting Energy Expenditure.

Beriberi

A disease, no longer prevalent, caused by a deficiency of the B_1 vitamin (thiamine).

Bioavailability

The bioavailability of a nutrient has been defined as the fraction of the amount ingested that is absorbed and is dependent on a large variety of factors. These factors have been groupd into host factors, such as the physiological and/or nutritional state of the consuming organisms, and dietary factors, including the chemical form of the nutrient, its level of intake, and the presence of other compounds in the diet that can increase or decrease absorption.

Bulk Population Method

A breeding method in which two known plants are crossed and the resulting seeds are sown together so that natural selection can then weed out weaker combinations while new combinations are created in the original stand.

Calories

The normally used unit of measurement for content of food energy and for daily energy requirement. When used in terms of Pcal% (protein calories percent) and Fcal% (fat calories percent), cereal calories percent, or sugar calories percent, it implies the proportion of the daily total calories coming from these dietary components.

Carotenoids

A variety of compounds found mainly in plant foods capable of being converted in the body into vitamin A activity. The degree of conversion possibly varies with the compound.

Consumer-Oriented Food Price Policies

There are certain governmental policies that aim to directly affect the prices consumers pay for food. These include subsidies, price ceilings, and ration coupons. They often have the politically desirable effect of lowering food prices, but can create disincentives for agricultural production.

Coronary Thrombosis

A type of heart attack caused by a blood clot that may have been induced by atherosclerosis (qv) in a vessel of the heart.

Deficit Farmer

A farmer who produces less than he consumes.

Developing Regions/Countries

Countries or regions that have a large number of people living at a subsistence level and on average that have a low standard of living in comparison to the rest of the world are frequently referred to as developing countries. Third World countries or LSCs (less developed countries) are often used to mean the same thing. These terms are somewhat subjective, although various measures have been used by the UN and others to indicate degrees of development. It is important that these measures, which depend on analysis for a whole country or region, take into consideration the distribution of wealth, income, and growth among different sectors and socioeconomic groups.

Digestibility

The proportion of a nutrient that is absorbed. In this book, digestibility mainly refers to protein or nitrogen digestibility, where it is defined as:

$$\text{Digestibility} = \frac{\text{Intake Nitrogen - Fecal Nitrogen}}{\text{Intake Nitrogen}}$$

The value may be expressed as a fraction or a percentage. Fecal nitrogen may or may not include a correction for endogenous nitrogen, which is excreted even if no protein is consumed, and originates from intestinal tissue and secretions. Digestibility is a form of bioavailability (qv).

Food Balance Sheets

These are comprehensive indicators of the pattern of the food supply to a specific country during a specified reference period. These are calculated, for all commodities potentially available for human consumption, as the difference between supply (production + imports + amount from stocks) and utilization (exported, used for seed, used for manufacture, losses and wastage and animal feed). The per capita supply is then obtained by dividing by the population. Data on per capita food supplies may be expressed both as total quantity and as sources of nutrients by use of appropriate food composition data.

Food Composition Tables

Tables of the nutrient contents of foods and food products obtained from food analytical data.

Goitre

A disease involving the thyroid gland caused by a deficiency of iodine. Endemic goitre refers to the disease state potentially present in an area and ready to appear at any time.

Gross National Product (GNP)

The monetary value of all goods and services produced by residents of a country, plus goods and services produced by residents abroad.

Household Behavior

Behavior of individual households depends on social, religious, ethnic, and economic determinants.

a) Household Food Allocation: This term refers to the distribution of food among family members; different levels of consumption will depend on age, sex, status, physical health, occupation, etc. of the members.

b) Household Food Acquisition: The production or purchase of food will vary among household members.

c) Household Food Acquisition Power: The determination of how much and what kinds of food will be produced or purchased by a family varies by family member. The decision is not always made by the same person who makes the acquisition.

Hunger

The deterioration of health status and/or productive performance arising from too low an intake of food by individuals or populations. Not identical with being hungry. There is a considerable degree of overlap with malnutrition (qv) when used to describe the results of a deficient intake.

Hyper-

A prefix meaning higher values for some appropriate index. For example, hyperglycemia means a higher than normal level of sugar (glucose) in the blood.

Hypo-

A prefix meaning lower values for some appropriate index. For example, hypothermia means a body temperature below normal, while hypovitaminosis-A implies deficient levels of vitamin A.

Infant Mortality Rate

The number of deaths at less than one year of age per 1000 live births. Neonatal mortality refers to deaths at less than one month of age, while perinatal mortality relates to still births and deaths under one week.

Junk Food

An undefined term implying disapproval of a specific food or foods. The term bears no relation to nutritional value, since it may be used for mixtures of high nutritional value, such as hamburgers, pizza, and fish and chips or for products of practically zero value such as low-calorie soft drinks. Use of term should be avoided.

Keratomalacia

An advanced form of vitamin A deficiency involving loss of substance of the cornea and consequent deformity ultimately leading to irreversible blindness.

Kwashiorkor

A severe form of protein-energy malnutrition (PEM) usually involving children between one and two years of age. Involves weight loss, edema (qv), and a liver highly infiltrated with fat. Often associated with consumption of diets of low protein to calorie ratio.

Life Expectancy

A statistical estimate for the expected residual length of life. Can be calculated for any age, but when used for comparisons between countries in relation to overall health and nutrition, it is normally life expectancy at birth. This index is highly influenced by the level of infant and childhood mortality and can thus show wide differences between developing and developed countries.

Limiting Amino Acid

The essential amino acid (qv) in a protein present as the least proportion of a reference (requirement) amino acid pattern. Should also be the essential amino acid that, when added to a protein fed to an animal under test conditions, will significantly improve the utilization of that protein. Because of limitations in knowledge of reference amino acid patterns, the limiting amino acid as defined by these two procedures is not alway identical.

Low Birth-Weight Infant

An infant whose birth weight is below 2,500 g. Includes infants whose low birth weight is because they are born prematurely as well as those who are low in weight at full term. The latter condition is more common in poor developing countries and reflects, inter alia, poor nutritional status of the mother.

Malnutrition

Strictly means bad (mal.) nutrition, which may be excess or deficit. Often only used to imply a nutritional deficiency situation. Should be distinguished from hunger (qv), although the two conditions overlap to a considerable degree.

Marasmus

More correctly called nutritional marasmus. A severe form of protein-energy malnutrition usually occurring in children before one year of age. Children with marasmus are severely wasted and are much below normal children in their weight-for-age. Less severe conditions can be diagnosed by anthropometric criteria.

Mineral Elements

Some 20 to 30 mineral elements are known to be present in the body, and of these the list of those known to be essential for life continues to grow with the development of more sensitive analytical techniques. They are sometimes separated into two groups -- the macronutrient elements such as calcium and phosphorus that are present in relatively large amounts in animal tissue, and the micronutrient or trace elements such as iron, zinc, and selenium present in much smaller amounts. The elements differ considerably in the forms in which they appear in food and the means by which they are absorbed and metabolized. The content of an element as determined by analysis often bears little relationship to the amount that may be absorbed, and thus the bioavailability (qv) can vary enormously among elements and among foods.

Pellagra

A now rare disease caused by a deficiency of nicotinic acid (niacin), one of the B vitamins, in the diet. Since part of the nicotinic acid requirements can be synthesized in the body from the amino acid tryptophan, the disease has also been associated with low-protein diets.

Production Function

A mathematical expression to describe a production process that shows the maximum output that can be produced given a specified amount of inputs. It is a functional form commonly used in agricultural research and is sometimes referred to as a logistic production function.

Protein

A major component of all living material and a necessary dietary constituent. All proteins, of which many thousands exist, contain nitrogen and are comprised of both essential and nonessential amino acids (qv). Protein quality is a term used to compare the abiity of different proteins to support growth and/or other physiological states and is a composite, inter alia, of digestibility and amino acid composition. Protein quality can be measured by a large variety of techniques, among which protein efficiency ratio (PER), net protein utilization (NPU), and nitrogen balance are some of the best known. These techniques all involve experimental animals or experimental subjects, but other techniques based on amino acid composition are also widely used.

Protein-Energy Malnutrition (PEM)

Formerly known as protein-calorie malnutrition (PCM). A spectrum of diseases involving deficiencies of intake of protein and/or calories. The range extends from kwashiorkor (low protein intake relative to calories) at one extreme to nutritional marasmus at the other. Marasmic kwashiorkor occupies an intermediate position.

Retinol

Vitamin A alcohol. The fully active form of the vitamin present in animal foods. Various carotenes (qv), found mainly in plant foods, can be partially converted to vitamin A. The sum total of vitamin A (preformed and formed from the various carotenes) is termed "retinol" equivalents" and is used to express the potential value of dietary sources. Vitamin A in its various active forms is not water-soluble and is transported in the blood in association with proteins, especially pre-albumins and retinol-binding protein. Because of the dependence on protein for transport, vitamin A deficiency (qv) is often associated with severe protein-energy malnutrition (qv).

Rust

A disease affecting parts of the plants above the ground, it forms initially on the lower surface of the leaflets or pods and spreads to the entire plant. Rust is probably the most common above-surface disease and can be a major problem in lentil-producing areas.

Scurvy

A now rare disease caused by a deficiency of vitamin C (ascorbic acid). The disease is of major historical interest because its causation was first understood by performing the first controlled nutrition experiments with human subjects.

Single-Seed Descent Method

A means of advancing populations while preserving genetic variance for later selection. The method uses less labour and space than bulk population breeding and back cross method (qv). A single seed is taken from each plant and used to propagate the next generation. Eventually, pure lines can be generated from existing lines.

Sitona

Insects that feed on the leaf margins and constitute the greatest insect threat to legume plants while they are growing. They may transmit some types of virus to the plants. The larvae attack root nodules and may do considerable damage beofe they mature.

Spectroscopy

A technique of analysis involving the absorption of light from solutions or surfaces. Used in a wide variety of procedures for the analysis of nutrients in foods. A recent technique, Near Infrared Reflectance Spectroscopy (NIRS), has been developed for the determination of protein and amino acids in cereal and legume samples.

Subsistence Farming

Many farmers do not produce enough to more than feed themselves and their families. Therefore it is difficult for them to adopt new technology because they cannot purchase the inputs that are required to improve production.

Sulphur Amino Acids (SAA)

A term used for methionine, cysteine, and cystine, because these three amino acids all contain sulphur. Only methionine is an essential amino acid (qv), but since it can be used to manufacture cysteine and cystine, the sum of the three is used in protein quality considerations and is termed "total sulphur amino acids" (Total SAA).

Vitamin A Deficiency

Also called hypovitaminosis-A. A nutritional deficiency disease associated with deficient intake of vitamin A and/or carotenes. In its most severe form (keratomalacia, qv) it causes partial or complete blindness. A less severe, but still serious, form is called xerophthalmia. Often found in children with protein-energy malnutrition.

INDEX